Handbook for the Assessment of Dissociation

A CLINICAL GUIDE

Handbook for the Assessment of Dissociation

A CLINICAL GUIDE

By Marlene Steinberg, M.D.

Associate Research Scientist
Department of Psychiatry
Yale University School of Medicine
New Haven, Connecticut

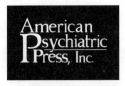

American Psychiatric Press, Inc.

Washington, DC
London, England

Note: The author has worked to ensure that all information in this book concerning drug dosages, schedules, and routes of administration is accurate as of the time of publication and consistent with standards set by the U.S. Food and Drug Administration and the general medical community. As medical research and practice advance, however, therapeutic standards may change. For this reason and because human and mechanical errors sometimes occur, we recommend that readers follow the advice of a physician who is directly involved in their care or the care of a member of their family.

Copyright © 1995   Marlene Steinberg, M.D.
ALL RIGHTS RESERVED
Manufactured in the United States of America on acid-free paper
98 97 96 95   4 3 2 1
First Edition

American Psychiatric Press, Inc.
1400 K Street, N.W., Washington, DC   20005

Library of Congress Cataloging-in-Publication Data
Steinberg, Marlene, 1953–
    Handbook for the assessment of dissociation : a clinical guide /
  Marlene Steinberg.
        p. cm.
    Includes bibliographical references and index.
    ISBN 0-88048-682-1
    1. Dissociative disorders—Diagnosis. I. Title.
    [DNLM: 1. Dissociative Disorders—diagnosis. WM 173.6 S819h
  1995]
  RC553.D5S73 1995
  616.85′23075—dc20
  DNLM/DLC
  for Library of Congress   94-24448
                                                                      CIP

British Library Cataloguing in Publication Data
A CIP record is available from the British Library.

To All the Silent Survivors

Contents

Part III: Clinical Applications

Preface

Voices mute for ever, or since yesterday, or just stilled;
If you listen hard you can still catch the echo.
Hoarse voices of those who can no longer speak,
Voices that speak and can no longer say anything,
Voices that think they're saying something,
Voices that speak and can't be understood:
Choruses and cymbals for smuggling sense
Into a senseless message.

—Primo Levi, "Voices"

we tried to tell you
in so many ways,
the pain, fear, despair, shame;
yet what came forth were
the silent screams.

it's not that we haven't tried—
you and us—to speak,
to hear, to understand,
to listen to these
silent screams.

there's no dramatics, no drama
no hysterics, no acting
yet we plead for help through
the silent screams . . .

—Peggy J., "Silent Screams"[1]

In their most recent monograph, Drs. Lyn Brown and Carol Gilligan (1992) describe a complex set of psychological problems: "the desire for authentic connection, the experience of disconnection, the difficulties in speaking, the feeling of not being listened to or heard or responded to empathically, the feeling of

---

[1] From Cohen et al. 1991, p. 11.

not being able to convey or even believe in one's own experience" (p. 5). Although the authors are primarily concerned with the maturational dilemmas of female adolescents, their description is a disturbingly accurate evocation of the inner world of a person who has a dissociative disorder. To the person trapped inside the machinery, as it were, of a childhood coping device gone awry and escalating out of control, the possibility of genuine communication and connection with the outside world, with caring and sympathetic others, is remote and unimaginable. If we understand the core symptoms of dissociation as the sequelae of childhood abuse, as the end results of a child's attempt to assimilate the incoherent jumble of love and pain that characterizes abusive families, we can begin to understand the dissociative disorders as a code language for communicating the unspeakable. The primary purpose of this book, *Handbook for the Assessment of Dissociation: A Clinical Guide,* is to provide clinicians with a guide to the "grammar" and "syntax" of this private language, and to introduce them to a diagnostic instrument that can help their patients find their real voices, perhaps for the first time in their lives. At the beginning, however, it is important for readers to understand not only the intensity of the suffering borne by dissociative patients but also the ways in which that suffering is compounded by their silence. To do that, we need to remind ourselves that people do not fall prey to mental disturbances in a cultural vacuum, nor do they recover without a renewed or improved ability to communicate their thoughts and emotions to others. The customary description of psychotherapy as "the talking cure" is itself a testimony to the power of language as a vehicle of healing. Thus this book proceeds from two premises: that diagnosis and assessment of the dissociative disorders are complicated by the silence of their human hostages, and that recovery begins when these patients discover that they can speak of their experiences, be heard, and be understood. Because the dissociative disorders are somewhat unusual across the psychiatric spectrum in that they have a good prognosis in most cases, the therapist who works with dissociative patients can have real hope that he or she is making a positive contribution by helping these patients to find their voices again. This book, therefore, is intended to help the reader become an informed and sensitive interpreter of dissociative symptomatology.

It must be added that the silent suffering of dissociative patients is only one of the problems involved in effective detection and treatment of the dissociative disorders; another is the collective silence of psychiatric professionals, broken only within the past 5 years. Because of the recent explosion of interest in the dissociative disorders, some researchers have finally begun to address the issue of professional denial. Because it is now generally recognized that dissociative symptoms and disorders are the sequelae of a history of childhood abuse, the incidence of these disorders in the general population points to a disquietingly high level of child abuse in North American society. The etiologic connection between childhood trauma and dissociative symptomatology in turn confronts clinicians with some realities that many prefer not to inspect too closely.

The first of these challenges has to do with the impact of dissociation as a coping mechanism on the patient's sense of adult identity or selfhood. Dealing with questions of human self-definition, however, has not been a significant aspect of most clinicians' training. The course of preparation for qualification in any of the health professions is sufficiently lengthy and stressful as to inhibit most students from exploring broad-based definitions of human identity or personality. Whereas Freud and Janet were the beneficiaries of a pattern of higher education that expected all graduates in any field of research to be conversant with the classical literature of the West and its reflections on the human condition, today's professional specialist may never have had to read any of the great poets, dramatists, philosophers, or theologians with an eye toward learning to ask basic questions about the form and content of human personhood, regardless of the answers one finally accepts. Because the dissociative disorders manifest as a fragmentation or dismembering of the patient's basic sense of selfhood and personal integrity, they pose questions that most clinicians tend to manage by referral to other specialists, as it were.

More disturbingly, the connection between childhood abuse

and the dissociative disorders challenges clinicians to look at themselves and their own personal histories from a new and potentially painful perspective. Briere's (1992) observation that "the majority of adults raised in North America, regardless of gender, age, race, ethnicity, or social class, probably experienced some level of maltreatment as children" (p. xviii) forces any reader to reexamine his or her background and upbringing for evidence of possible maltreatment. No matter what the results of such introspection, some discomfort is predictable. For therapists who can honestly conclude that they were fortunate enough to be reared in a relatively healthy family, the necessities remain of learning to identify the symptoms of childhood abuse in their patient population as well as the more crucial matter of confronting their own attitudes toward abuse survivors. The unfairness of human life forces the privileged—in any category of privilege—as well as the deprived or marginalized to question the unequal distribution of goods and benefits, whether material or psychological. Just as research into a variety of prejudicial attitudes in the general population has indicated that persons who belong to advantaged groups tend to blame members of subordinate or excluded groups for their disadvantages, so too those who benefited from the love and nurture of mature and responsible parents need to examine themselves for any tendency to "blame the victim" of parental abuse for his or her suffering.

On the other hand, clinicians who see their own faces reflected in Briere's mirror have an equally difficult set of challenges to confront. To some extent, it is easier in the current social climate for those in the helping professions to acknowledge the presence of trauma in their own histories. The pioneering work of Timmen Cermak and others, who discovered that they were attracted to the helping professions in the first place because they had learned to be caretakers in alcoholic families, has been followed by monographs written by clinicians whose families may not have been damaged by substance addiction specifically but that were nonetheless abusive (Farmer 1989). Thus those in the helping professions who have had to acknowledge themselves to be abuse survivors no longer need fear that the presence of this long-the same patient to be assessed by clinicians of various back-grounds with a high degree of consistency. However, it is recommended that therapists who are unfamiliar with the instrument not only acquaint themselves with the *Interviewer's Guide to the SCID-D* (Steinberg 1993a, 1994a) but, in addition, acquire training or supervision in its administration and interpretation. Workshops in the use of the SCID-D are offered annually at a number of sites.

■ Outline of the *Handbook*

The body of the material in this book is organized as follows: In Chapter 2, I review the general literature on dissociation and trauma. The purpose of this overview is to provide clinicians with a practical framework for assessing dissociative phenomenology during initial interviews as well as for gaining a clearer understanding of a patient's subjective experiences.

Chapters 3 through 11 focus on each of the five dissociative symptoms in depth, first presenting the available literature on each symptom and then reviewing their assessment by introducing the questions in the SCID-D that are relevant to differential diagnosis. Chapter 12 then describes the relationship between severity and symptoms and differential diagnosis. Chapter 13 describes the assessment of intra-interview cues of dissociation. Chapter 14 overviews the SCID-D in relation to the nondissociative disorders and is followed by a sample SCID-D interview in Chapter 15. The book concludes with a summary chapter that includes some reflections on future clinical applications and research.

suppressed motivation for wanting to help others disqualifies them from continuing to serve as therapists, social workers, clergy, or teachers. There is a growing body of material explicitly addressed to the personal and professional problems of therapist/survivors. Gil (1988) and Briere (1992), for example, have both included sections explicitly intended for therapist/survivors in their monographs on treatment issues of abuse survivors. Both writers point out that whereas the therapist/survivor is in a position to empathize with his or her patient and to understand the economic, educational, and social difficulties that the patient must face, he or she must also confront a possible tendency to impose his or her beliefs about abuse and recovery on the patient, to project his or her emotional issues on the patient, or to become involved in boundary confusion with the patient (Gil 1988). With respect to the dissociative disorders in particular, the therapist/survivor will want to work through his or her own issues about selfhood and a sense of personal identity in order to assist patients with self-work.

■ About the *Structured Clinical Interview for DSM-IV Dissociative Disorders*

A word about the theoretical background and orientation of the *Structured Clinical Interview for DSM-IV Dissociative Disorders* (SCID-D; Steinberg 1993b, 1994b): it is a semistructured instrument designed for clinical diagnosis and assessment of the presence and severity of dissociative symptoms and disorders. Its open-ended format enables practitioners working with a patient subpopulation overwhelmingly composed of abuse survivors to elicit information relevant to a trauma history even though the instrument does not ask direct questions about abuse as such. Moreover, the SCID-D is intended for use by clinicians trained in any school or tradition of psychotherapy; because it does not rely on paradigms or concepts specific to one particular therapeutic approach it can be used by any professional with sufficient sensitivity and clinical experience. The SCID-D's theoretical neutrality has the advantage of allowing

Acknowledgments

I want to give priority in these acknowledgments to the 125 women and 53 men who participated as subjects in the SCID-D pilot study and National Institute of Mental Health–funded field trials. The pilot study group was made up of a set of "normal" control subjects, a subgroup of persons diagnosed with nondissociative psychiatric disorders, and another subgroup of persons diagnosed with dissociative disorders. The field study subjects included patients with a variety of psychiatric disorders, both dissociative and nondissociative. The field trials included approximately 340 interviews with 130 subjects over a 3-year period, yielding over 800 hours of videotaped interviews. The citations in the body of this book are drawn from verbatim transcriptions of the videotapes used with the informed consent of the subjects. With respect to issues of patient confidentiality, I have followed the guidelines of accepted professional practice in disguising the identities of patients by altering circumstantial details. In transcript excerpts dealing with alter personalities, the names of the alters have also been changed but in such a way as to maintain the tone or "flavor" of the name supplied by the patient. I hope that readers of this book will come to understand my gratitude to these courageous subjects, who were willing to share their once-silent suffering with me and allowed me to record their stories so that others might be instructed by their experiences and struggles. These case studies of the dissociative disorders offer evidence of the admirable capacity of the human spirit to resist and overcome undeserved abuse and suffering, and are painful testimonies to the high incidence of such abuse.

Second, I would also like to express my appreciation to two colleagues whose collaboration was essential to the refinement and field-testing of the SCID-D: to Bruce Rounsaville, M.D., who served as methodological consultant; and Domenic Cicchetti, Ph.D., who supplied statistical analysis and expertise. They have generously shared their respective areas of expertise with me during the past 10 years, and their contributions have helped to bring the dissociative disorders into the mainstream of psychiatric research.

Next, I wish to thank my senior colleagues in the field who contributed advice, suggestions, and critiques. They include Robert Spitzer, M.D., and Janet Williams, D.S.W., authors of the *Structured Clinical Interview for DSM-III-R* (SCID; Spitzer et al. 1990), together with Michael B. First, M.S.W., and Miriam Gibbon, M.S.W., who allowed me to use their diagnostic instrument as a prototype for the SCID-D; Richard P. Kluft, M.D., who has supported the research from the outset and generously agreed to participate in the multicenter field trials; and Philip M. Coons, M.D., Elizabeth Bowman, M.D., Catherine Fine, Ph.D., David Fink, M.D., and Pamela Hall, Psy.D., for contributing their time and expertise to the multicenter field trials of the SCID-D in Philadelphia, Indianapolis, and Summit, New Jersey. In addition, I want to thank Francine Howland, M.D., my former clinical supervisor, who introduced me to the dissociative disorders during my Yale residency in 1982; and David Spiegel, M.D, who has been supportive of SCID-D research since my participation in his dissociative disorders advisory committee for the revisions for DSM-IV. I am also grateful to Morton Reiser, M.D., and George Mahl, M.D., former clinical supervisors at Yale, who were supportive of my work at a time when the dissociative disorders were not regarded as being in the purview of mainstream psychiatry. I would also like to thank Boris Astrachan, M.D., John Docherty, M.D., Lillian Gross, M.D., Harold Ratner, M.D., Rochelle Schreibman, M.D., and Moshe Torem, M.D. Lastly, my special thanks to two women who have been generous in their friendship as well as with collegial support—Pamela Hall, Psy.D., and Olivia Hall, M.Div.

In addition, I want to acknowledge the contributions of the interviewers who assisted in the pilot study and field trials to evaluate the instrument's interrater reliability. They include Christine Amis (who also corated the tapes of the preliminary study), Jean

Bancroft, Geanine Peck, and Susan Wharfe. Their high level of clinical skills and sensitivity helped greatly in the compilation of a sizable collection of instructive interviews.

Moreover, I am grateful to my staff over the years, whose varied skills have contributed to the final form of this book: Josephine Buchanan, SCID-D Project Coordinator, and Karen Zych, who recruited the subjects and matched them with the interviewers as well as overseeing the many daily activities of the office; and the SCID-D research staff, including Gerald Melnick, Aysha Corbett, and Susan Macary. Lastly, I want to acknowledge the contributions of Jonathan Lovins, research assistant, for his computer expertise, and Rebecca Frey, research and editorial assistant, whose background in the humanities brought a holistic perspective and a concern for clear style, which proved invaluable in shaping the form of the final manuscript. I would also like to thank Martin Lynds, project editor at the American Psychiatric Press, for guiding the manuscript of this handbook through the publication process. In conclusion, a word of special thanks to my sister, Annie Steinberg, M.D., who has provided professional feedback as well as personal support.

PART I

Introduction

CHAPTER 1

Escape From Consciousness

Five Core Dissociative Symptoms

God created me to be a child, and He caused me always to remain a child. But why did He cause life to buffet me about, and take away my toys? Why did He abandon me at school during recess, leaving me to tear my smock—which was filthy with my flowing tears—with my weak little hands? If I could not live except with tenderness, why was tenderness left out of my life? Ah, every time I see a child weeping in the streets, a child exiled from playmates, the pain from the unforeseen horror within my exhausted heart is greater than the child's sadness. I feel pain with all the stature of experienced life, and the hands that twist the corner of the smock are mine, the mouths twisted by real tears are mine, the weakness is mine, the solitude is mine, and the laughter of the adult life that passes by uses me like the light of matches struck on the sensible tissue of my heart.

—**Fernando Pessoa,** *The Book of Disquiet*

The floor is cold.
The wall at which I plead
Denies me, whitely.
I want one thing: to be
Part of the plaster.
The man I cringe from
As you cross to comfort me was larger;
His squat arms cradled his paunch lightly,
Furred,
Willing to strike.
There is nowhere
That this three-, this thirty-year-old,
Can crawl to escape him.

—**Lynne Yamaguchi Fletcher,** "Again"

The etiologic relationship between the dissociative disorders and childhood trauma is now generally accepted within the helping professions. It is appropriate to open this chapter with a pair of literary reflections on the impact of adult insensitivity and unkindness toward children. These two writers express in their own anecdotal and descriptive fashion the hard statistical evidence that is making its way into the medical literature regarding the connection between the dissociative disorders and the emotional and physical abuse of children. The pioneering work of Alice Miller, beginning with *Prisoners of Childhood* (1981) and continuing through *For Your Own Good* (1983) and *Thou Shalt Not Be Aware* (1984) to *The Untouched Key* (1988), has called attention to the genuine suffering inflicted on children by widespread social assumptions about the right of adults to exploit, humiliate, deceive, and mistreat children in a variety of ways. Although Miller is not herself a specialist in the dissociative disorders, other clinicians have followed up on her work to draw explicit connections between childhood trauma and adult dissociative pathology. The "white light in the back of [the] mind" that Louis MacNeice (1993) once described as every child's birthright, to serve as an inner guide or monitor in the perplexities of adult life, can be obscured or even extinguished by sufficiently severe mistreatment in the early years. Clinicians who must assess and evaluate the growing population of patients who have one or another of the dissociative disorders, or a dissociative disturbance coexisting with another form of psychiatric disorder, need to recognize and understand a number of troubling facts:

1. **The shocking incidence of childhood abuse.** Russell's (1986) often-cited figures that 16% of women in the general American population are sexually abused by a relative before their 18th birthday, and 31% are sexually abused by a nonfamily member, have been followed by other depressing statistics. In terms of the hospitalized population, 50%–75% of general psychiatric patients endorsed histories of childhood trauma (Bryer et al. 1987; Ellerstein and Canavan 1980; Emslie and Rosenfelt 1983; Husain and Chapel 1983; Myers 1991; Sansonnet-Hayden et al. 1987). The reader is referred to Tables 1–1 through 1–4 for a statistical summary of recent studies of abuse.

2. **The growing body of research indicating a causal connection between a history of trauma in childhood and dissocia-**

tive pathology in adult life. Dissociative symptoms and disorders are now considered to be posttraumatic in origin (Fine 1990; Kluft 1985b; Spiegel 1991; Terr 1991). Some studies have noted histories of abuse in 82%–98% of all reported cases of dissociative disorders (Coons et al. 1988; Hornstein and Tyson 1991; Kluft 1988a; Putnam et al. 1986; Schultz et al. 1989).

3. **The clinical professional's own tendencies toward self-protective incredulity in the face of this material.** As Goodwin (1985) has explained, incredulity functions to 1) distance the clinician from threats to emotional homeostasis, 2) protect the clinician from coming to grips with his or her own painful memories, and 3) shield the professional from the patient's (or the patient's family's) pain and rage. Although it is true that empathic overidentification with a patient can cloud professional judgment, it also is important to remember that dissociative disorders are more than ordinarily subject to misdiagnosis because of the opposite form of professional overreaction. Kluft (1990b) has pointed out that incest in

Table 1–1.   Sexual abuse among psychiatric outpatients

	Outpatients			
	N	Percentage sexually abused		
Study	(male/female)	Male	Female	Total
Swett et al. 1990	125[a,b]	13	—	13
Gale et al. 1988	202[c] (101/101)	9	27	18
Sheldon 1988	115[a,d]	—	21	21
Surrey et al. 1990	140[a,d]	—	37	37
Threlkeld and Thyer 1992	117[e] (53/64)	11	49	30

[a]Adults (≥ 18 years old).
[b]Sample of men only.
[c]Children (≤ 9 years old).
[d]Sample of women only.
[e]Children and adolescents (≤ 17 years old).

particular is a form of abuse that causes extreme coun-
tertransferential difficulties for therapists:

> we further detoxify the impact of the patient's account by wrap-
> ping ourselves in speculations that the incest may not have oc-
> curred. The "objectivity" of the clinician who takes an
> incredulous stance is not objective; it is a retreat from anxiety-
> provoking issues and candid exploration of countertransference
> concerns into the realm of wishful (or even magical) thinking
> (p. 33).

Table 1–2.   Sexual abuse among psychiatric inpatients

| | Inpatients | | |
| | *N* | Percentage sexually abused | | |
Study	(male/female)	Male	Female	Total
Jacobson and Herald 1990	100[a] (50/50)	26	54	40
Kohan et al. 1987	110[b]	16	48	32
Neisen and Sandall 1990	201[a] (151/50)	42	70	56
Livingston 1987 (no sex breakdown in article)	100[b]	—	—	13
Bryer et al. 1987	66[a,c]	—	54	54
Sansonnet-Hayden et al. 1987	54[d] (29/25)	24	38	31
Chu and Dill 1990	98[a,c]	—	36	36
Sandberg 1986	150[b] (99/51)	4	37	20
Jacobson and Richardson 1987 (no sex breakdown in article)	100[a] (50/50)	—	—	35

[a]Adults (≥ 18 years old).
[b]Children and adolescents (≤ 17 years old).
[c]Sample of women only.
[d]Adolescents (between 10 and 17 years old).

This book is not intended to address the theoretical questions raised by recent statistics, such as whether there has been an increase in the actual incidence of abuse and of the dissociative disorders, or simply an increase in reporting of the former and more accurate diagnosis of the latter. Rather, this work is designed to serve as a reference guide to the dissociative disorders as a group, and as a practical introduction to their evaluation, assessment, and treatment strategies. We proceed in this chapter to a comprehensive overview of the five dissociative symptoms assessed by the *Structured Clinical Interview for DSM-IV Dissociative Disorders* (SCID-D; Steinberg 1993b).

Originally developed to incorporate DSM-III-R criteria, the SCID-D was updated in 1993 to incorporate DSM-IV criteria for

Table 1–3. Sexual abuse among nonpsychiatric subjects (control subjects)

	Control subjects			
	N	Percentage sexually abused		
Study	(male/female)	Male	Female	Total
Finkelhor et al. 1990	2,626[a] (1,145/1,481)	16	27	21
Goldman and Goldman 1988	991[a]	9	28	18
Risin and Koss 1987	2,972[a,b]	7.3	—	7.3
Cameron et al. 1986	4,339[a] (1,605/2,734)	—	—	16
Baker and Duncan 1985	2,019[c]	8	12	10
Kercher and McShane 1984	1,065[a]	—	—	7.4
Russell 1983	930[a,d]	—	38	38
Fritz et al. 1981	952[a]	4.8	7.7	12.5
Bagley 1991	750[a,d]	—	32	32
Russell 1984	> 900[a,d]	—	16	16

[a]Adults (≥ 18 years old).
[b]Sample of men only.
[c]Adolescents and adults (≥ 10 years old).
[d]Sample of women only.

the dissociative disorders. Preliminary field trials and National Institute of Mental Health (NIMH)–funded field trials of the SCID-D at Yale University have indicated good-to-excellent reliability and discriminant validity for each of the five dissociative symptoms as well as for the dissociative disorders (Steinberg et al. 1989–1992; Steinberg et al. 1990). These results have been replicated by Goff et al. (1992) at Harvard University and by Boon and Draijer (1991) in a cross-national replication study in Amsterdam. In addition, findings from three of the four sites in the multicenter field trials of the SCID-D (involving expert researchers from New Haven, Connecticut [Drs. Cicchetti, Rounsaville, and Steinberg]; Philadelphia, Pennsylvania [Drs. Fine, Fink, and Kluft]; Indianapolis, Indiana [Drs. Bowman and Coons]; and Summit, New Jersey [Dr. Hall]) also indicate good-to-excellent reliability and validity (Steinberg et al. 1989–1993).

■ The Five Dissociative Symptoms

The dissociative symptoms considered in this theoretical framework are the following: 1) amnesia, 2) depersonalization, 3) dereal-

Table 1–4.   Child abuse among patients with dissociative identity disorder (DID)

	DID patients			
Study	N (male/female)	Percentage physically or sexually abused	Percentage physically abused	Percentage sexually abused
Putnam et al. 1986	100 (92/2)	97	75	83
Ross et al. 1989c	236	89	75	79
Coons et al. 1988	50 (46/4)	96	60	68
Schultz et al. 1989	355 (319/36)	98	82	86

Note.   All subjects studied were adults (≥18 years old).

ization, 4) identity confusion, and 5) identity alteration. An understanding of these five core symptoms is essential to adequately diagnose and assess dissociative disorders, for two reasons: 1) the five dissociative disorders (i.e., dissociative [formerly psychogenic] amnesia, dissociative [formerly psychogenic] fugue, depersonalization disorder, dissociative identity disorder [DID; formerly called multiple personality disorder], and dissociative disorder not otherwise specified [DDNOS]) can all be defined in terms of different constellations of the five core symptoms, and 2) the variety of external manifestations of dissociation, such as flashbacks, out-of-body experiences, auditory hallucinations, and the like, can be understood as clinical indicators of the five core symptoms. Figures 1–1 and 1–2 provide a visual summary of the five symptoms; Figure 1–3 shows the five core symptoms in relation to a number of manifest behaviors and symptoms.

Amnesia

Amnesia may be regarded as the foundational symptom of the five dissociative symptoms in that it is the "building block" on which the others rest. Amnesia is usually described as "gaps" in the patient's memory, ranging from minutes to years, and is sometimes described as "lost time." Patients with severe amnesia are often unable to recall the frequency or duration of their amnestic episodes. In addition, they may "come to themselves" away from home, unable to remember how they got there, or have trouble remembering their name, age, or other personal information. Severe amnesia of psychogenic origin in adult life is often an indication of childhood trauma. In addition, trauma can both eliminate and intensify a memory. Patients who have a history of trauma and who seem to be amnestic for their traumatic experiences may experience sudden intrusive memory fragments, or *flashbacks*. These flashbacks represent portions of the traumatic experience. Patients may also demonstrate implicit memory for experiences beyond the reach of conscious recollection exhibited by behaviors "cued" by responses to seemingly innocuous objects having a symbolic connection to past trauma. Furthermore, self-destructive behavior is a common consequence of abuse in that amnestic patients may "awaken" with self-inflicted wounds and be unaware of their origin. SCID-D research indicates a spectrum of amnesia ranging from normal, occasional forgetfulness to recurrent or persistent episodes of amnesia in patients who reported histories of recurrent childhood abuse.

Depersonalization

Depersonalization manifests in a variety of ways in trauma survivors. It may be related to amnesia in that patients may be amnestic for depersonalization, and this amnesia may occur because the symptom itself is initially frightening to many people who experience it. Patients report depersonalization in terms of their feeling detached from the self, feeling that the self is strange or unreal, feeling physically separated from part(s) of their body, feeling detached from their emotions, or feeling that they are an automaton or robot. Difficulty in describing the nature of the episode and fear

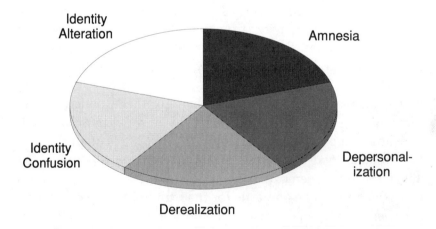

Figure 1–1. Manifestations of dissociation: five core components.

of negative reactions from others are factors in the connection between amnesia and depersonalization. For this reason, the SCID-D has been designed to elicit reports of depersonalization by indirect as well as direct questions. In some instances, depersonalization episodes may echo memories of verbal abuse; for example, patients may experience a mirror image of themselves insulting them. Some patients recall episodes of depersonalization during past abuse, such as one woman with DID who remembered feeling her body rise to the ceiling while being raped. Depersonalization sometimes induces patients to inflict pain on themselves to regain the feeling of being alive. Lastly, depersonalization may manifest in the form of ongoing internal interactive dialogues between an observing and participating self in patients whose childhood trauma resulted in a dissociative disorder.

Derealization

The relationship between *derealization* and amnesia is similar to that between depersonalization and amnesia in that patients are

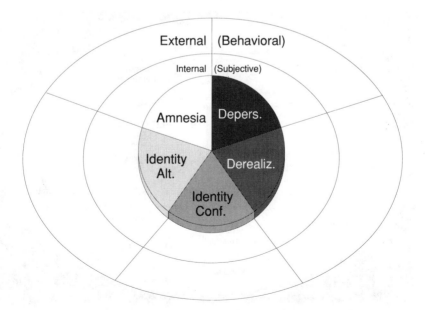

Figure 1–2. Manifestations of dissociation.

often amnestic for episodes of derealization and for the same reasons as depersonalization. Again, just as with depersonalization, derealization is common in patients with histories of severe trauma. This symptom includes feelings of estrangement or detachment from the environment, or a sense that the environment is unreal. Patients who have experienced recurrent emotional, physical, and/or sexual trauma frequently endorse derealization episodes in which close relatives or their own home seem unreal or foreign to them. These feelings are often associated with traumatic memories of childhood events, which patients may spontaneously share when describing intense derealization experiences. Patients with histories of trauma also may report flashbacks and age-regressed states in which the contemporary environment becomes unreal while a past experience is relived. As with depersonalization, the SCID-D's format is designed to encourage patients to describe experiences of derealization in a nonthreatening and open-ended manner.

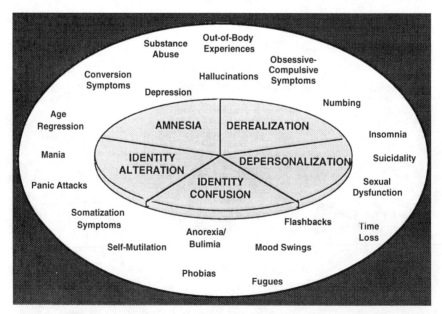

Figure 1–3. Manifestations of dissociation: internal and external.

Identity Confusion

Identity confusion is defined by the SCID-D as a subjective feeling of uncertainty, puzzlement, or conflict about one's own identity. Patients who report histories of childhood trauma characteristically describe themes of ongoing inner struggle regarding their identity; of inner battles for survival; or other images of anger, conflict, and violence. SCID-D research has found that patients who have been sexually abused may experience severe identity confusion regarding their own sexual identity.

Identity Alteration

Identity alteration is defined in the SCID-D as a person's shift in role or identity, which is observable by others through changes in the person's behavior. Manifestations of identity alteration include the use of different names, the possession of a learned skill for which one cannot account, and the discovery of strange or unfamiliar personal items in one's possession. These transitions in role or behavior may be connected with amnestic episodes in which a person is unable to remember events that occurred while undergoing a personality switch. Identity alteration in DID is characterized by its complexity, its distinctness, the ability of alters to take control of behavior, and the interconnection with other dissociative symptoms. In addition, this symptom usually causes the patient significant distress or anxiety because of its actual or potential effects on employment and interpersonal relationships. Many patients with severe identity alteration have lost jobs or close relationships because their behavioral shifts are confusing and upsetting to others.

▌ Some General Observations for Clinicians

Difficulties in Assessing the Dissociative Disorders

Clinicians should note that assessment of dissociative symptoms and disorders is frequently complicated by the fact that the symptoms are found in patients with a wide range of psychiatric disorders, including obsessive-compulsive disorder, eating disorders, substance use disorders, and borderline personality disorder (Goff et al. 1992; Kluft 1988a; Spiegel 1984; Stone 1990; Torem 1986). Instances in which dissociation is primary, such as in the dissociative disorders and posttraumatic stress disorder, may be far more common than previously realized (Bliss and Jeppsen 1985; Helzer et al. 1987; Kluft 1988a; Loewenstein 1991; Ross and Norton 1988; Spiegel 1991; Steinberg 1991; Tucker et al. 1973). However, until recently, dissociative disorders have not been considered routinely in the differential diagnoses of psychiatric patients.

Assessment of dissociative disorders is further complicated by the nature of the symptoms involved. Isolated symptoms may mimic a spectrum of psychiatric conditions, including psychotic, affective, and character disorders (Braun and Sachs 1985; Coons 1984; Kluft 1984a, 1987c; Putnam et al. 1986; Rosenbaum 1980; Steinberg 1994b). These posttraumatic, dissociative defenses initially evolved as the patient's self-protection, to seal off memories of traumatic experiences. A patient whose major defense is dissociation may be amnestic for his or her symptoms (e.g., identity alteration, depersonalization) and for the trauma itself. Lastly, clinicians should be aware that because reality testing remains intact in patients with dissociative disorders, they may be reluctant to discuss or describe their experiences for fear of being judged as "crazy." The chief exception is depersonalization: this symptom often goes unreported because the absence of affect characteristic of chronic depersonalization may seem "normal" to the patient.

Consequences of Inadequate Diagnosis

Because of the complications discussed in the preceding subsection, the dissociative disorders are frequently misdiagnosed. Several researchers have found that the misdiagnosis and consequent ineffective treatment of dissociative disorders may be perpetuated for years (Coons 1984; Kluft 1988a, 1991; Putnam et al. 1986; Ross and Norton 1988; Spiegel 1986). For example, an investigation of 100 patients studied at NIMH revealed that, on the average, DID patients had received 3.6 psychiatric diagnoses (range = 0–11) and spent 6.8 years (range = 0–23 years) in therapy before accurate diagnoses were made (Putnam et al. 1986). Often, cases of dissociative disorders that are initially treatable on an outpatient basis may end in unnecessary hospitalization because of incorrect diagnosis.

On the positive side, other studies indicate that patients receiving appropriate therapy specific for dissociative disorders have good prognoses (Coons 1986; Kluft 1984c, 1991; Putnam 1989a). In a study of 32 patients who ultimately received treatment for DID, Kluft (1984c) found that 47% required hospitalization before receiving the correct diagnosis compared with 19% who were hospitalized during treatment subsequent to accurate diagnosis.

■ History Taking and Diagnostic Assessment

With respect to history taking and diagnostic assessment, the SCID-D is a time- and cost-effective instrument with a variety of clinical applications. In addition to diagnosis for treatment and identification of symptoms for treatment planning, it can be used for long-term follow-up of patients' symptoms. A clinician can administer the instrument at 6-month or yearly intervals to monitor changes in symptomatology and reassess treatment strategy accordingly. The SCID-D may be particularly useful to practitioners of hypnosis, in that it can be administered to patients prior to the induction of formal hypnotic trance in order to establish the patient's dissociative symptom baseline. Moreover, the SCID-D is a tool that can be used for patient education (during a follow-up session with the subject) regarding the nature and significance of the patient's dissociative symptoms. Many patients have reported therapeutic benefits from the opportunity to discuss their symptoms with the interviewer, as the case study in Chapter 15 indicates. Lastly, because the instrument is designed to be filed with patients' charts, it secures easily accessible documentation of symptoms for record keeping and psychological reports (Hall and Steinberg 1994). This feature is particularly beneficial to clinicians who are expert witnesses in forensic cases, in that SCID-D results can be submitted as evidentiary material that is less controversial than amobarbital interviews, hypnosis, or the results of projective psychological tests.

CHAPTER 2

Dissociation and Trauma

Where is my mind? My thoughts? They race each other until I can only see the places they have been. All blurred like a cartoon car taking off in a chase. I can't slow them, I can't even see them anymore. I just stand back and look where they usually are projected.

Then it stopped. A lady reached out her hand to touch mine. She told me there are lots of men like me. She said that in time the terror would end. She said the pain wasn't my fault, or the abuse either. I believed her. Months later I knew I wasn't losing my mind, insanity wasn't tearing at my face. I had nothing to lose in this madness. It was something coming out, not going in.

Crazy isn't some place to go, for me it was where I had been.

—Gregory B., "Running"[1]

As the introductory chapter has indicated, recent investigations suggest that dissociative disorders and symptoms are much more prevalent than previously realized (Bliss and Jeppsen 1985; Coons et al. 1988; Fine 1990; Kluft 1988a; Spiegel 1991; Steinberg 1991, 1994b; Tucker et al. 1973). Researchers' estimates of the incidence rates of dissociative disorders and symptoms in clinical and community populations vary widely. Their accuracy has been limited until recently by the lack of valid and reliable diagnostic tools. With respect to the symptom of depersonalization in particular, Cattell and Cattell (1974) ranked depersonalization as the third most common clinical symptom among psychiatric patients, exceeded only by depression and anxiety. Of psychiatric patients without a primary diagnosis of depersonaliza-

---

[1]From Cohen et al. 1991, p. 57.

tion, 12% were described as having experienced one or more "severe and lasting" episodes of depersonalization (Brauer et al. 1970). A history of the symptom "was only elicited from detailed examination of the patient" and had not been included in the initial psychiatric evaluation (Brauer et al. 1970). Noyes et al. (1977) reported that transient depersonalization syndrome developed in "nearly one-third of [control] persons exposed to life-threatening danger" (e.g., accident victims) and in nearly 40% of a group of hospitalized psychiatric patients. With respect to amnestic syndromes, dissociative amnesia is regularly seen in hospital emergency rooms (Nemiah 1985). One study (Kiersch 1962) reported that 20% of all hospital admissions for amnesia are of dissociative origin. Croft et al. (1973) found dissociative amnesia or fugue in approximately 10% of patients referred for neurological consultation. The incidence of dissociative identity disorder (DID) among psychiatric inpatients has been found to range from 6% to 10% (Bliss and Jeppsen 1985; Kluft 1991). Lastly, from a sample of 345 college students, Ross et al. (1991) estimated that the prevalence DSM-III-R dissociative disorders among college students was 11%.

The conceptual model underlying discussion of the dissociative disorders in this book was developed through research with the SCID-D (Steinberg 1993b, 1994b). Most of the previous discussions in the literature on these disorders list a bewildering variety of dissociative and nondissociative symptoms. Moreover, they treat dissociation in the context of other nondissociative symptoms, such as anger, shame, or anxiety. This book, following the SCID-D, conceptualizes the dissociative disorders as being made up of five core symptoms: 1) amnesia, 2) depersonalization, 3) derealization, 4) identity confusion, and 5) identity alteration. The five dissociative disorders (i.e., dissociative amnesia, dissociative fugue, depersonalization disorder, DID, and dissociative disorder not otherwise specified [DDNOS]) can then be distinguished from each other according to their characteristic constellations of the five core symptoms. Moreover, the dissociative disorders can be differentiated from other disorders by use of standard diagnostic criteria. The dissociative disorders also have unique diagnostic signs and symptomatology that are best elicited by a series of direct and indirect questions that are not routinely asked in mental status examinations. These questions are essential to compiling a reliable patient history and arriving at accurate diagnosis.

The clinician's use of the five core dissociative symptoms as a basis for assessment and evaluation minimizes the possibility of misdiagnosis. Although the dissociative symptoms as described in this book may occur in other disorders, such as schizophrenia or borderline personality disorder, they possess clear, diagnostically discriminating features when they occur in the dissociative disorders. These features are connected with the maintenance of reality testing during dissociative episodes.

This book also emphasizes the posttraumatic nature of the dissociative disorders as being the cognitive, affective, and behavioral sequelae of severe emotional, physical, and/or sexual abuse in the patient's childhood. This book is intended to increase the sensitivity and awareness of professionals to the high prevalence of child abuse and its etiologic relationship to the dissociative disorders.

■ Dissociation: Definitions and Classification

Despite ongoing theoretical controversies regarding the psychological processes underlying dissociative phenomena, there appears to be agreement among researchers concerning the general phenomenology of dissociation. DSM-IV defines *dissociation* as "a disruption in the usually integrated functions of consciousness, memory, identity, or perception of the environment" (American Psychiatric Association 1994, p. 477). Nemiah (1991) describes dissociation as "the exclusion from consciousness and the inaccessibility of voluntary recall of mental events, singly or in clusters, of varying degrees of complexity, such as memories, sensations, feelings, fantasies, and attitudes." Maintained in an unconscious state, these mental events may intrude into consciousness spontaneously or affect consciousness in the form of ego-dystonic symptoms. Spiegel and Cardeña (1991) define dissociation "as a structured separation of mental processes (e.g., thoughts, emotions, conation,

memory, and identity) that are ordinarily integrated." Other definitions in the recent literature include the following:

1. "To sever the association of one thing from another" (Braun
   1984).
2. "The separation of an idea or thought process from the main
   stream of consciousness" (Braun 1988).
3. "A process whereby certain mental functions, which are ordinarily integrated with other functions, presumably operate in
   a more compartmentalized or automatic way, usually outside
   the sphere of consciousness or memory recall" (Ludwig 1983,
   p. 93).
4. "A method of coping with an experience that would otherwise
   be overwhelming; it is a process through which the person
   compartmentalizes various parts of his personality, emotions,
   or body, and sees them as separate from his 'true' self"
   (Hunter 1990, p. 61).
5. "The process whereby a coordinated set of activities, thoughts,
   attitudes or emotions becomes separated from the rest of the
   person's personality and functions independently ... thoughts
   or memories that produce anxiety are cut off from consciousness ... each of the dissociated aspects maintains its integrity"
   (Reber 1985, pp. 208–209).
6. "Discontinuity in one's perception of self and environment"
   (Goff et al. 1992, p. 332).

Frankel (1990) has argued that these preceding definitions are
too inclusive. However, their lack of clarity may result from the
complexity of dissociative phenomena themselves. For clinical
purposes, it is best to consider the global concept of dissociation in
terms of interdependent but discrete components.

Classification of Dissociation

Until 1980, dissociative disorders were classified as a subcategory
of hysteria, conversion disorders being the other major subcategory. In 1980, DSM-III (American Psychiatric Association 1980) in-

troduced the term *dissociative disorder*, thus breaking from previous psychoanalytic definitions. The five disorders included under the heading in DSM-III-R were 1) psychogenic amnesia, 2) psychogenic fugue, 3) depersonalization disorder, 4) multiple personality disorder, and 5) DDNOS (a residual category). In addition, DSM-III-R separated these disorders from the conversion disorders, which, however, are also thought to involve some dissociative processes (Nemiah 1991). DSM-IV has included *dissociative trance disorder* as a subcategory of DDNOS to accommodate dissociative disorders that occur in specific cultural contexts and involve "an involuntary state of trance that is not accepted by the person's culture as a normal part of a collective cultural or religious practice and that causes clinically significant distress or functional impairment" (American Psychiatric Association 1994, p. 727).

The International Classification of Diseases (ICD; World Health Organization 1992) (which is the European counterpart of the DSM) followed the lead of the United States in including the category of dissociative disorders in its 10th revision (ICD-10), replacing the term *hysterical neurosis* (Garcia 1990). Dissociative disorders, according to the ICD, include 1) dissociative (conversion) disorder, 2) dissociative amnesia, 3) dissociative fugue, 4) dissociative stupor, 5) trance and possession disorders, 6) dissociative disorders of movement and sensation, 7) dissociative motor disorders, 8) dissociative convulsions, 9) dissociative anesthesia and sensory loss, 10) mixed dissociative and conversion disorders, 11) other dissociative disorders including Ganser's syndrome and multiple personality disorder.

Varieties of Dissociative Phenomena

Any human psychological or behavioral function may become dissociated from consciousness. Braun (1988) proposed the *BASK* mnemonic and model, in which dissociation can be regarded as involving any or all of the following processes: Behavior, Action, Sensation, and Knowledge. According to Braun, these four elements function along a time line.

The three functions singled out by DSM-IV as the primary mental capacities affected by dissociative disturbance, namely *identity, memory,* and *consciousness,* are interrelated in complex ways (Ensink 1992). William James (1890) stressed the interdependence of consciousness and identity when he defined consciousness as "self reference," or "I feel, I think," rather than "feelings and thoughts exist." *Identity* may be defined as a function of a higher order, encompassing memory and consciousness. However, discussion is complicated by the fact that there seem to be two distinct usages of *identity: identity* in common usage, and *sense of identity,* which is more aligned with self-consciousness.

Consciousness

Consciousness is a difficult abstraction to define, yet it is central to the concept of dissociation. Moreover, if one accepts reflective consciousness as one of the most highly prized dimensions of human life, the impact of the fragmentation of consciousness by a dissociative disturbance on a person's sense of selfhood or basic humanity is readily understandable. One can think of consciousness as a structured experiential process that functions to encode, process, and communicate information. Its components include memory storage and retrieval, a sense of orientation to reality, and the more general levels of awareness of one's existence and identity. In normal circumstances, human beings integrate these components into a global experience accessible to introspection in the present moment and recall in the future. There is also an inexpressible subjectivity composing one particular level of consciousness—what Kihlstrom terms *phenomenal awareness*—which is the presence of information in the brain, along with a *feeling*—an affect that confers an internal reality on human thoughts.

The literature of the human sciences contains a variety of definitions of consciousness. Some adopt a functionalist perspective. For example, Kihlstrom (1984) sees two principal functions associated with consciousness: 1) monitoring of self and environment to ensure accurate representations of percepts, memories, and thoughts in phenomenal awareness; and 2) control of self and environment in order to voluntarily initiate and terminate thoughts and behaviors. Other writers favor a more organic interpretation. William James (1890) claimed over a century ago that the fundamental aspect of consciousness was the continuity of experience, underscoring the essential underlying features of integration, organization, and singularity in consciousness. From a clinical perspective, the most general usage is perhaps the most useful, namely that consciousness is a mental domain containing the sensations, perceptions, and memories of which a person is momentarily aware. Its connection with the mechanism and phenomena of dissociation are the subject of the following sections.

Dissociation as Fragmentation of Consciousness

In the context of this book, *dissociation* will be used to mean the dissociation of *consciousness* from some other personal aspect or capacity that is normally integrated with consciousness. This usage explains why dissociation can be considered an altered state of consciousness. During a dissociative episode, the mental contents that are dissociated from full consciousness remain on some peripheral level of awareness; from this perspective, dissociation can also be defined as a fragmentation of consciousness. In other words, not only does dissociation imply the separation of a *process* from consciousness, it also implies the separation of a "part-consciousness" from a "main-consciousness" (or phenomenal awareness). The actual *mechanisms* of dissociation are related to a variety of phenomena, including habitual and automatic activities, parallel processing, neuropsychophysiologic state-dependent learning, and divisions between executive and monitoring functions or between mental representations of the self and representations of experience, thought, and action (Braun 1984; Hilgard 1986; Kihlstrom 1987; Kihlstrom and Hoyt 1990).

Normal Dissociative Processes

Certain dissociative processes fall well within the normal spectrum of experience. Depersonalization and derealization, for instance, are common occurrences before or after sleep, in periods of unusual fatigue or emotional stress, after drug or alcohol consumption, or during some forms of meditation or trance (Castillo 1990; Dixon 1963; Fewtrell 1986; Guttmann and Maclay 1936; Keshaven and Lishman 1986; Moran 1986; Roberts 1960; Steinberg et al. 1990; Szymanski 1981; Trueman 1984b). These normal experiences of derealization and depersonalization involve isolated, brief episodes, usually associated with stress (Dixon 1963; Roberts 1960; Steinberg et al. 1990; Trueman 1984b). With respect to the symptom of amnesia, nonpathological varieties include childhood amnesia, sleep and dream amnesia, and hypnotic amnesia (Schacter and Kihlstrom 1989). An example of identity confusion falling within the normal range for adults would include the need many people feel to integrate their various familial and social roles (e.g., wife, professor, registered voter) (Steinberg et al. 1990). A "normal" person experiences identity alteration in terms of integrating these different roles, is aware of the role transition, and understands it as being within his or her conscious control (Steinberg et al. 1990). Another type of dissociation that falls within the boundaries of normal experience is dissociation during therapeutic hypnosis (Bliss 1986; Frankel 1990; Frischholz 1985; Kihlstrom and Hoyt 1990; Spiegel 1990; Sutcliffe and Jones 1988). *Hypnosis* is defined by Spiegel (1990) as "controlled dissociation elicited in a structured setting" (p. 247). Clinicians should note that hypnosis is a more inclusive term than dissociation, in that it also comprehends absorption (preoccupation with a particular stimulus; in this case, the hypnotist's instructions) and suggestibility (Hammond 1990).

The final category of "normal" dissociation is dreaming. While dreaming, humans exhibit dissociative symptoms (Gabel 1990; van der Kolk et al. 1984). Gabel (1990) mentions several aspects of dreaming that are dissociative: 1) there is a narrowed focus of consciousness; 2) thoughts and feelings are symbolic *(hallucinatory symbolism);* 3) dreamers are usually amnestic for their dreams upon awakening; and 4) the dream state contains components of derealization, depersonalization (including seeing oneself in the dream), and identity alteration.

Lastly, clinicians should be aware that the range of "normal" dissociation varies according to the stages of the human life cycle. In particular, the range of dissociation is apparently wider in children than in adults in that children dissociate more freely than adults (Putnam 1985).

The Functions of Dissociation

It will be helpful for professionals to understand the functions that the processes of dissociation serve, whether in normal or in pathological contexts. This understanding will enable clinicians to refine their ability to distinguish between normal, threshold, and pathological experiences of dissociation during patient interviews. Ludwig (1983) proposes six main functions for the mechanism:

1. **Automatizing behavior.** Dissociation permits a person to perform some actions or thought processes without direct conscious attention in order to increase efficiency. An example would be the mild dissociation that allows a skilled driver to perform routine maneuvers while driving without having to devote full attention to them.
2. **Resolution of irreconcilable conflicts.** Dissociation allows a person in a condition of cognitive dissonance to keep the conflictual desires or a conflict between attitudes and behavior on a different level of consciousness so that the person can function. For example, a medical student who "knows" that smoking is harmful to health but is addicted to the habit would dissociate from knowledge of the bad effects of smoking while lighting up a cigarette.
3. **Escape from reality.** In some instances, dissociation induces people to imagine that they have some kind of mastery over intractable environmental difficulties. Dissociation is often implicated in magical thinking or self-induced trance states. This aspect of dissociation is frequently found in abuse survivors. It is not uncommon for abused children to engage in magical thinking to retain an illusion of control over the situation (e.g., believing that they "cause" the perpetrator to act out).
4. **Isolation of catastrophic experiences.** Dissociation may function to seal off overwhelming trauma into a compartmentalized area of consciousness until the person is better able to

integrate it into mainstream consciousness. This function of dissociation is particularly common in survivors of combat, political torture, or natural or transportation disasters.

5. **Cathartic discharge.** In cultures that have rituals for the periodic release of pent-up emotion (e.g., Mardi Gras or the German *Karneval* and *Oktoberfest)*, the ritual serves to dissociate the inhibitions that normally block the feelings.

6. **Enhancement of human bonding.** Dissociation seems to aid in interpersonal bonding or group solidarity by increasing suggestibility to charismatic leaders and causes. This function of dissociation also serves to explain the particular vulnerability of abuse survivors to revictimization by a trusted member of the helping professions or to sectarian cults or ideological programming or "brainwashing" of any kind.

Dissociation and Repression

The terms *dissociation* and *repression* were introduced by Janet and Freud, respectively, toward the close of the nineteenth century. Dissociation and repression have sometimes been used loosely or interchangeably in the literature. One difference in usage, however, has to do with the source of the pain that the person is seeking to minimize or avoid. *Repression* is more often used to refer to pain that is intrapsychic in origin, whereas *dissociation* is used more frequently to refer to the avoidance of pain from an external source. In addition, Spiegel (1990) has noted that Freud originally introduced the concept of repression to connote the banishment of unacceptable libidinal desires rather than of traumas or of memories of traumas. Freud saw the unconscious as a source of pleasurable but disturbing impulses rather than of painful memories. As a result, he construed that the function of ego defenses was to repress these conflictual impulses from consciousness to protect the person from anxiety.

Another distinction between dissociation and repression concerns the relative activity or passivity of the mental capacities involved. Generally speaking, dissociation is a passive process, repression an active one. Janet's conception of dissociation depicted a passive splitting of the mind due to a weak ego, whereas Freud's concept of repression implied an active rejection of unacceptable ideas from consciousness "by an ego strong enough to banish [the idea] from sight." (Nemiah 1979, p. 317). Otherwise put, repression is the removal of material by the ego, whereas dissociation is the ego's allowing itself to fall apart (i.e., passive fragmentation.

The remaining major distinction between repression and dissociation has to do with the nature and complexity of the material that is being warded off. In repression, certain mental contents are separated from the mainstream of the person's consciousness, but the psychological processes themselves are not affected (Kernberg 1984). Put slightly differently, repression preserves the patient's "sense of self," whereas dissociation causes the person to experience the self as fragmented (Fink 1988). The dissociated parts of the mind may be perceived by the patient as a semiautonomous entity, whereas repressed material tends to be less complex and less likely to reemerge into full consciousness as a separate personality fragment. The *dissociative unconscious* (ideas that are dissociated from awareness) is capable of organized and logical thinking, whereas the unconscious as Freud defined it is primitive and chaotic. The relevance of these distinctions to differential diagnosis is that they help to explain 1) the connection between the mechanism of dissociation and the fragmentation of personality and identity that characterizes the dissociative disorders as a group, and 2) the source of the anxiety and emotional distress that patients in this category experience. One can readily understand that a person experiencing several different centers of consciousness would be more anxious than a person who is simply out of touch for the time being with some undifferentiated memories or perceptions.

Dissociation as a Posttraumatic Symptom

The Dissociative Aftereffects of Trauma

As has been mentioned (in the introductory sections of this book), the causal connection between a person's history of trauma and development of dissociative symptomatology is an important reason for taking a complete history. In addition, one should be aware that the dissociative defenses used to cope with trauma in early life tend to be maintained throughout life to cope with stress arising from nonabuse factors (Gelinas 1983). These findings indicate that trauma not only triggers dissociative defenses at the time of its infliction but causes long-term damage to the survivor's psyche in that he or she tends to interpret life in general as being a negative or traumatic experience long after the initial abuse has ended. Moreover, survivors of abuse are often involved in reenactments of the early abusive relationship in their adult life. This pattern of revictimization is described in various ways by therapists of different theoretical orientations. Some use the term *repetition compulsion* to describe a survivor who is understood to be engaging in reenactments of the original abuse to gain mastery over it (Herman 1981). Others use the terminology of *life scripts* and other phrases of Gestalt psychology to imply that abuse survivors learn to act out a *victim script* or self-fulfilling prophecy, and that this can be changed by a cognitive and perceptual reorientation (Stone 1989). Some researchers maintain that humans have biologic responses to trauma, such that abuse survivors only feel "normal" under conditions of hyperarousal. Specifically, as van der Kolk (1989) stated, "people who were neglected or abused as children may require much higher external stimulation of the endogenous opioid system for soothing than those whose endogenous opioids can be more easily activated by conditioned responses based on good early caregiving experiences" (p. 401). In sum, however, whatever explanatory model a clinician may favor, he or she should be prepared for the presence of dissociative symptomatology in adult survivors of trauma. Because, as was mentioned in a preceding section, children are prone to dissociate more freely than adults (Kluft 1985b), it stands to reason that a child who resorts to dissociation as a means of coping with overwhelming pain will continue to employ that mechanism during stressful periods in later life.

Although the SCID-D is not a trauma questionnaire as such, its open-ended questions regarding dissociative symptoms frequently elicit accounts of trauma from patients. SCID-D research indicates that all five symptoms of dissociation can be connected to traumatic histories (Steinberg 1993b, 1994b). In amnesia, the person may forget aspects of the self, the perpetrator, and the traumata; in DID, one personality may be amnestic for the very existence as well as the behaviors of another. In depersonalization, a person dissociates from his or her sense of self to detach from a painful state of consciousness connected with the actual physical encounters with the abuser. Experiences of derealization typically involve the patient's home, parents, and spouses, often indicating the relationship between derealization as a symptom and intimate family traumas. In identity confusion, the person may dissociate aspects of the self that remember the abuse with fear and anger, and other aspects that are confused, or retain some fondness for the perpetrator. Finally, in identity alteration, a person can dissociate entirely from personality fragments involving memories of the abuse or from residual feelings of love for the abusive relative.

The Assessment of Traumatic History

Dissociative disturbances pose special problems from the outset for the diagnostician. Even at the level of the initial interview, dissociative disorders complicate the taking of the patient's history. It may be difficult for a subject whose major defense is dissociation to volunteer an accurate history; some patients will be amnestic for their symptoms, whereas others will seek to hide episodes of depersonalization or problems with their identity (Kluft 1988a). The close connection between the dissociative disorders and severe trauma, child abuse, or incest may also complicate assessment because patients may deny or be amnestic for these specific stressors. When child abuse and its sequelae are the underlying causes of the mental illness, other issues are often substituted. For instance, patients mention difficulties relating to others and feelings of worthlessness, fear, and depression (Hunter 1990). One reason for reticence with respect to the dissociative symptoms themselves is fear of the interviewer's incredulity or negative judgment (Goodwin 1985). As this book will mention in a number of contexts, the symptoms of dissociation often manifest in ways that are difficult for the patient to describe at all.

Even for patients who are not amnestic regarding past abuse, frankness and honesty with the interviewer are often compromised by shame issues. Our culture's tendency to blame victims for their own suffering, to maintain that they either "ask for it" or enjoy it on some level, encourages survivors of abuse to deny their own victimization. Furthermore, Nathanson (1989) has observed that the very exposure of sexual trauma that is involved in psychotherapy is itself felt to be a shaming experience by the patient. Acknowledgment of abuse issues is particularly difficult for male survivors, insofar as male socialization in Western societies regards victimization as a compromise of masculine sex identity. Male survivors of abuse may manifest a severe degree of sexual identity confusion as well as other dissociative symptoms (Myers 1991). Lastly, patients' experiences of revictimization by previous therapists may hamper full disclosure during the taking of the patient's history. Kluft's (1990a) findings agree with Rutter's (1991)—not only that the incidence of revictimization of incest survivors (of either sex) by therapists is alarmingly high but that the illicit sexual contact often begins *shortly after the incest is revealed* to the therapist. Kluft's conclusion is that the survivor's admission means that she or he is "no longer seen as deserving respect or protection." Although incidents of survivor revictimization by members of the helping professions are in the minority, users of this book should be aware that they occur frequently enough to be a possible factor underlying acute dissociative symptomatology. In some cases, the patient may have been reabused by a professor, lawyer, or member of the clergy rather than a medical professional, but the same traumatic violation of personal boundaries is involved, and the same dissociative reactions may result.

As a diagnostic instrument, the SCID-D does not ask explicit questions regarding a history of trauma, but its semistructured format is designed to allow the patient to expand on the patient's dissociative experiences in such a way that descriptions of abuse often emerge spontaneously.

PART II

The Five Dissociative Symptoms

CHAPTER 3

Amnesia

The Black Hole of Dissociation

Think about the last time you forgot someone's name or a minor detail. Did trying to remember drive you nuts? MPD is like that, but there are many, many more things you don't remember. Add to that the fact that you don't remember, or that when you do finally remember, you FORGET that you remembered, etc. . . .

—Patricia M., *Multiple Personality Disorder From the Inside Out*[1]

As the epigraph above illustrates, amnesia is a "negative symptom." As with a black hole, the very nature of amnesia entails the affected person's lack of awareness of it. Neither amnesia nor a black hole can be directly observed; we can only infer their existence and nature from their effects. Patients usually become aware of their amnesia only after it begins to cause disruption in their social or work environments.

Unlike other physical or psychiatric symptoms, such as headaches, muscle cramps, or the delusions and hallucinations that typify psychosis, a patient may have no subjective awareness of amnesia. Ensink's (1992) study of women who experienced "time gaps" found that most of them learned about their amnesia from others informing them about behaviors that they did not recall. Additional clues included physical evidence of forgotten actions, such as notes and diaries, or environmental differences or changes, such as finding themselves in a strange place (sometimes even a different city or state). Some of Ensink's subjects also stated that they had a history of having had "a bad memory."

In order to get a better understanding of the many implications

---

[1] From Cohen et al. 1991, p. 24.

of memory loss, let us first review the functions that amnesia disrupts.

■ Memory and Consciousness

Memory is one of the most essential functions of the human mind, and if lost in its entirety, it renders a person completely dysfunctional. Dysfunction due to memory loss is not solely a matter of the patient's impairment in employment and interpersonal situations, although these may be the manifestations most visible to others. With specific regard to cognitive functioning, memory can be thought of as an information processing system in the mind that stores, represents, and manipulates all of the experiences acquired in a person's lifetime through the physical senses as well as through the internal processes of thought or imagination. As early as the fifth century A.D., Augustine of Hippo described memory as "a great field or a spacious palace, a storehouse for countless images of all kinds which are conveyed to it by the senses. In it are stored away all the thoughts by which we enlarge upon or diminish or modify in any way the perceptions at which we arrive through the senses, and it also contains anything else that has been entrusted to it for safekeeping" (Augustine 1961, p. 214). Memory is quite possibly the most essential part of human consciousness in that persons require a sense of memory retention and continuity to maintain a realistic awareness of the occurrence of events before they can attach significance to the events. We can think of memory as the "language of identity" because our sense of self is dependent in large measure on how we remember our history of personal events, relationships, and beliefs, and on how we expect ourselves to respond to situations based on past experience. Loss of memory is frequently experienced as an assault on one's sense of identity. To begin with, verbal and symbolic memory are mental functions that distinguish humans from other primates. Moreover, in our present society, in which people's sense of selfhood is typically constructed around a personal history, gaps in the continuity of this history are often perceived by amnestic subjects as worrisome or frightening. Memory also mediates a sense of corporate or collective identity through the recollections we share with others, the sense of familiarity we have with others, and the personal connection we retain to values in the wider society that we find meaningful.

Pierre Janet (1859–1947) was one of the pioneers in the scientific study of memory. Janet described the two primary functions of memory as follows: 1) the processing and storing of sensations, and 2) the organization of incoming data (internal and external) according to previous memories (van der Kolk and van der Hart 1989). What Janet described as the "stream of consciousness" is maintained by a sense of familiarity with one's surroundings, which in turn is mediated by the retention of memory for what one experiences. Consciousness, then, is maintained by a memory system that is constantly interpreting new experiences in terms of earlier ones. In terms of abstract cognition, any understanding of an idea is dependent on the individual's recognition of both the linguistic symbols as well as the simpler concepts used to construct or convey a more complex idea or concept. Thus memory, as Janet conceived it, is quintessential for understanding, whether of one's immediate physical surroundings or of a highly abstract conceptual domain.

For Janet, consciousness consists of a memory that draws together and unifies all facets of experience. He considered a capacity for rich association and identification, with one's memories as essential to emotional health and full identity. Furthermore, Janet saw memory as "the action of telling a story"—that is, as an active narrative reconstitution of past experiences. In the period since Janet, researchers in many different fields have expanded the boundaries of his pioneering work. The findings from studies of early childhood development, cultural anthropology and historiography, the neuroanatomy and neurophysiology of the brain, biochemistry and pharmacology, as well as general psychology and psychotherapy, have added to our understanding of the functions of memory, its development within the individual from birth to old age, and its abnormalities and dysfunctions.

To turn to the work of the cognitive psychologists, memory can be encoded in three different ways: enactively, iconically, and linguistically. These methods of encoding parallel Piaget's developmental stages of sensorimotor, concrete operations, and formal operational functioning (Kihlstrom 1984). Infants and small children encode experiences enactively, or "through action," integrating memory with sensorimotor experiences, such as for nursing, looking at a face, touching brightly colored objects, defecating, and so on. As the child develops, memory is then encoded iconically. Eventually, the normal human arrives at a stage at which he or she is capable of linguistic encoding or operations requiring abstract thought, such as arithmetical calculations, reading and writing, and the like. The more primitive developmental levels of encoding can be accessed through special states, experiences, or techniques, which include trauma, spontaneous age regression, hypnosis, and other means.

In addition to specifying the developmental stages of the human acquisition of memory, Kihlstrom (1992) differentiates implicit memory from explicit memory. Implicit memory is the encoding of information that is temporarily inaccessible to consciousness. This is akin to hysterical blindness, a state in which a person is registering visual stimuli but is not conscious of them. Kihlstrom writes that "explicit memory refers to the person's conscious recollection of some previous event—the ability to say that THIS EVENT HAPPENED TO ME or I DID THIS THING AT SUCH-AND-SUCH A TIME AND IN SUCH-AND-SUCH A PLACE. . . . Implicit memory, by contrast, is revealed by any change in experience, thought, or action that is attributable to some past episode" (p. 10). For instance, explicit memory would include the kinds of detail surrounding an event that a courtroom witness might describe during a trial, such as the timing of his or her discovery of a crime, the objects he or she saw at the scene, the suspect's physical appearance, and so forth. Implicit memory might be manifest in such things as an abuse survivor's phobic reactions to objects or to environments that trigger anxiety resulting from the abuse, even though the person may not make a conscious connection between the original abuse and the later setting or stimulus.

■ Amnesia: Severity, Etiology, and Context

Some researchers consider amnesia to be the easiest symptom to simulate and the most difficult symptom to disprove (Kiersch 1962). *Amnesia* may be defined as the absence from memory of a specific and/or significant segment of time (Steinberg 1993a; Steinberg et al. 1990). Benson (1978) defines amnesia as a failure of recall or impaired ability to learn, with preserved cognitive characteristics.

When we speak of memories being forgotten, we normally do not mean the permanent loss of that stored information, as would occur in the formatting or accidental erasure of a computer disk. Such a situation may occur in brain trauma. However, dissociative amnesia represents a *displacement* of the memory from awareness to unawareness. The need for localizing these dormant but still dynamic memories led to the institutionalization of the concept of the "unconscious" (Frankel 1990). The continued activity or influence of these "forgotten" memories represents unconscious processing—that is, psychological activity that takes place without conscious cognitive awareness.

In amnesia, memories are not "available"—that is, they can only be retrieved under special conditions. They may be involuntarily triggered by environmental cues, such as in a flashback, or they may be voluntarily retrieved through hypnosis, psychotherapy, or the administration of certain drugs (e.g., amobarbital, Amytal interview).

Amnesia occurs across a spectrum of severity. (See Figure 3–1 for a description of the varied manifestations of amnesia.) Forms of amnesia in the general population include dream amnesia, infantile and childhood amnesia, the "tip-of-the-tongue" phenomenon, and amnesia associated with mild to moderate substance use or other altered states (e.g., religious meditation, self-induced trance). Severe amnesia is more typical of dissociative disorders and organic mental disorders. Amnesia can also be categorized according to etiology as well as severity. Schacter and Kihlstrom (1989) subdivide functional amnesia into amnesias that have *pathological* and *nonpathological* etiologies. Nonpathological amnesias include childhood amnesia, sleep and dream amnesia, and hypnotic amnesia. Pathological amnesias include *functional retrograde amnesia,* which entails "loss of personal identity and large sectors of one's personal past." Lastly, amnesia can be categorized as either episodic or chronic. Kopelman (1987) distinguishes between *discrete episodes* of amnesia, which occur in epilepsy, blackouts, or fugue states, and *persistent impairments* of memory, which occur in drug toxicity or pseudodementia.

People who are aware of periods of time that they cannot account for often speak of *time gaps* in their memory. Time gaps are commonplace occurrences in dreaming, when we may be in dream-consciousness for hours and yet can usually remember only brief sequences from the dream (Ensink 1992). Time gaps also occur when we temporarily lose our recall of what we were doing at some point in the day or the week. They are not called amnesia if the events or activities are recalled with some intentional effort. This kind of normal time gap was noted by Augustine (1961), who commented that "memory produces some things immediately; some are forthcoming only after a delay, as though they were

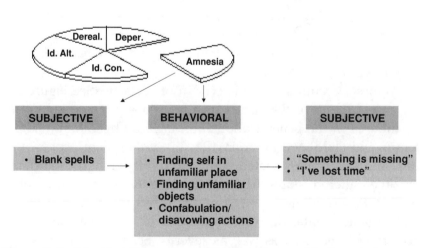

Figure 3–1. Manifestations of amnesia in patients with dissociative disorders.

being brought out from some inner hiding place" (p. 215). Most of us have had the experience of having a time gap accounted for when our memory is "jogged" by a reminder of some kind, such as coming across a ticket stub from a journey, or a friend's mentioning something that happened during the time period in question.

If we look at the categories of amnesia specified in DSM-IV (American Psychiatric Association 1994), we find four general types. *Localized* amnesia is the failure to recall all events that occurred during a circumscribed period of time; *selective* (or systematized) amnesia is the failure to recall some events during a circumscribed period; *generalized* amnesia consists of a loss of all memory of one's life prior to a given event; and *continuous* amnesia is the failure to encode events as they occur. This fourth type of amnesia is usually organic.

Amnesia can be categorized by etiology and context. *Functional* memory loss can be distinguished from *ordinary forgetting* on the one hand and *organic* amnesia on the other (Schacter and Kihlstrom 1989). Dissociative amnesias fall into the functional category and can be conceptualized in a variety of ways. Amnesia that is nonorganic is almost always *retrograde* (loss of information about the past), whereas organic amnesias are often *anterograde* (inability to remember events occurring after the amnestic onset) (Keller and Shaywitz 1986).

Numerous mechanisms have been cited as potential causes of amnesia. Kopelman (1987) lists the possibilities of faulty encoding, faulty consolidation (transfer from short- to long-term memory), accelerated forgetting, faulty retrieval, and faulty temporal or spatial context retrieval. Dissociative or functional amnesia is most likely caused by faulty encoding/retrieval (state-dependent learning) and/or *motivated forgetting,* such as occurs in repression, dissociation, and forgetting the commission of a crime (Christianson and Nilsson 1984; Kopelman 1987).

Normal Amnesia

Nietzsche (1874/1980) once said: "Without forgetting it is quite impossible to *live* at all." There are many conditions in which amnesia is natural or even necessary. If the mind were constantly required to process all the data accessible to memory on a conscious level, the result would be an overwhelming stimulus overload. To begin with a developmental account of ordinary amnesia, researchers have discovered that human memory for the first three years of life is usually absent. Schachtel (1947) explains this phenomenon by arguing that in infancy and childhood, experiences are encoded primitive, prelinguistic schemata. Because of state-dependent learning limitations, these infantile experiences cannot normally be retrieved by the adult, who is in a more highly developed, linguistic encoding state most of the time. The ability of hypnosis to alter an adult's state of consciousness to more primitive levels may be related to reported memories of infantile experiences.

Another common form of nonpathological amnesia is found at the other end of the human life cycle, namely amnesia associated with aging. Amnesia is the most serious cognitive impairment connected with geriatric mental disorders. In normal aging, elderly people have problems with recent memory, rather than *immediate* or *remote* recall, and are less adept in encoding memories than younger people (La Rue 1982).

Amnesia is very common in hypnosis and was frequently observed in early studies of subjects with hysteria (Janet 1907; Nemiah 1979). In hypnosis, many remarkable memory-related phenomena can manifest. Hypnotists can easily induce instantaneous amnesia, posthypnotic amnesia, and *source amnesia* (forgetting the source of learned information). The opposite, namely repristination of memory, can also be observed; hypnosis can break through amnestic barriers so that the subject can recall memories more vividly (Spiegel 1990).

Amnesia of Organic Etiology

Amnesia is a common clinical symptom that occurs in a variety of organic disorders. Some of the most common organic amnestic disorders include Korsakoff's psychosis, amnesia secondary to head trauma, amnestic stroke, postoperative amnesia, postinfectious amnesia, and transient global amnesia (Benson 1978). Other less common forms include epileptic seizures, cerebrovascular disease, metabolic abnormalities, toxic states (including poisoning), and drug and alcohol abuse (including alcoholic blackouts) (Croft et al. 1973; Kopelman 1987). The distinguishing features of organic amnesias are as follows: 1) they do not normally involve recurrent alterations in one's identity; 2) the amnesia is not selectively limited to personal information; 3) the memories are not circumscribed around a stressful or emotionally traumatic event; and 4) the amnesia is often more anterograde than retrograde. Organic amnesia is commonly associated with toxic confusional state, head injury, epilepsy, alcoholic blackout, hypoglycemia, post-ECT, drug toxicity, migraine, viral encephalitis, and global dementia (Croft et al. 1973; Kopelman 1987).

Transient global amnesia (TGA) is a common term applied to a syndrome of circumscribed, mainly anterograde amnesia of organic etiology. It is thought to result from a stroke or epileptic seizure. TGA is characterized by sudden onset; impaired memory encoding; variable retrograde memory loss; intact immediate recall; preserved self-identity; up to a 24-hour duration; full, gradual recovery; and low recurrence rate (Miller et al. 1987; Rowan and Rosenbaum 1991). After an attack of TGA, the patient is usually amnestic for the episode itself. Patients usually realize during the episode that their memory has deficits, and they may repeatedly ask questions in an attempt to orient themselves (Croft et al. 1973). People with TGA can also perform complicated actions, such as driving a car (Deisenhammer 1981).

TGA is thought to result from cerebrovascular disturbances and epileptic seizures, and is often associated with unusual EEG recordings (Croft et al. 1973; Deisenhammer 1981). Its precise etiology is controversial; in some cases, it may result from both cardiovascular disease *and* a seizure, since a stroke can cause a seizure (Gilbert 1978). Attacks of TGA are known to be precipitated by emotional stress, strenuous exertion, hot showers, and sexual intercourse (Gilbert 1978; Miller et al. 1987); however, these are thought to be merely the precipitating causes of the organic dysfunction. It is important to differentiate TGA from dissociative amnesia (Hall and Steinberg 1994).

Amnesia that occurs in the context of epileptic seizure is called *ictal amnesia*. In these instances, there is often anterograde amnesia during the seizure and retrograde amnesia following the seizure (Croft et al. 1973). In ictal amnesia, the person appears otherwise normal and retains a sense of his or her identity. The event is circumscribed and brief, and recovery is expected (Rowan and Rosenbaum 1991). Amnesia that occurs during an epileptic seizure would be characterized by short duration and epileptiform EEG (Rowan and Rosenbaum 1991).

In patients with head injuries, there is usually a brief period of retrograde amnesia and a longer period of anterograde amnesia (Kopelman 1987). Blackouts during alcohol intoxication involve partial to complete amnesia for events occurring during the intoxicated state, and this may be related to amnesia following criminal behavior (Kopelman 1987). In Korsakoff's syndrome, there is significant anterograde amnesia and variable retrograde amnesia; other cognitive functions are usually left intact (Kopelman 1987). In dementia, the memory loss occurs in combination with multiple cognitive deficits, and many different kinds of memory are disturbed, including remote memory (Kopelman 1987).

Confabulation is common in both normal and abnormal memory impairment (Kopelman 1987). It can range from *provoked* confabulation, which involves fleeting distortions and additions to minor memory loss, to *spontaneous* confabulation, which involves fantasy weaving. Amnesia in senescent dementia, a serious organic disorder that can be associated with aging, is characterized by both retrograde and anterograde amnesia, confabulation, and disorientation, as well as by serious disturbances in the recall of recent memory (La Rue 1982).

To differentiate between the different categories of amnesia, it is important to obtain a complete history of the patient's behavior during the episode, and its onset, as well as physical examinations, laboratory tests, and an EEG record as soon as possible (Croft et al. 1973). Abnormal EEG readings may not be noticeable by normal measures. Therefore, sleep-deprivation EEG or nasopharyngeal recordings may be more likely to show deviant spikes (Gilbert 1978).

Amnesia in Depression

Moderate amnesia is a common cognitive impairment characteristic of major depression. *Depressive pseudodementia*, a *functional* depression, is affective in nature (e.g., fear of isolation) and is treatable with therapy. Depressive pseudodementia involves amnesia that is less severe than that in senescent dementia and is characterized by "I don't knows" rather than near-misses or confabulations (La Rue 1982). Patients who have dementia of depressive origin are also more likely to complain about their amnesia than those who have dementia of organic etiology (La Rue 1982).

Amnesia in the Dissociative Disorders

In the dissociative disorders, amnesia is functional; that is, it results from dissociative rather than organic factors. Amnesia in dissociative disorders is intercorrelated with other dissociative symptoms (Steinberg et al. 1990). Ensink (1992) reported that among women who experience time gaps, some experienced forms of *depersonalized* consciousness during the time gaps or at their beginning and end. These dissociative alterations of consciousness included perceptual disturbances such as autoscopy, darkness, sinking, and feelings of unreality. One of the main cognitive processes contributing to amnesia in dissociative disorders is *state-dependent learning* (e.g., Putnam 1989a). According to this theory, information encoded in one mental state is most easily retrieved at a later time under that same state. If experiences occur in sufficiently disparate and dissociated states, information available to a person in one state will not be available to the same person in another state (Ludwig 1966; Swanson and Kinsbourne 1979). Organizing experience according to previous memories is essentially what occurs in state-dependent learning. If, as in dissociative identity disorder (DID), different memories are available to the patient at different times, incoming data will be organized differentially according to those state-dependent memories.

When applying state-dependent learning theory to the phenomenon of DID secondary to abuse, one finds that experiences encoded in the psychological state of abuse can chain together into a complex and consistent personality if the abuse is sufficiently severe and persistent (Braun 1988). These particular alter personalities may not remember facts that other alters remember. In less severe cases of abuse, the abuse state is disparate enough from other states that memories of the abuse cannot be retrieved; however, different personality states may not be formed. Experiences of overwhelming pain and fear are very distinct from other more tolerable states of being.

❚ Trauma and Amnesia

Janet was one of the earliest researchers to emphasize the role of trauma in cognitive impairments. He recognized that traumatic experiences leave deep scars on human memory and that the pain and fear of these memories may persist throughout one's life. The fear associated with traumatic memories must be made more manageable for a person to function normally. When anxiety-provoking memories cannot be neutralized, they may be dissociated from the stream of consciousness (Janet 1925).

Memories incapable of being knitted into the fabric of mental narrative create a phobia of memory and an inability to fully recite narrative memory. Also, traumatic memories impair the integration of new experiences, causing the personality to fixate at the time of the trauma. Traces of the painful memory tend to linger and intrude as flashbacks, obsessions, and attempts to reenact the trauma, which are incomplete attempts to integrate the memory (van der Kolk 1988). Many instances of this "repetition compulsion" are better understood as the patient's attempts to come to terms with intrusive recollections of traumatic experiences (Goodwin 1990).

Janet stressed the role of one's particular emotional reaction to a trauma as a factor affecting one's inability to integrate memories, rather than the impact of the actual traumatic event by itself. His perspective seems similar to contemporary psychoanalytic emphasis on the power of fantasy and wishes in determining the extent of the traumatic effect of an event (e.g., Ulman 1988). In explaining hysteria in his adult patients, Freud moved from a focus on exter-

nal and interpersonal dynamics to internal and intrapsychic explanations after his renunciation of the seduction theory. Rather than
following through on the implications that his patients' symptoms
resulted from child abuse perpetrated by their parents, Freud decided to concentrate on the child's unacceptable libidinal impulses
toward his or her parents. According to Freud's revised theoretical
model, the child's own impulses of lust and anger had the power
to determine the strength of a "trauma." For example, Freud wrote
of one of his patients that

> the patient's neurosis could then be equated with a traumatic
> illness and would come about owing to inability to deal with an
> experience whose affective colouring was excessively powerful
> ... on the one hand, a little girl's being in love like this with her
> father is something so common and so frequently surmounted
> that the term "traumatic" applied to it would lose all its mean-
> ing ... her erotic fixation appeared to have passed off without
> doing any damage, and it was only several years later that it
> reappeared in the symptoms of the obsessional neurosis. (Freud
> 1922/1966, p. 275)

The interpersonal dimension of the patient's situation receives
minimal attention in Freud's description.

In reaction to Freud's tendency to minimize external factors,
other psychologists argue that the nature of a particular trauma is
more important than the person's subjective reaction to it. For instance, Spiegel and Cardeña (1991) state that "dissociative processes ... [are] associated to actual traumatic events or particular
attentional strategies (e.g., meditation) rather than to ward off unacceptable unconscious ideas or fantasies" (p. 367).

Current experimental work in psychology has not added significantly to our understanding of the relative importance of external
and intrapsychic factors in a given patient's response to trauma.
Most recent studies of the relationship between trauma and amnesia are case studies or postfacto statistical studies. Manipulative
experimental studies have been attempted (Christianson and Nilsson 1984), but the types of "trauma" induced in these studies are
understandably mild and thus not generalizable to the extreme ex-

periences reported by patients in therapy. On the other hand, recent clinical research (Williams 1994) indicates a high incidence of amnesia in adults with documented histories of childhood abuse.

In addition to traumas inflicted on individuals by other individuals, we should consider the type of corporate or collective trauma involved in group persecution or genocide, such as the Turkish mass slaughter of Armenians in the 1920s or Hitler's proposed extermination of the Jews. The link between trauma and amnesia is clearly visible in a major social trauma such as the Holocaust (Jaffe 1968; Langer 1991). For Jews, the Holocaust is a cataclysmic event that many survivors prefer not to remember. One can detect specific aspects of traumatic amnesia in a community affected by the social trauma as well as in individual survivors. The Holocaust offers a particularly instructive example of collective and individual amnesia. Langer (1991) summarizes the traumatic experiences of Holocaust survivors as "wounded time": "As memory plunges into the past to rescue the details of the Holocaust experience, it discovers that cessation plays a more prominent role than continuity. One surviving victim speaks of . . . [a] childhood that has passed during his 'absence'" (p. 75).

In addition to a numbing of memory, survivors may manifest a compartmentalization or encapsulation of traumatic recall. Langer (1991) points out that the experiences of Holocaust survivors become memories that are kept separate from normal life. One survivor said: "Everything that happened to this other 'self,' the one from Auschwitz, doesn't touch me now, *me*, doesn't concern me, so distinct are deep memory and common memory" (p. 5). This person's reference to *deep memory* has to do with buried memories of the trauma; conversely, *common memory* refers to memories that are part of the survivor's ongoing everyday life. We see here one form of correlation between amnesia and identity disturbance in a dissociative reaction to the social trauma of the Holocaust.

The Return of the Repressed

The irony of amnesia is that the material it removes from consciousness can resurface involuntarily and often forcefully. Freud

(1920) recognized the ultimate failure of repression as a mechanism when he said that the neurotic person "does not *remember* anything of what he has forgotten and repressed, but *acts* it out" (p. 150, emphasis added). Freud stated that repressed, amnestic material was like a coiled spring that pressured people to repeat repressed material in the form of physical symptoms.

Spiegel (1989) maintains that the infliction of trauma causes a loss of control over one's memories and an inability to ward off reexperiencing the traumatic memories. He has used hypnosis to help victims of abuse regain control of their memories and integrate their painful experiences into their wider senses of identity.

In some instances, the repressed memories return to the patient's consciousness in symbolic form. As an example, van der Kolk et al. (1987) present the case of a young woman who had survived a deadly nightclub fire. The fire had spread through the building's wiring system, and a revolving door had become stuck in the rampage, preventing scores of people from escaping death. The patient in question developed amnesia for her traumatic experiences, but the forgotten experiences emerged through symbolic delusions and similar symptoms. The patient claimed that her body was being invaded by gases and electrical currents. These delusions were fairly transparent descriptions of the spread of the fire in the nightclub. The young woman's behavioral reenactments included screaming "Fire!" in a supermarket and in a hospital. It was later learned that she had been physically abused as a child and had endured a year of severe polio, during which she had full-body paralysis. Memories of the later trauma of the nightclub fire were particularly intrusive. Relevant visual cues relating to the fire triggered phobic behavior; for example, the patient had a fear of electrical wires and revolving doors, and panicked on one occasion when she saw steam issuing from her radiator.

In theory, the patient's symptoms represented the isolation or compartmentalization of painful, anxiety-provoking, and overwhelming memories. Although this isolation protected most of her personality from damage caused by eruption of the memories, these warded-off memories came back in dissociated forms (e.g., dreams, acting out, irrational fears, delusions). The patient's delusions were manifestations of helplessness and magical thinking. Delusion-like symptoms can occur as a part of a response to trauma, when the delusions occur in the context of symbolic dissociative reenactments of repressed traumatic memories.

Most accounts of amnestic sequelae of trauma concern adult survivors. Longitudinal follow-up studies of child survivors of trauma are relatively uncommon. However, Terr (1988) studied 20 children who were under the age of 5 at the time that they had a traumatic experience. Witness reports, photos, and other evidence corroborated the children's ordeals. The specific traumas included sexual abuse, physical injury/deformation, evisceration, a plane crash, kidnapping, and being stuck in an elevator. Children who underwent the trauma before approximately 3 years of age did not have the capacity for full verbal recollection. Instead, they retained *behavioral memories.* Behavioral memories mirrored traumatic events at any age. The general accuracy of the children's memories was high, and the children were more likely to have verbal recall of short, isolated episodes than of protracted or multiple events. The children's behavioral memories included posttraumatic play (i.e., reenactment of the trauma), personality changes related to reenactments, and trauma-specific fears. These behavioral memories were quite accurate, as measured by corroborating evidence. Recollections of this type do not require the subject's conscious awareness and so are well-tolerated. As was mentioned earlier, Freud argued that behavioral reenactments and flashbacks represent the patient's attempts to master the trauma. However, in these cases involving children, the reenactments did not succeed in conferring a sense of mastery. Therefore, reenactments of physical overreactions, like a scar, attempt to heal and then create an overgrowth (Terr 1988).

Flashbacks

Flashbacks are sometimes referred to as *intrusive recall* (Schetky 1990). The fact that they occur as dissociative symptoms poses a theoretical paradox in terms of their connection with amnestic episodes. As Greenberg and van der Kolk (1987) have stated, "Failures of recall can paradoxically coexist with the opposite, intruding memories and unbidden repetitive images of the traumatic events" (p. 191). This peculiar situation may arise from overcompensation, as follows: Traumatic experiences are dissociated from the person's normal integration of memory. Either because the mind attempts to integrate the experiences into previously existing memories, or precisely because of the lack of integration, the experiences involuntarily reemerge into consciousness (van der Kolk et al. 1984). Flashbacks secondary to trauma suggest that the traumatic experiences were encoded in the enactive and iconic modes described by Kihlstrom (1984), and so are likewise remembered in these modes. These regressive memories are difficult to retrieve linguistically but are triggered by affective or sensory cues.

Holocaust survivors report an amnestic barrier produced by their traumatic experiences. One survivor used the metaphor of a skin or hide: "The skin covering the memory of Auschwitz is tough" (qtd. in Langer 1991, p. 6). Another survivor described it similarly:

> You can't excise it, it's like—there's another skin beneath this skin and that skin is called Auschwitz, and you cannot shed it, you know. And it's a constant accompaniment, and though a lot of the survivors will deny this, they too feel it the way I do, but they won't give expression to it. . . . Probably a greater number will deny it—these memories—than not. . . . I see the crematorium and I see all of that. And it's too much. (qtd. in Langer 1991, pp. 53–54)

In this instance, we also encounter the *return of the repressed*—involuntary flashbacks of repressed and dissociated memories that the person experiences as unwanted intruders into the routines of day-to-day existence as is shown in the following comments by the first survivor mentioned above:

> Sometimes, however, [the skin] bursts, and gives back its contents. In a dream, the will is powerless. And in these dreams, there I see myself again, *me*, yes, *me*, just as I know I was: scarcely able to stand . . . pierced with cold, filthy, gaunt, and

the pain is so unbearable, so exactly the pain I suffered there, that I feel it again physically . . . I feel myself die. (qtd. in Langer 1991, pp. 6–7)

Dissociative symptoms have been directly investigated with respect to posttraumatic stress disorder in Holocaust survivors. For example, Jaffe (1968) focused on dissociative states in which dissociated traumatic material emerged in trancelike, daydreaming states that ranged from flashbacks to quasidelusional episodes. In such conditions, the patient may experience a dual consciousness in which part of the mind is oriented toward present reality and part is recalling the time, place, and context of the trauma. In some instances, the second dimension of consciousness overlaps with the first; as a result, impressions of the past episode superimposed on the present produce a quasidelusional state.

Dreaming

Intrusive recollections of past trauma can also take the form of nightmares (van der Kolk et al. 1984). The dream state in general has much in common with other dissociative states; while dreaming, we exhibit dissociative symptoms (Gabel 1990). Amnesia is prominent among the aspects of dreaming that resemble dissociation. Typically, we are amnestic for most of the dreams we have each night; in adults, extensive recollection of dreams, particularly nightmares, is considered sufficiently unusual as to be noted by therapists. Essentially, most of us have significant time gaps for the several hours each night that we spend in sleep. We may experience minor flashbacks, when a chance thought or object reminds us of a dream we had the night before. From this perspective, dreaming is a memory phenomenon (Reiser 1990). When a person has a history of trauma, memories of the pain may well take the form of recurrent nightmares.

Credibility of Trauma Memories

The issue of the credibility of trauma survivors' memories has aroused increased controversy in the past several years. In December 1993, the American Psychiatric Association (APA) Board of Trustees (1993) issued a formal statement on memories of sexual abuse, summarizing "information about this topic that is important for psychiatrists in their work with patients for whom sexual abuse is an issue" (p. 1). The APA's statement briefly describes the current consensus regarding reliability of traumatic memories:

> It is not known what proportion of adults who report memories of sexual abuse were actually abused. Many individuals who recover memories of abuse have been able to find corroborating information about their memories. However, no such information can be found, or is possible to obtain, in some situations. While aspects of the alleged abuse situation, as well as the context in which the memories emerge, can contribute to the assessment, there is no completely accurate way of determining the validity of reports in the absence of corroborating information. (p. 2)

The present controversy has resulted from a combination of factors, including 1) a documented increase in reports of child sexual abuse; 2) the hypothesized connection between childhood trauma and adult psychopathology, including the dissociative disorders; 3) a rise in litigation involving allegations of childhood abuse; and 4) recent research involving the nature and limitations of human memory (Bourne 1994; Frankel 1993; Ganaway 1989; Gutheil 1993).

It is important, first of all, that clinicians understand the distinction between the ethical and the epistemological dimensions of questions of memory. As Bok (1978) has stated,

> There is great risk of a conceptual muddle, of not seeing the crucial differences between two domains: the *moral* domain of intended truthfulness and deception, and the much vaster domain of truth and falsity in general. The moral question of whether you are lying or not is not *settled* by establishing the truth or falsity of what you say. In order to settle this question, we must know whether you *intend your statement to mislead.* (p. 6)

Bok goes on to observe that

> the several meanings of the word "false" only add to the ease of confusing the two domains. For whereas "false" normally has the larger sense which includes all that is wrong or incorrect, it takes on the narrower, moral sense when applied to persons. A false person is not one merely wrong or mistaken or incorrect; it is one who is intentionally deceitful or treacherous or disloyal . . . . To further complicate matters, there are, of course, many uses of "false" to mean "deceitful" or "treacherous," which do not apply directly to persons, but rather to what persons have intended to be misleading. A "false trail," a "false ceiling," or a "false clue" carry different overtones of deceptiveness. (p. 7)

It will be seen from Bok's examples that *false memory* is a phrase that carries pejorative overtones—that is, the implication that the subject may be intentionally misleading as well as mistaken. Some researchers have attempted to deal with the issue of veracity by appealing to a distinction between the "true" and the "real," as is shown in the following comment by Gutheil (1993): "Something may be true for a person, in the sense of deeply held, strongly believed, and expressed with conviction; yet that very thing may not be real, in the sense of objectively determined and available for empirical proof or consensual validation" (p. 528). This distinction between subjective "truth" and objective "reality" tends to focus attention on documentary verification of reports of child abuse. Frankel (1993) holds that "only rarely has the [patient's] history [of abuse] been compellingly corroborated" (p. 958). His opinion has been contradicted by statistics for three northeastern states published in *The New York Times* ("Pulse: Child Abuse" 1994), indicating that between 22% and 65% of government-mandated child abuse reports between 1989 and 1993 were corroborated. In an earlier study, Herman and Schatzow (1987) reported independent corroboration of 74% of their subjects' reports of abuse. A recent prospective study by Williams (1994), involving 129 women with documented histories of sexual victimization in childhood, found that 38% were amnestic for abuse reported to authorities 17 years earlier. The author concludes that "long periods with no memory for abuse should not be regarded as evidence that the abuse did not occur" (p. 2). Furthermore, a rigid conceptual distinction between subjective "truth" and objective "reality" does not accommodate the clinical finding that many abuse survivors experience periods of emotional confusion in which they doubt the credibility of their own memories.

Another dimension of the question of credibility of memory is its social/interpersonal dimension. Humans are social creatures whose sense of personal identity is shaped and confirmed through interactions with other people in their environment. Though memory has individual characteristics, in the sense that no two people have identical sets of memories, humans learn the skills of encoding, storing, and retrieving their memories from experiences shared with others. In addition, one of the functions of memory is to facilitate communication with other people; people who cannot identify themselves, remember learned skills, or recall recent activities will have serious difficulties in their day-to-day existence. The third and fourth factors that Kluft (1984b) postulated in his discussion of the etiology of dissociative disturbances reflect this social dimension of memory. Kluft has stated that dissociative defenses may be "shaped toward personality formation" by implication in "normal and abnormal intrapsychic structures," and by the failure of others in the child's environment to provide "nurturing and healing experiences" (p. 130). Children whose recall of events is repeatedly invalidated by the adults around them are at risk for developing dissociative amnesia. Williams (1994) found that her subjects were more likely to recall sexual abuse by strangers than abuse by perpetrators within their families: "[S]uch abuse may be more likely to be ignored or hidden by family members. This may send a powerful message to the child to forget about it" (p. 14). Also, dysfunctional families are often characterized by problematic feedback loops and projective distortions of reality. Schuman (1987) has called attention to the impact of the group process on children's perceptions of significant events in the family: "At the end of such cycles, children . . . can be 'shaped' toward 'true' beliefs that are not valid but which are not 'lies' either . . . childhood accommodation to adult attitudes is misleading [to clinicians] and common" (p. 244).

The interpersonal dimension of human memory is connected to the third factor that complicates the question of the validity of traumatic memories, and that is that human memory operates along affective as well as cognitive axes. Williams (1994) found that children who were 4–6 years old at the time of their abuse were just a likely to be amnestic for the abuse as those age 3 or younger at the time of their victimization: "These findings suggest that factors other than cognitive development and language acquisition (factors associated with so-called infantile amnesia) play a role in forgetting" (p. 10). Terr's research on traumatized children indicates that recall of traumatic events is affected by the duration and repetition of the trauma. Children older than 28–36 months usually retain verbal memories of painful events. Brief, single-event traumas, such as transportation accidents or falls and similar injuries, are recalled with greater completeness and accuracy. Terr (1990) found, however, that lengthy or repeated traumas, such as ongoing abuse within the child's family, may be forgotten entirely, retained as spot memories, and/or inaccurately remembered. Terr (1994) has subsequently classified "false" memories of trauma into four categories: 1) strongly imagined memories (e.g., child hears others describing a traumatic event and "sees" the event in his or her own mind); 2) totally distorted memories (e.g., child "remembers" an adult's account of a nonexistent event as a true occurrence); 3) deliberate lies; and 4) misconstructed impressions (e.g., child confuses a surgeon's operation on her urethra with a relative's touching of her genitals). Terr advises clinicians to evaluate each case "for its particular truth" and check patients for specific symptoms and signs of trauma. These symptoms and signs include reenactments of the painful or frightening episode, sleep disorders, physical symptoms similar to those felt during the episode, and pessimism about the future (Terr 1994). Children who do not manifest this cluster of symptoms and signs are more likely to be describing false memories. Knoepfler and Knoepfler (1994) have added the category of vicarious abuse (e.g., a child's witnessing the rape or other abuse of a parent, sibling, or even a stranger) to the list of circumstances that may lead to posttraumatic, abuse-like symptoms in adults, including intrusive memories.

Recent studies of human memory indicate, at most, that *some* of the traumatic memories mentioned by patients may be mis-constructed and/or elaborated. These studies do not support the hypothesis that survivors fabricate these memories from whole cloth, as it were. Briere and Conte (1993) have summarized the present state of the question as follows: "Although clinical experi-ence leads the present authors to doubt that abuse confabulation is a major problem in abuse research, only further study and empiri-cal data in this area will resolve this question" (p. 29).

Self-Injury and Amnesia

Self-mutilation is a phenomenon frequently encountered in abuse survivors. It may represent either a symbolic repetition of past abuse, as when an incest survivor selectively attacks the parts of the body that drew the perpetrator's attention, or an attempt to integrate the traumatic memory into the fabric of experience (Krugman 1987). Instances of self-mutilation may thus also be an-other form of the "return of the repressed" (Miller 1984). Further, self-mutilation or associated forms of self-destructiveness (e.g., ac-cident-proneness, revictimization) may be implicit or screen mem-ories of the abuse and may serve to keep memories of abuse out of direct consciousness. Some researchers (e.g., Briere 1992) have de-scribed self-mutilation as a short-term device for tension reduction in that the abuse survivor seeks to relieve the psychic tension asso-ciated with self-loathing, guilt, and anxiety, by self-cutting, self-burning, and the like. Briere (1992) notes that the behavior is cyclical in many patients, consisting of a repetitive pattern of self-injury, subsequent calm, and the gradual escalation of tension leading to another episode of violence directed against the self.

Amnesia may occur in connection with many forms of self-destructive behavior. Self-wounding, like dissociative symptoms in general, is an adaptation to childhood abuse and trauma. Self-injury, including suicide attempts, is a signal to the attentive clini-cian that a patient may have been abused. One patient in an interview in the SCID-D (Steinberg 1993b) reported an attempt to commit suicide by poison. On awakening in a hospital emergency room, she was so confused by her failure to recall trying to kill herself, that she refused to believe that she had taken the poison:

Interviewer: So though you have memory gaps that occur frequently, you find you are able to function?

Patient: I would say I function, yeah. I mean, you know, I function until I don't function. The only bad part about it is, like, I have ended up in the hospital, you know, for supposedly trying to kill myself, and like how much can your body take? You know what I mean? I was in the hospital, and I don't even know how I got there, from drinking—do you know what oil of wintergreen is? Are you aware of that? It's obviously very toxic. And I apparently drank this whole bottle of oil of wintergreen. And like they thought my kidneys were going to shut down and everything. And I'm there and the doctor says, "Well, you know, geez, you almost died," and all this, and "They don't keep people in intensive care for nothing." You know, it was serious. And I'm like, "Oh well, I would like to leave now." And he was like, "You have to be crazy." I'm like, "I'm fine." He said, "What are you, depressed?" [I said,] "No."

Interviewer: Then why did you drink the oil of wintergreen?

Patient: I didn't drink it.

Interviewer: Why did you take it?

Patient: I didn't take it. I don't *remember* drinking it, I don't *remember* taking it. I only know that they kept insisting that I did, when I was in the hospital.

Interviewer: So who drank it?

Patient: I don't know!

Interviewer: ... Do you have any thoughts of how that might have occurred? That you felt you didn't take it but apparently you were told you did?

Patient: Obviously, well yeah, it was obvious, I mean it was in my system. Although I didn't have any—this doctor's trying to tell me like I almost died, and my kidneys were shutting down, and I'm saying, "Well I feel fine. You know, I don't even feel weak. Nothing's wrong." (SCID-D interview, unpublished transcript)

The reader may well raise questions about the mental mechanisms that are sufficient to induce amnesia for life-threatening events. Suppression of memories of abuse may arise within dysfunctional family systems dominated by shame and secrecy, systems in which the abuse is hidden from the outside world and often even from others in the home (Wise 1989). Added to this are attempts by abusers to convince victims that the abuse never happened, or that it was an expression of love (i.e., instead of what it really was, abuse). "Letting out the secret" of abuse can disrupt the homeostasis of a family that is unstable to begin with, and repression of the abuse then becomes a survival issue for all concerned (Wise 1989). Furthermore, representatives of other institutions in the community surrounding the family (e.g., teachers, clergy, medical practitioners) may also have a vested interest in maintaining denial of abuse. For example, a physician who suspects that a child's injuries are the result of abuse may hesitate to report the case in spite of legal requirements if the child belongs to a prominent or influential family. Or a pastor or rabbi might not want to believe reports of abuse from the son or daughter of a leading member of the congregation. Self-destructive acts may reinforce the family's concern for secrecy (Miller 1984). Because self-mutilation is a form of "the return of the repressed," amnesia may be a reaction to the *surfacing effect* that self-mutilation and suicide can bring about (Wise 1989). Self-mutilation brings the memories of the trauma into consciousness in many ways: Injury inflicted on one's own body can serve as an attempt to reinforce the reality of the past abuse and the present pain, both of which have been avoided through dissociation and persistent denials by other family members. The effect of reality-testing through self-inflicted injury can be literal, as when the sensation of pain restores the feeling of being alive (Gil 1984), or can function on a more abstract or symbolic level, as when the feeling of pain reinforces a patient's conviction that he or she was in fact abused as a child. Self-injury is a way to *behaviorally recall* (i.e., reenact) the abusive events of the past. It can provide a memory link to the scars of the past.

In a patient who is amnestic for much of his or her childhood, the presence of self-mutilation strongly suggests a forgotten history of child abuse (Coons and Milstein 1990). Because patients with DID almost invariably have a history of persistent sexual and/or physical abuse, the presence of self-mutilation and suicidal behaviors in this population is not surprising. Coons and Milstein (1990) found that of patients with DID in their study who injured themselves ($N = 50$), 58% had amnesia for the act of mutilation itself, and all of the mutilations were carried out by an alter personality. In many of these cases, patients report that they "find themselves" with cuts, scratches, or burns on their bodies, in the same way that they find themselves in strange places without knowing how they got there.

Self-destruction reaches its culmination in suicide attempts. In a patient with DID, alter personalities may think that they can kill other personalities and survive the suicide by themselves (Fine 1990). Often, some of the patient's alters will not remember suicide attempts made by other personalities. Fugue states can sometimes be a "flight from suicide" (Kopelman 1987), in that the person may have an episode of amnestic fugue under the influence of one personality as a way of forestalling suicidal impulses coming from another alter. Lastly, self-mutilation that escalates toward suicide is a frequent behavioral manifestation in patients who believe themselves to be survivors of cult programming. Glass (1993) interviewed one patient whose self-wounding progressed from the cutting and skinning of her ankles, to banging her head and face on concrete surfaces, to an outright suicide attempt on Halloween eve by cutting her throat. The patient maintained that she had been programmed by a cult to perform blood sacrifices, including attempts on her own life.

■ Compensatory Techniques

Because of the disabling effects of amnesia, people who are affected by it devise ways of adapting to the problems it causes them. Common techniques include confabulation, note-making, diary-keeping, screen memories, unobtrusively acquiring information from others, and sheer denial.

Compensation for normal memory loss includes the substitution of reports from others for real memories or of cold facts for more emotion-laden memories. In one instance, a patient in the SCID-D study remarked the following:

> Even what I remember doesn't seem like I remember it. So it is like saying I have no memory because I am not really too connected to it. It is like the memory is what I have been told is the memory. Like we will help you fill in the blanks, read the book, or look at a movie, you watch the movie and then that is your history there. And I say oh—sort of looks like it—but like I don't really remember. (SCID-D interview, unpublished transcript)

Another patient, who had global dissociative amnesia, relied on his friends and relatives to restore the information that he had lost:

Interviewer: How often did that occur, that you were unable to remember your address or your age? Did that last for several weeks in a row?

Patient: No. It was only a couple of weeks.

Interviewer: A few weeks?

Patient: After being told, I mean, are you asking me if I ever remembered?

Interviewer: No, just how long it lasted.

Patient: It only lasted until someone kept telling me. As far as remembering where I actually live, no. I still don't recall. Ok. I know I live now on 56 Longhill Drive, but I have been told. As far as remembering I live there, no. (SCID-D interview, unpublished transcript)

Although confabulation and the other methods that patients use to compensate for amnestic episodes or chronic amnesia may allow them to get by in everyday life without too many embarrassing or awkward moments, the need to compensate is still a source of significant distress to many. Not only are they fearful of the potential for serious misunderstandings on the job or in personal relationships, but many patients also feel a sense of moral or ethical discomfort with the dishonesty involved in confabulation or outright denial of memory loss. This aspect of the impact of amnesia on a person's sense of self (i.e., his or her sense of character integrity) should not be overlooked.

■ Hypermnesia

William James (1890) once said, "If we remembered everything, we should on most occasions be as ill off as if we remembered nothing." An enhanced memory can sometimes be more of a curse than a blessing and can also be an aftereffect of trauma. Single or acute traumas are more likely to be remembered in full detail. This characteristic of recall is as true of children as it is of adults. In her study of traumatized children, Terr (1991) writes, "Verbal recollections of single shocks in an otherwise trauma-free childhood are delivered in an amazingly clear and detailed fashion. Children sometimes sound like robots as they strive to tell every detail as efficiently as possible" (p. 14), whereas memories of prolonged abuse develop into amnesias. The experience of hypermnesia may be similar to flashbacks in that there is a replay of memory that is vivid and precise.

Photographic memory can also occur in the context of dissociative states. Attention to the surface details of an event can result from or lead to the misallocation of attention to the event's emotional dimension. Similarly, a person may deliberately concentrate attention on superficial details to avoid the painful emotional repercussions of a traumatic experience.

One DID patient described her use of hypermnesia as a defense against abuse. In this case, objectifying her memories permitted her to depersonalize without detaching completely from her memories:

Patient: I have a photographic memory . . . I can look at a page and read it and then when it's time for the exam I could read the sentence off the page and write it down on the paper word for word. . . .

Interviewer: How did you learn to memorize so well?

Patient: . . . 'cause we move all the time and so my mother says that she was going to leave us and so I had to memorize where we lived in case she left me or if she gave me away, so I could get back home again. And the other thing is that I used to go with my Daddy when I was six . . . We used to take the D train and my Daddy would get very drunk and I'd have to bring him home and if you have to know how to get home you have to memorize how you got there in the first place.

Interviewer: How old were you?

Patient: Six . . . He left on Saturday morning about three o'clock in the morning and he was drunk by nine-thirty and he wanted to leave me that night . . . I was trying to memorize when we were driving in the car all the street names so that I'd know how to get back to the train station . . . to get back because I couldn't trust my Daddy.

[In another situation] I used to get separated from all my toys. So the only way to remember them was to memorize them all on the shelves. I know exactly where they're all sitting and then if we happened to leave those toys, 'cause when we left my Daddy broke all the toys . . . He gave them away and so I could memorize my toys and when I was by myself in my mind I could play with them . . . Gotta take pictures in my mind. A picture's worth a thousand words.

Interviewer: Uh huh.

Patient: But pictures have no emotions.

Interviewer: Uh huh.

Patient: It's much easier to take a picture of a scene than to be there.

Interviewer: Uh huh.

Patient: So I guess I decided I wanted to be a camera . . . instead of a little girl. Cameras have film, right . . . and you could save the picture.

Interviewer: Uh huh.

Patient: But pictures, they tell stories, but they don't feel. You never see a picture crying, do you?

Interviewer: No.

Patient: But you could look at the photograph of someone crying, but you don't have to cry yourself. You just have a photograph somewhere of yourself crying and when you have a chance you can look at it. (SCID-D interview, unpublished transcript)

Hypermnesia can be induced by hypnotic and/or pharmacological intervention in cases where amnesia needs to be reversed and lost memories revealed. Such situations include therapy for trauma victims as well as court cases in which amnestic material is crucial to the outcome of a trial. Hypnosis is useful in uncovering these lost memories via hypnotic regression, recall, and revivification (Dwyan and Bowers 1983; Hilgard 1986; Hovec 1981; Spiegel 1990). The use of hypnosis, interestingly, results in both enhanced ability to recall memories, and enhanced ability to confabulate (Dwyan and Bowers 1983). This error factor increases with increased use of hypnosis and with more highly hypnotizable subjects. In sum, although clinicians can obtain a kind of hypermnesia with hypnosis, the "fantastic memories" elicited by it may not be genuine. For this reason, Coons (1991) maintains that the use of hypnosis in forensic contexts is contraindicated: "If at all possible, defense experts should generally eschew use of hypnosis to avoid introduction of hypnotic artifact in an extremely suggestible individual or someone predisposed to malingering to avoid criminal responsibility" (p. 763).

Use of short-acting barbiturates (e.g., amobarbital) has been described as facilitating recall in patients with dissociative amnesia (Ruedrich et al. 1985). Such pharmacological measures may be employed when more traditional methods of therapy are unsuccessful.

■ Conclusion

In sum, amnesia is the inability to bring memories to consciousness. Amnesia as a dissociative symptom arises from the overwhelming pain and anxiety associated with traumatic events, and the dissociation of consciousness from those memories. Amnesia can be very difficult to assess because occurrences that cannot be recalled cannot be reported. Many patients with amnesia are unaware of it and may attribute their time gaps to other factors, such as "spaciness" or "stupidity." Because amnesia is a "negative symptom," some observers have called the credibility of trauma memories into question. Although it is true that confabulation sometimes occurs under hypnosis and with DID, it is also the case that almost all patients with severe dissociative symptomatology have some abuse history. Though it may not be possible to validate all memories of trauma, it is true that many survivors' memories are all too sadly accurate.

CHAPTER 4

Assessment of Amnesia

Amnesia is the first dissociative symptom assessed by the SCID-D (Steinberg 1993b). As a symptom, *amnesia* may be defined as the absence from memory of a specific and significant segment of time. Amnesia can be caused by organic factors, such as head injury and epilepsy, or by psychological factors, such as severe psychic trauma. Amnestic episodes may occur in a variety of psychiatric disorders; however, amnesia that occurs in dissociative disorders has distinctive diagnostic features. Clinically, amnesia as a dissociative symptom may take the form of a history of blank spells, "blacking-out" or "spacing-out" in the absence of temporal lobe epilepsy, drug or alcohol use, or other organic etiology. One patient with DID in the SCID-D study compared her amnesia to a broken TV:

Interviewer: Have you ever felt as if there were large gaps in your memory?

Patient: Yeah, I have, I really have.

Interviewer: What are those like?

Patient: Like a blank hole. It's like turning on a TV, only the TV doesn't work and there's just a blank screen. That's exactly what it's like [chuckles]. (SCID-D interview, unpublished transcript)

Dissociative amnesia is not a dysfunction of cognitive or logical capacities. As one woman with DID put it,

I have an excellent memory. But I don't remember anything much about myself. I could probably read a book, take an exam on it, and remember all the details that are in it. Academically in school I did very well. Like a 4.0 average. (SCID-D interview, unpublished transcript)

■ The Elusiveness of Amnesia

Of the five dissociative symptoms evaluated by the SCID-D, amnesia is the most difficult to assess. Amnesia is to symptomatology as the black hole is to cosmology. Neither can be observed directly; rather, the presence of amnesia, like that of the black hole, is usually ascertained indirectly, in terms of its effects on other aspects of the patient's personality and functioning. Amnesia involves the absence or privation of memory, as opposed to a distortion or embellishment of memory. In this sense it resembles a *negative* symptom in schizophrenia, such as flat affect, rather than a *positive* symptom, such as an intrusive thought. Precisely because amnesia is the negation of memory, patients may be unaware that something is missing from their recall; that is, they may be amnestic for their amnesia (Kluft 1988a). One patient evaluated by the SCID-D described her time gaps as follows:

> It's a sense of nothing. There's a feeling of nothing. And that's when I think of time sometimes. It's a feeling of nothing. (SCID-D interview, unpublished transcript)

As a result, it is difficult for clinicians to obtain reliable estimates from patients of the frequency and extent of their amnestic episodes. The task of assessment becomes even more difficult with patients who have experienced chronic amnesia and may have learned to adapt to, or compensate for, their memory lapses. Individuals with chronic amnesia often confabulate replies in an attempt to patch the holes in their memory.

■ Signs Suggestive of Amnesia

Patterns suggestive of amnesia may be deduced from both verbal responses and nonverbal behaviors during the SCID-D interview.

A pattern of vagueness or inconsistency in answering questions, or generalized difficulty in providing a coherent history of past events by an otherwise cooperative patient may suggest amnesia. Evidence of sudden disorientation as to time, place, or person during the course of an interview, including the patient's attempts to orient him- or herself after talking with the interviewer for a while, may also indicate amnesia. For example, the disoriented patient may ask the interviewer "Where am I?" as a way of covering confusion as to the interviewer's identity or the location of the interview. Other clues indicative of amnesia include a history of finding oneself in a place and not knowing how or why one got there, finding unfamiliar objects in one's possession, disavowing actions that are confirmed by observers, and a history at any time of having lost one's identity. If the clinician fails to ask appropriate questions about these multifaceted manifestations of amnesia, reports of memory problems may not surface.

Because patients are often amnestic for their amnesia, the symptom by itself is rarely the presenting problem. Initially, patients are likely to report that they have been experiencing "blank spells" as well as anxiety or depression. They may also report occurrences that puzzle them. For example, one person with previously undetected DID presented with the report that personal items of clothing were appearing and disappearing; she attributed this phenomenon to recurrent break-ins by a burglar who transferred these items around the house without actually stealing them. After evaluation with the SCID-D interview, this patient not only was assessed as having severe amnesia, but the patient in fact met the DSM-IV criteria for dissociative identity disorder (DID). The "burglar" turned out to be an alter personality who moved her underwear and other items from one room to another. People will describe their amnestic episodes as "gaps," "holes," or "spacing out," and may not think of them as serious problems. Then, as patients become aware of other behavioral manifestations connected to their amnestic episodes, they gain a better understanding of the significance of the symptom.

One complicating social factor that clinicians should keep in mind when evaluating patients' explanations of memory deficits is widespread popular interest in science fiction, the occult, New Age thought, and paranormal phenomena. People who read these materials may well adopt their vocabulary and thought patterns, and thus describe their amnestic experiences in terms of out-of-body, UFO, and channeling experiences—all of which may complicate assessment (Richards 1991). Further research using the SCID-D in these populations should allow clinicians to separate persons who are both interested in these materials *and* suffer from dissociative disorders, from the larger population of individuals who dabble in New Age and similar thought systems without necessarily manifesting a dissociative disorder. For example, someone may report that they lost time due to space aliens "stealing" their time. The patient might well have DID and be amnestic for periods of time in which an alter is in control and seeking to account for the lost time by using the language of science fiction ("space aliens"), if the dominant personality is interested in that kind of literature.

It is difficult on initial assessment to determine the quantity or nature of the material that is inaccessible on account of the patient's amnesia. Therefore, SCID-D questions use a variety of strategies to enable the clinician to assess the situation indirectly, without raising the patient's anxiety level by making straightforward inquiries about forgotten material. In fact, one reason that the SCID-D begins with amnesia, besides the fact that amnesia is a symptom that contributes to the others, is that the interviewer can open with a series of general questions that elicit not only information about the amnesia itself but also spontaneous elaboration regarding the other dissociative symptoms.

■ The SCID-D's Assessment of Amnesia

The SCID-D is structured to approach the symptom of amnesia by a series of indirect and direct questions. The first question dealing with amnesia, question 1: "Have you ever felt as if there were large gaps in your memory?" is followed by questions tapping into identity confusion as well as amnesia, such as question 11: "Have you ever found yourself away from your home and been unable to remember who you were?" and question 15: "Have you ever been unable to recall your name, age, or address or other important information?" Question 15 is a diagnostically discriminating question in this interview, in that patients with dissociative disorders will supply distinctive responses to it. Patients in this category tend to endorse this question by describing episodes of memory loss of important personal information, such as their name, age, address, or phone number. Patients with other types of personality disorder do not usually report difficulties with recall of this kind of basic personal information. Moreover, persons who have dissociative disorders commonly describe repeated or chronic amnesia, as opposed to isolated episodes, and they typically manifest emotional distress and dysfunction. The SCID-D rates confusion about age or name as indicative of a severe level of amnesia. The following transcript excerpt from an interview with a subject diagnosed with DID is an example:

Interviewer: Have you been unable to remember your name, age, address, or other personal information?

Patient: Yes.

Interviewer: What sort of information did you forget?

Patient: I never, I didn't remember my address. I remember my name, not my address or anything else that goes along with it. Like my zip code.

Interviewer: Your age?

Patient: I remember my age.

Interviewer: . . . So that when somebody said to you what is your address or what is your age, what would you say?

Patient: For a while I said, I didn't know. But after a while, 42; you don't forget your age when someone tells you. I even doubted how old I was, in the beginning.

Interviewer: You had questions about your age.

Patient: Questions about everything.

Interviewer: What sort of questions did you have?

Patient: Do I really live here, is this really my family . . . all those questions. (SCID-D interview, unpublished transcript)

It is not unusual for a person with amnesia to describe an amnestic episode in terms that resemble accounts of fugue states. The patient suddenly becomes aware, as if he or she had not been previously fully awake, that he or she is in the middle of a purposeful and/or complex task (e.g., driving a car, cooking a meal), yet unable to remember its inception. Feelings of disorientation are commonly expressed, as the following excerpt illustrates:

> There's just a blank there. You just have no recollection of existing at all. I can sometimes all of a sudden be in the middle of doing something, and the last memory I have was in the middle of something else totally unrelated and I could be in a different car, a different location, I could be any place that would happen. (SCID-D interview, unpublished transcript)

Another woman with DID reported episodes of unaccountable travel, sometimes to other states, that made her aware of missing time:

Patient: When you end up in another state 5 days from the time that you last saw, or the date that you last saw, and you don't know how you got there or what you're doing there, and you have absolutely no recollection of it.

Interviewer: How often has that occurred?

Patient: Well, it happens quite frequently. It makes it very difficult to keep a job . . . how about this morning for instance. I was supposed to be meeting some people to sell a pedigreed dog and I started at the right time. I got up and I left home and drove my car and I started driving, only to end up in Northampton instead of Boston.

Interviewer: You ended up in Northampton this morning?

Patient: This morning.

Interviewer: Did you have a reason for going to Northampton?

Patient: I was supposed to be going to Boston. (SCID-D interview, unpublished transcript)

In the SCID-D, each positive response to a question in the amnesia section has follow-up questions designed to help the patient explore the symptom further in her or his own words. If a patient endorses the existence of large gaps in his or her memory, follow-up questions, such as "What was that experience like?" or "Can you describe what makes you aware of your memory gaps?" can help the clinician specify the nature and extent of the amnesia. In addition, endorsements of amnesia symptoms are followed by questions regarding frequency, duration, and course. The following transcript excerpt from an interview of a woman with DID opens with the first question in the amnesia section of the SCID-D:

Interviewer: Have you ever felt as if there were large gaps in your memory?

Patient: Oh yeah.

Interviewer: What sort of gaps have you experienced?

Patient: Um, days, segments . . . it's like segments of time. When I go back and I think about school, I can remember thinking, "When did I learn that? I don't remember learning that."

Interviewer: Have there ever been hours or whole days that were missing, that you couldn't account for?

Patient: [Nods]

Interviewer: What was the longest period of time that you ever lost?

Patient: When I was in school, as I look back on it, there [was] probably . . . maybe a month of time that would go by that I couldn't account for.

Interviewer: And how often would that occur, that you would lose blocks of time like that?

Patient: Maybe two or three times a year. (SCID-D interview, unpublished transcript)

The SCID-D is also designed to elicit information from the patient concerning his or her acquisition of awareness of amnestic episodes. Many times, people are confronted with gaps in their memory because of comments from others in their life, or awkward or embarrassing events. The interviewer is advised to ask what made the person aware of missing time, as in the following example of a woman diagnosed with DID:

Interviewer: What makes you aware of the gaps?

Patient: People tell me.

Interviewer: What do they say?

Patient: You know, they say, "Remember when we did this?" and I don't. And that I change, sort of. I act different, but then I don't remember doing that, and I don't remember what I was doing when I acted different. Sometimes I just go in and out really quick. Like when I watch TV. I can watch the same program as my boyfriend and my daughter, and ask what just happened. I'm always doing that. They get really mad.

Interviewer: And you think that that may be related to some of the gaps?

Patient: Oh yeah. (SCID-D interview, unpublished transcript)

In some instances, the patient may be made aware of the missing time by a combination of personal self-monitoring and feedback from others. The following example is taken from an interview of a patient diagnosed with DID:

Interviewer: When you say that you used to lose time, what do you mean by that?

Patient: Well, I would be aware that people around me were responding to something that I had no memory of, something that I had done, for example . . . OK, and telling me I had done stuff and I had no memory of it. Or I would simply sort of realize that I didn't know what I had been doing for, you know, the previous hour or day or something—things like that. (SCID-D interview, unpublished transcript)

■ The Spectrum of Amnesia

SCID-D research indicates that amnesia occurs across a spectrum, ranging from normal occasional forgetfulness and no psychological dysfunction, to occasional or frequent memory difficulties of patients with a variety of psychiatric disorders, to recurrent or persistent episodes of amnesia (lasting days or longer) in patients who have dissociative disorders (Steinberg et al. 1990) (see Figure 4–1 and Table 4–1). Frequent episodes of amnesia are often associated with impairment in social or occupational functioning, are not necessarily precipitated by external stress, are prolonged, and are usually associated with dysphoria. The SCID-D's severity rating definitions were developed to operationalize assessment of severity (see Appendix 1).

Mild amnesia is nonpathological and is widespread in the general population. Familiar examples include the "tip-of-the-tongue phenomenon," such as forgetting the name of an acquaintance; "blanking out," such as not being able to remember the Pledge of Allegiance when asked to recite it; or missing a doctor's appointment.

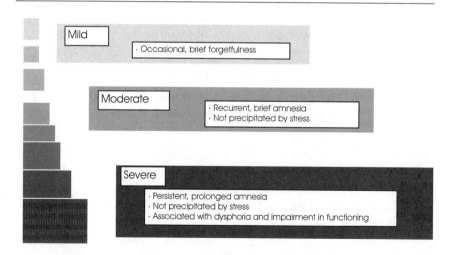

Figure 4–1. The severity range of amnesia.

Moderate amnesia, by contrast, involves recurrent brief episodes, few prolonged episodes, or experiencing one or two "blanks" in the interview. It may be associated with dysphoria or distress. Although few people are likely to be made anxious by the everyday examples of forgetfulness that characterize mild amnesia, a significant section of the population will be disturbed by episodes of moderate amnesia. This is particularly true for people whose occupational functioning is affected by it. A teacher who experiences momentary "blanking out" during a lesson, for example, may well be concerned about what the pupils were doing during the "blanks."

Severe amnesia involves at least one prolonged gap in memory that results in severe dysfunction. Finding oneself in a strange place without knowing how one got there and inability to recall important personal information are additional examples of severe amnesia. A gap of months or years in one's memory and forgetting learned talents or skills also is an indication of severe amnesia. For example, one subject interviewed in the SCID-D study mentioned

Table 4–1.   The spectrum of amnesia in the SCID-D

	No psychiatric disorder	Nondissociative and personality disorders	DID and DDNOS
Forgetfulness	Minor forgetfulness associated with stress	Rare memory gaps; forgetfulness of a minor nature	Gaps for hours–years
Presence/ absence of fugues	No fugues	No fugues	Associated with fugues
Frequency of episodes	None–isolated episodes	Isolated episodes	Recurrent– persistent episodes

Note. SCID-D = Structured Clinical Interview for DSM-IV Dissociative Disorders; DID = dissociative identity disorder; DDNOS = dissociative disorder not otherwise specified.

the loss of a talent for woodworking that he had discovered in high school:

> **Interviewer:** Have you ever . . . forgotten skills that you used to know, or talents?
>
> **Patient:** Yeah. Yeah.
>
> **Interviewer:** What kinds of things?
>
> **Patient:** I used to be pretty good with [stutters] tools and stuff. I'm not good with that stuff no more. I used to make like little wooden bowls with legs. I couldn't do that no more. . . . . . Back in high school I used to make big beautiful salad bowls. I used to give them away. I didn't ask for money, just gave them away. . . . I feel that I can't get it in me to do it now. (SCID-D interview, unpublished transcript)

Finally, the association of significant distress or dysphoria and the occurrence of significant intra-interview amnesia indicate the presence of severe amnesia.

As an example of severe amnesia, the following patient with DID presented with extensive symptoms:

> **Interviewer:** Have you ever felt as if there were large gaps in your memory?
>
> **Patient:** Yes, definitely.
>
> **Interviewer:** What sort of gaps have you experienced?
>
> **Patient:** Well, I can just fuse different bits and pieces of my childhood. Very vague memories. A lot of gaps. Just through my whole life. A lot of gaps. I can't tell you dates, I can't tell you my age, I can't tell you a lot of things. I just don't remember.
>
> **Interviewer:** How often does it occur that you feel as if there are gaps?
>
> **Patient:** It happens to me all the time . . . I forget where I'm going, I forget . . . I forget everything.
>
> **Interviewer:** This is something that you've been aware of for quite a while?

Patient: Oh yeah. Most of my life has been just a haze . . . most of my past is gone. (SCID-D interview, unpublished transcript)

| Manifestations of Amnesia

Confabulation and Self-Monitoring

The occurrence of amnesia in day-to-day life can disastrously affect a patient's relationships, employment, education, or family life. To maintain relationships, hold jobs, or stay in school, people with chronic amnesia have to develop numerous adaptive strategies. One such strategy is confabulation, or the invention of the data of a particular event as "cover" for a memory gap. In some cases, patients confabulate when they sense that honest admissions of amnesia are straining valued relationships. One subject with DID spoke of tension in her marriage caused by her husband's reaction to her amnestic episodes:

Interviewer: Have you ever had a time when you had difficulty remembering your daily activities?

Patient: Uh huh . . . when Charlie and the kids were infants and I would have to wonder if I fed them—wonder what I did with them—wonder where we went. Often, as I think of it, I couldn't figure out what we had done. When my husband would come home from work and he'd say, "Gee, what did he have for lunch? How did he eat? How many times did he eat?" I wouldn't be able to tell him.

Interviewer: What would you say?

Patient: After a while I began to lie because if I said to him, "Gee I'm not sure," then he—because of the relationship we had— he began to say, "Well, what do you mean you don't know? How could you not know? This is your son. You didn't take care of him?" So he would accuse me—if he cried at night it would be because I didn't feed him. And now I'm sure that I fed him because he grew, he thrived. He did fine. There was probably a different reason why he was crying. But at the time, I figured it was because I didn't feed him. Oh, God, it was terrible. (SCID-D interview, unpublished transcript)

In this case, confabulation protected the patient from her husband's criticism. Clinicians should be aware of the importance of explaining confabulation as a response to memory loss to members of the patients family or, when appropriate, to close friends. Relatives of patients who have amnestic episodes may need counseling on the varied manifestations of this symptom. One husband of a woman with DID has written a helpful first-person account of his difficulties, in coping not only with his wife's amnesia but with the negative reactions of other family members, friends, and even medical personnel (see Cohen et al. 1991).

One subject with DID in the SCID-D study described a painful history of employment problems resulting from her amnesia, culminating in her decision to be her own boss:

Interviewer: Do your memory gaps affect your ability to work?

Patient: Yes, very much. Fortunately I work for myself so I have more leeway than someone else would have who was working for someone else. You know, I can try to arrange my time around myself easier than other people.

Interviewer: What kind of work are you doing?

Patient: I'm a free-lance artist. . . . The only problem with that is, you know, you do have clients who want so much done by such and such a time, and sometimes there is a time factor. . . . I'm supposed to meet them there and I don't show up or they can't reach me and I've lost a few dozen accounts on account of it. But I can't be fired so I'm lucky.

Interviewer: Because you're independently doing this. Have there been other jobs that you've worked at?

Patient: Well, I tried to be a computer programmer—forget that. I tried to . . . um . . . I was going to school for awhile, but I kept missing all the classes. It's just . . . it goes on and on. I tried to work with my girlfriend who is setting up an interior decorating business, and when you tell clients you're going to be there, you have to be there and after awhile excuses, I don't care what you say, they don't cover it anymore. (SCID-D interview, unpublished transcript)

In addition to confabulation, persons with amnesia may resort to a variety of forms of self-monitoring to protect themselves from potential negative consequences of memory loss. The following patient with identified DID had a number of techniques and tactics for reinforcing her frighteningly unreliable memory. She relied on reminiscences from friends and kept a scrapbook of the things that she did.

> The other thing that I think is even more confusing is my sense that even what I remember doesn't seem like I remember it. So it's like saying I have no memory. Because I'm not really too connected to it. It's like the memory is what I've been told is the memory. Like we'll help you fill in the blanks, here, read the book or we'll look at a movie. You watch the movie and that's your history there. And I'll say "Oh, sort of looks like it." But like I don't *really* remember. People tell me things, sometimes, and it's like I heard it for the first time. They'll say, "Remember I told you this?" And we sat and discussed it, and I'll be like [sigh]. Stuff like I shouldn't forget . . . I tend to collect things to prove that I did things, like I can kind of like retrieve them and say this is what I did. So this is what I do. I have about 20 or 25 scrapbooks, and in it are things, because if they didn't exist— I just kind of like take them out and, "Oh yes"—without them I have this thinking that I wouldn't remember a *thing*. (SCID-D interview, unpublished transcript)

Self-monitoring for many people is preferable to collecting information from others because the latter involves direct admission of an embarrassing problem. In an "information age" such as our own, in which information collection and retrieval is critical to success in many fields, problems with memory carry a real stigma. Thus a person who enlists friends or relatives to help recover forgotten events or details may find their assistance helpful and painful at the same time. There are many ways, however, in which a person can elicit needed information from others while concealing the nature of his or her intentions. One patient with DID indicated a pattern of striking up conversations with people who are similar in age as a way of covering for amnesia related to date of birth:

Interviewer: Have you ever been unable to remember important personal information?

Patient: I can never remember my birthday, never.

Interviewer: So if somebody asks you when your birthday is . . .

Patient: I have to struggle to remember. I've learned to associate. If I'm with someone, I'll find out what day they were born and I tend to ask them if we're in the same group.

Interviewer: You tend to ask them?

Patient: I'll find somebody who is close to my age and I'll say, "When were we born?" (SCID-D interview, unpublished transcript

In another instance, a patient with DID described a strategy of conversational passivity intended to obtain information from others that would "jog" her out of her amnesia, without telling her friends the true nature of her situation:

Patient: The feeling of everything being foreign and everything is real common, but usually I fake it pretty good with the friends and everybody else.

Interviewer: How do you manage to fake it? What do you do if you don't recognize somebody that you think you should?

Patient: Well, I just sort of keep my mouth shut and hope they'll let me, they'll say enough about themselves or about something that I'll . . . that something will click in. (SCID-D interview, unpublished transcript)

With regard to self-monitoring, patients may demonstrate considerable ingenuity in providing themselves with records of participation in events that they may not recall later. Alternately, they may detach from others somewhat to avoid confrontations or embarrassment regarding missed appointments. For example, a person might give up certain customary activities with friends rather than risk "standing up" a friend because of an amnestic episode. Clinicians should be aware that a missed therapy hour may indicate the presence of amnesia rather than avoidance of therapy. As an example of a self-protective self-monitoring device, one patient with DID and severe amnesia notes the number of miles on her odometer each evening and each morning to detect any amnesia for her use of the car during the night. Another patient once reported writing down her address in case she forgot it:

> **Interviewer:** Your address? Have you ever had trouble remembering that?
>
> **Patient:** Mmm. I don't think so. For a long time I thought I would . . . I used to write down my old address, my home address, on a lot of things and, you know, I'd just see it there and I'd think, "Oh, that's not right," and I'd cross it out. (SCID-D interview, unpublished transcript)

Distortions in Time Perception

Amnestic episodes are frequently characterized by the patient's subjective misperception of elapsed time. When a person suddenly comes to full consciousness without remembering what transpired in the moments immediately preceding, he or she often feels "transported" from the last moment of fully remembered consciousness to the present. This usually generates a distorted sense of the rapid passage of time. A subjective distortion of this type can be a very frightening experience because it leaves the person with the impression that events can occur outside his or her consciousness and therefore, by implication, out of his or her control. As one woman with DID recounted:

> All of a sudden I'll be standing some place. It happened to me recently, so I'm thinking of standing at the sink. I all of a sudden realized I was standing at the sink and I thought, "What time is it?" and I looked at the time and then I go through a process of figuring out what time it is, what day it is, and then I start thinking, "What happened?" So I just all of a sudden find myself someplace. (SCID-D interview, unpublished transcript)

Clinicians should be careful to ask appropriate follow-up questions whenever a patient endorses distortions in time perception, because discussion of this particular symptom often yields additional indications of the symptoms of derealization and depersonalization. One subject in the SCID-D field trials, later diagnosed as having depersonalization disorder, described her perception of discontinuity in time as analogous to using drugs: "It feels like when you're high on drugs, you know, 5 minutes may seem like an hour, uh, or things just don't flow in a regular pattern of time" (SCID-D interview, unpublished transcript). The following excerpt from a patient with DID also illustrates the value of such follow-up questions:

Interviewer: Have you ever felt that time was discontinuous? By that I mean the flow of time seems very choppy?

Patient: Oh yeah.

Interviewer: What does that feel like?

Patient: Um, it feels like a feeling of going in and coming out. Um, it's . . . that's the best way I can describe it—a feeling of going in and coming out.

Interviewer: By going in and coming out, what do you mean?

Patient: I mean it feels like retreating. It feels like going inside.

Interviewer: Of yourself.

Patient: Yeah.

Interviewer: So to speak having a different level of awareness to what's going on around you. Is that what you mean by going in and coming out?

Patient: An awareness? Um [pauses], I guess so. I don't think about it as awareness. It's a physical feeling of joining. (SCID-D interview, unpublished transcript)

The following two patients indicated a distorted sense of the passage of time. In the first case, the person lost awareness of the course of a weekend. In the second, the distortion extended to the seasons of the year.

It will seem to me that it's still a Friday and then I'll realize that it's Monday and I'll search my memory to figure out what happened over the weekend. (SCID-D interview, unpublished transcript)

I get the months mixed up. Why do you think it's January? It's like I'm wearing a sleeveless outfit, it's 80 degrees out! . . . I can go into the mall to go shopping, walk by a sign that said, "Summer Sizzling Sale," and my reaction would be, "Gee, they should take down that sign because it is January. . . . They've made a mistake, that is the dumbest sign, they shouldn't be advertising summer clothes in January." And then the message coming in, "No, it's not January, it's July," and then my saying, "Oh, right. Why am I so confused to think it's January?" And then it will come to me that it's not January. But my initial response is like it's January. . . . (SCID-D interview, unpublished transcript)

The emotional impact of time distortions should not be underestimated. To lack memory of significant portions of one's life can leave one with an eerie sense of personal abbreviation (i.e., of not having fully "tasted" or experienced one's elapsed span of life). One may express feelings of loss or may worry about having "wasted" the missing months or years. The following example, from a patient with DID, is typical:

Patient: It's like I have specific things that flash on the screen, specific, I'm only talking about minutes, hours at the most. It's like my whole, from the time I was not quite 5 till not quite 13, it seems like my memory is in an hour's time. Then from the time I am like 14 through high school seems pretty . . . I can remember all that. In between like from the time I'm through high school till I'm 21 that seems pretty clear. And from the time I am 21 forward there sometimes seems to be entire years like I arrived, I feel like I arrived at this age.

Interviewer: At 43.

Patient: Yes. I would say, "Wow, where was I at 30?" (SCID-D interview, unpublished transcript)

Intra-interview Amnesia

The observation of intra-interview cues of amnesia during a clinical interview provides important information in the assessment of this symptom. SCID-D item 265 assesses the occurrence of intra-interview amnesia, which is defined by the following characteristics: 1) the subject suddenly forgets the topic of conversation, 2) the subject is amnestic for previous replies, or 3) the subject is disoriented as to time, place, or purpose.

The patient in the following transcript excerpt entered into an autohypnotic state in which she closed her eyes, lapsed into silence, and then "awoke." She was very disoriented and appeared paranoid. She then attempted to orient herself by asking the interviewer what time it was, and indicated ignorance of her reasons for being in a doctor's office. In spite of the dramatic nature of this switch and its associated amnesia, she did not admit to losing memory, nor did she believe she had DID. Instead of complaining about the amnesia, she tried to cover up for her behavioral switch. She was not forthcoming in telling the interviewer that something unusual had occurred; rather, she tried to regain her composure indirectly. Before this point in the interview, she had been talkative, generally composed, and self-controlled.

> **Interviewer:** OK. Have you ever found yourself in a place and you are unable to remember how or why you went there?
>
> **Patient:** [Eyes flutter and then partially close. Eyes are moving rapidly under eyelids, which are partially closed. Head rocks back and forth. This continues for about a minute.]
>
> **Interviewer:** What are you feeling now?
>
> **Patient:** [Eyes jar open, breathing heavily, wide open eyes scanning room and interviewer anxiously.]
>
> **Interviewer:** Do you understand what's going on here? You look a little surprised.
>
> **Patient:** [Continues to scan room silently.]
>
> **Interviewer:** Do you have any questions for me?
>
> **Patient:** [Looks at interviewer suspiciously.]

Interviewer: Do you know why you are here now?

Patient: [Quietly] What's your name?

Interviewer: My name is Dr. Steinberg. Do you remember coming in here just a few minutes ago and talking with me?

Patient: *I* talked to you, on the phone.

Interviewer: You did talk to me on the phone. Do you remember just being here for the last 5 minutes?

Patient: [Looks around the room with rapid eye movements] What time is it? (SCID-D interview, unpublished transcript)

Amnesia and Memories of Abuse

It is important for clinicians to be aware of the connection between a history of trauma in a person's life and the symptom of amnesia. Paradoxically, trauma can both conceal and intensify a memory. Patients with dissociative disorders are typically amnestic for much of the abuse that they endured as children. However, during stressful periods in later life, such as military service, preparation for academic examinations, or being fired from a job, or because of a sensory "trigger," a person can experience intrusive traumatic memories. Sometimes, a trace element of a past traumatic experience may trigger anxiety in a person without his or her conscious understanding of any historical connection. The following example concerns a person diagnosed with DID, who reacted to a symbolic reminder of sexual abuse:

> I'm paranoid of handkerchiefs. I was scared to death. My mother married a guy who uses a handkerchief. She had me washing white clothes. I could not touch one. I was afraid of a handkerchief. When I finally traced my mind and forced myself to remember and everything else, I remember why now. At, I don't know, I guess 4 years old, a baby-sitter used to *gag* me with a handkerchief, shove it down my throat, and rape me. No wonder I'm afraid of them, you know? It's like things like that. I'm afraid of libraries, places with high bookshelves, because that's the room I was in. Things like that. It's like after a while

> you learn to remember it. I don't want to remember it, but in order to help myself I knew I had to. God, I was afraid of the things that I was learning, because it's like totally new. Your mind blanks it out. I didn't remember it and now I know why . . . too painful. (SCID-D interview, unpublished transcript)

People who have been abused often do not trust their memories because their childhood perceptions and memories were invalidated by their abusers. Children run the risk of disbelief, criticism, or additional punishment when they complain about abuse from an adult. The perpetrators of the abuse frequently threaten their victims with extreme penalties for disclosure; it is not unusual for adults to threaten to kill or abandon the child. Alternately, the victim may be told that the abuse is an acceptable form of parental love. A survivor's constant struggle to validate memories, to "believe" in experiences that he or she is not sure really occurred, can cause genuine confusion about the past. The existence of multiple personalities often accentuates this struggle to gain a sense of reality, and the person is left with significant identity confusion as well as deficits in memory. One survivor gives a graphic account of the experience of both dissociative symptoms:

> Because I can't really remember things and [the personalities] are telling me what the memory is, or telling me what *my* memory is, well I end up feeling for example, I could end up thinking, "Well, yes, I'm a multiple, yes I was abused," then I'll get a "No, I'm not a multiple, no I'm not abused," so what's the truth? The truth is both of them? I don't know. I end up with an I don't know, I don't know. (SCID-D interview, unpublished transcript)

Amnesia and Suicide

The most tragic consequence of abuse is that it may be perpetuated by the victim, either in the form of victimizing others or in the form of self-destructive behavior. Patients with DID are especially likely to present with serious difficulties in these areas. Because the alter personalities of the DID patient developed originally in the context of repeated severe trauma, their very sense of identity may be constructed around the abuse. The patient's original sense of worth and right to parental attention was contaminated by the need to gratify the perpetrator's sadistic desires. Patients with DID experience severe identity confusion; as a result, their self-destructive behavior may take the form of one personality trying to eliminate another alter. In the trance-distorted logic of identity alterations, one alter's wish to destroy the body that was the passive vessel of the original abuse is not always identified by the patient's healthier personalities as the irreversible destruction of all the personalities. Putnam (1989a) advocates therapeutic contracts with DID patients whose systems include suicidal alters to minimize the possibility that an alter might harm the patient.

As we see in clinical observations of DID, time gaps are usually not really empty because the different personalities typically manifest during these episodes. Self-destructive alters may attempt to hurt or kill the patient, and the dominant personality may regain consciousness in a hospital with no recollection of the previous behavior. One patient in the SCID-D study diagnosed as DID referred to an episode in which she was driving and one of her more responsible alters apparently restrained a suicidal alter from using the car as a means of self-destruction:

Interviewer: Can you give an example of something that you did that you felt was not in your control?

Patient: Before I came up here, I was very suicidal and I almost [smashed] myself up in my car; and I didn't think I had any control over that, because it was almost as if I stopped existing and something else took over.

Interviewer: What do you think it was that took over?

Patient: I don't know [laughs]. To tell you the truth, it just happened. I just totally numbed out and I was sort of pulled towards doing something. (SCID-D interview, unpublished transcript)

As a result, if a patient has a history of suicidal and/or self-destructive behavior associated with amnesia, one should seriously consider the possibility of a dissociative disorder, more specifically DID. The patient in the following transcript has DID, of which she was unaware at the time of the interview. Her awareness was confined to experiencing episodes of amnesia. She reported instances of dissociative fugue combined with self-inflicted injury:

Patient: Is there ever a chance that one, well, I come to with cuts on me. Is there a way um, like, um, I guess, could commit suicide without knowing? Is there a way, do you know what I mean?

Interviewer: What do you mean?

Patient: Do different sides ever do things to each other?

Interviewer: It is possible. Have you ever had the experience of finding yourself hurt and not knowing how it happened?

Patient: Yeah.

Interviewer: What sort of experience have you had?

Patient: Like, um, cuts on my stomach. Underneath, uh, the left, um, what is it, part of the chest, left part of the chest, um, arms and leg.

Interviewer: What would you find on your arms and leg?

Patient: Uh, slashes. Not really—just enough to leave a mark, but not enough for stitches.

Interviewer: And did you injure yourself in that way?

Patient: I don't know. I don't know how it happened. I don't know.

Interviewer: What would make you aware that it *had* happened?

Patient: Um, come to in the shower, and the soap would sting on those cuts. Or, wake up, you know, with blood, on the arm.

Interviewer: And you would have no recollection of how the blood got there?

Patient: Um hm. Well, from the cuts, but I don't know how the cuts got there. (SCID-D interview, unpublished transcript)

Another patient with DID had a similar experience. Members of this clinical population find it very difficult to believe that they are the agents of their self-destructive behavior:

> **Patient:** Sometimes I'd be hospitalized for suicide attempts, which I don't remember doing. I just did them ... I know when I woke up one time I was on a life-support machine, and I had been in a coma for about a week. But I don't remember doing the suicide attempt. And then, my boyfriend told me I was hospitalized about a year ago for taking too many Klonipins, but I don't remember that either.
>
> **Interviewer:** I see. And you said when you were in the coma for a week ... what had you done to arrive at that state?
>
> **Patient:** They said that I took a bottle of chloral hydrate and some valium. . . .
>
> **Interviewer:** And when you say that you don't remember taking the pills, were you depressed prior to those events?
>
> **Patient:** I don't know. Evidently I was.
>
> **Interviewer:** So when you woke up, you found yourself in the hospital?
>
> **Patient:** Yeah, with this big thing going down my throat.
>
> **Interviewer:** And how did you understand why you were there?
>
> **Patient:** The doctor came and told me, and he kept the life support in—I remember 'cause it was really painful—for about 3 or 4 more days, until my lungs would start working.
>
> **Interviewer:** ... How do you understand that occurring to you?
>
> **Patient:** I guess I just do it spur of the moment. I don't plan. They always ask me, "Do you feel suicidal?" and I always say, "No," and when they say that I had suicide attempts in the past, they always ask me, "How do you plan to do it?" and I don't. I guess I just do it. 'Cause I don't really remember doing it.
>
> **Interviewer:** So it's a puzzling experience.
>
> **Patient:** It's real frustrating. (SCID-D interview, unpublished transcript)

❙ Summary

Amnesia is a fundamental dissociative symptom, the pathway into the others, as it were. In its most severe forms, it inflicts grave dysfunction and distress. Amnesia is a natural consequence of severe abuse, insofar as the human organism will banish painful and overwhelming experiences from consciousness. In DID, amnestic barriers function to separate or distinguish the personalities. Events that a specific person (or personality) cannot remember are processed as having happened to someone else.

Amnesia can range from mild, as in the "tip-of-the-tongue" phenomenon, to severe, as in failure to recall one's name or place of residence. The frequency and duration of amnestic episodes also contribute to determination of the severity of the amnesia. Duration may include the length of the time gap itself and also as the length of time that the person remains amnestic for information.

CHAPTER 5

Depersonalization

The Detached Self

One had to lose oneself in the crowd, melt into the night. To survive one needed not to exist.

—**Elie Wiesel**, *The Fifth Son*

If I find myself, I lose myself . . . As if I were strolling, I sleep, but I am awake. As if I had fallen asleep, I wake up, and I don't belong to myself. Life, ultimately, is one grand insomnia, and there is a lucid disorientation in everything we think or do.

—**Fernando Pessoa**, *The Book of Disquiet*

Depersonalization, the second symptom assessed by the SCID-D (Steinberg 1993b), was first described in the late nineteenth century, but it was not until the mid-twentieth century that advancements were made in its systematic description. Ackner (1954) defined four salient features of depersonalization that continue to be generally accepted today: 1) a feeling of unreality or strangeness regarding the self, which the patient perceives as different from her or his normal experience; 2) a retention of cognitive insight and corresponding lack of delusional elaboration, 3) an emotional disturbance resulting in a loss of all affective response except discomfort in regard to the depersonalization itself, and 4) an unpleasant quality that may vary in intensity inversely with the patient's familiarity with the symptom.

Depersonalization is reported by a number of researchers to be a normal response to life-threatening events (Noyes et al. 1977). It frequently occurs among victims of sexual abuse, political imprisonment, and torture (Jacobson 1959; Spiegel 1984). As was stated by Noyes and Kletti (1977a): "The data presented suggest that depersonalization is, like fear, an almost universal response to life-threatening danger" (p. 382). It is important for clinicians to note the connection between abuse and experiences of depersonalization, insofar as the majority of patients who have dissociative disorders report histories of trauma. In addition, depersonalization often accompanies altered states of consciousness. Such states include hypnosis (Wineburg and Straker 1973), transcendental meditation (Castillo 1990; Kennedy 1976), hypnagogic and hypnopompic states, sleep deprivation (Bliss et al. 1959), sensory deprivation (Reed and Sedman 1964), and drug or alcohol use (Good 1989). The material that follows will focus on depersonalization in its specific connection with the dissociative disorders.

■ The Phenomenology of Depersonalization

Current literature describes depersonalization as a sense of detachment from the self. This sensation has commonly been experienced as a feeling of strangeness of the self, a sense that one is observing oneself from the outside, and a flattening of affective response (Ackner 1954; Edwards and Angus 1972; Fewtrell 1986; Galdston 1947; Levy and Wachtel 1978; Mayer-Gross 1935; Saperstein 1949; Steinberg 1991) (See Figure 5–1).

One patient with DID in the SCID-D study was quite explicit about the loss of affect in her experiences of depersonalization:

> **Interviewer:** Have you ever felt that you were going through the motions of life, but you really felt detached from your behavior?
>
> **Patient:** Almost all the time.
>
> **Interviewer:** Can you describe what that is?
>
> **Patient:** Well, it's like . . . I don't know. It makes things easier in a way, 'cause things are detached so I'm not as involved, I'm not as likely to get as emotionally involved and stuff like that, but I also never feel real feelings. You know, I don't get either real upset or real happy. There's always a distance there. (SCID-D interview, unpublished transcript)

Other patients describe depersonalization as a feeling of being unreal, of being dead, of being like a ghost, or of watching a movie of the self. A SCID-D subject reported an episode of feeling watched or observed by her reflection in a mirror:

Interviewer: Have you ever felt that you were able to observe yourself from a point outside of your body as if you were seeing yourself from a distance?

Patient: Um hmm. Once. That happened before I was sick.

Interviewer: Can you describe what that experience is like?

Patient: I was looking in the mirror, and all of a sudden it just felt as if the image in the mirror was looking back out upon myself.

Interviewer: And that occurred one time?

Patient: Right. (SCID-D interview, unpublished transcript)

Still other manifestations may include feelings of bodily numbness and of parts of the body being disconnected. Pessoa (1991),

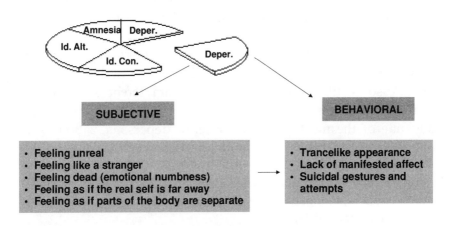

Figure 5–1. Manifestations of depersonalization.

the Portuguese poet cited in the epigraph opening this chapter, noted in his diary that "months have passed without my being alive. . . . For a long time, I haven't existed. I am extremely calm. . . . Perhaps tomorrow I will wake up to myself and again take up the course of my existence. . . . For a long time, I haven't been myself" (pp. 105–106). However, as Pessoa's remarks indicate, a person experiencing depersonalization is not delusional; reality testing tends to remain intact, as the subject often describes the symptom in "as if" terms, rather than as a literal division of the self (Ackner 1954; Fewtrell 1986; Saperstein 1949). In one study (Steinberg et al. 1990), a patient described her depersonalization this way:

> It's really weird. It's sort of like I'm here, but I'm really not here and that I kind of stepped out of myself, like a ghost . . . I feel really light, you know. I feel kind of empty and light, like I'm going to float away . . . Sometimes I really look at myself that way . . . It's kind of a cold, eerie feeling. I'm just totally numbed by it. (SCID-D interview, unpublished transcript)

Although depersonalization often involves a loss of emotion, patients who describe depersonalization experiences often do so with great expressions of emotion. The tendency for patients to elaborate with vividness and detail may involve such accompanying affect.

Feelings of detachment from the body and perceptual distortions in body image often occur simultaneously in depersonalization. Pessoa's (1991) diary contains frequent references to difficulty in recognizing himself or photographs of himself. More specifically, one of the most common forms of depersonalization is the out-of-body experience. One subject described this as follows:

Interviewer: Have you ever felt that you were watching yourself from a point outside of your body, as if you were seeing yourself from a distance?

Patient: Um hmm.

Interviewer: Can you describe that, or give me an example?

Patient: It's like I can step outside of this body, and go behind it or above it, or next to it. It's the body that gets watched. So I'm watching the body that I'm supposed to be in. (SCID-D interview, unpublished transcript)

Ackner (1954) identified a feeling of unpleasantness as one of the main features of depersonalization. He qualifies this by remarking that the unpleasantness can vary inversely to the familiarity of the symptom. Among people who experience depersonalization to a pathological degree, *chronic* depersonalization may lead to a sense of habituation and even comfort because of the symptom's familiarity (Steinberg 1991). Recent studies of non-psychiatric subjects have also provided examples of depersonalization experienced as a *pleasant* experience. For example, the type of depersonalization that characterizes meditative experiences is often ego-syntonic (Kennedy 1976). Additionally, depersonalization that may occur with therapeutic progress may be experienced as pleasurable, as was noted by Bonime (1973): "A woman was disturbed by the strangeness of her reflection in a mirror, but liked what she saw" (p. 111). Ego-syntonic depersonalization may not manifest the numbness that is usually associated with depersonalization. In fact, the dissociation that is associated with meditation and hypnosis may be characterized by enhanced affective response or even intense euphoria (Bliss 1983; Castillo 1990; Kennedy 1976).

The following comments from a patient in the SCID-D field study, diagnosed as having dissociative identity disorder (DID), serves as an example of chronic depersonalization leading to diminished distress from the symptom:

Interviewer: Have you ever felt as if you were watching yourself from a point outside of your body, as if you were seeing yourself from a distance or watching a movie of yourself?

Patient: Uh huh. Yes Frequently.

Interviewer: How does that feel to you?

Patient: Now it's OK. I guess because I know what's going on. Before the diagnosis, I was concerned, worried. Now it doesn't bother me . . . In most cases it's not frightening. In the beginning it was. Now it's not. It's like you're observing life. (SCID-D interview, unpublished transcript)

Another instance from SCID-D research concerned a woman who had found depersonalization to be useful as a form of self-anesthesia. She suffered chronic physical pain due to a blood disorder and resorted to depersonalization as a way of coping with it:

Patient: I always refer to my body as third person and, um, I always have. . . . It's great in a way. It has some advantages because I can cope with a lot of pain that I have because I just dissociate from my body and I don't feel it.

Interviewer: In the same respect does it feel as if part of your body was disconnected or detached from you?

Patient: The whole body seems disconnected. . . .

Interviewer: Can you describe what that experience is like?

Patient: Well, it's like, sometimes it is just sort of floating away, like when I was a child and I had a lot of pain in my legs and stuff. Um, I just kind of severed things at the waist and my lower body would just kind of float away. It's a neat trick. (SCID-D interview, unpublished transcript)

▋ The Etiology of Depersonalization

The chief theories about the origin of depersonalization involve psychophysiological, psychological, and psychoanalytic explanations (Lehman 1974; Sedman 1970). Mayer-Gross (1935), for example, considered depersonalization to be primarily a physiological response of the brain that could be triggered by biological or psychological antecedents. He termed this a "preformed functional response of the brain," suggesting that depersonalization is governed by the more primitive regions of the brain. The occurrence of depersonalization in physiological states (e.g., sleep, organic illnesses such as epilepsy) and its universality in the general population (Dixon 1963; Roberts 1960) give some credibility to the "preformed-process" hypothesis (Sedman 1970). However, the interaction of the brain's lower centers with the higher centers of the cortex, as well as with psychosocial stimuli, requires further examination.

Analytic theories generally consider depersonalization as a defense against painful affects (Cattell and Cattell 1974; Frances et al. 1977; Shraberg 1977). Some researchers have viewed depersonalization as a regressive state (Stewart 1964). Depersonalization is more widely seen as a response to anxiety, which results in a loss of affect (e.g., Oberndorf 1950). Secondary anxiety may result from the person's fear of going crazy or being labeled as crazy. The poet Pessoa (1991) concludes a description of one of his experiences of depersonalization with the words, "I was afraid of going mad, not of madness itself, but of going mad. My body was a latent scream" (pp. 105–106). In fact, this secondary anxiety contributes heavily to the "silent suffering" inflicted on people by the dissociative disorders. Because experiences of depersonalization, as well as some of the other dissociative symptoms, are difficult to put into words or explain to others, many patients either do not understand the occurrence or fear negative reactions from others.

Related etiologies for depersonalization focus on the split between the observing and participating self (e.g., Arlow 1966; Noyes and Kletti 1976). Noyes and Kletti (1976) note that "in the face of mortal danger we find individuals becoming observers of that which is taking place, effectively removing themselves from danger" (p. 108). In addition, splits between the observing and the participating self are extremely common in incest survivors (Braun 1990).

■ Transient Depersonalization Syndrome

Depersonalization commonly occurs in response to life-threatening dangers, such as sudden accidents, cardiac arrests, and serious illnesses (Noyes and Kletti 1977a; Noyes et al. 1977). Noyes et al. (1977) found that a transient depersonalization syndrome developed in "nearly one third of [normal] persons exposed to life

threatening danger (accident victims)" (p. 401). Three features associated with depersonalization appear to be more common in experiences associated with this type of external danger than in
depersonalization as encountered in psychiatric patients: 1) panoramic memory, 2) isolated episode whose onset occurs immediately following trauma, and 3) the pleasurable nature of the
episode.

Panoramic memory, which is often described as "seeing one's
life pass before one's eyes," is the instantaneous retrieval of a mul-
titude of life memories. This tends to occur under the stress of
life-threatening situations, such as drowning, confrontation with
an armed criminal, or other near-death experiences (Noyes and
Kletti 1977b). Because of its relationship to single-trauma incidents,
panoramic memory is more common in transient depersonalization syndrome than in chronic depersonalization disorder. Panoramic memory seems to be a fairly organized response; thus its
function is most likely adaptive rather than a random by-product
of the trauma. There are three possible explanations for panoramic
memory:

1. **Scanning and retrieval of past adaptations.** Panoramic
   memory may represent the mind's attempt to recall previous
   encounters with danger and the coping strategies that came
   into play. An approximate match with the present dilemma
   may supply clues to survival.
2. **Therapeutic function.** Panoramic memory allows the person
   to reexperience the most meaningful parts of his or her life to
   reinforce its value to themselves. This positive reinforcement
   could aid in the survival of the trauma by increasing the
   person's will to survive.
3. **"Famous last words."** Scanning meaningful experiences and
   people in one's memory may increase the chance that the person who is about to die will say something "adaptive," that is,
   he or she may say something that will have a positive impact
   on a relative or friend, or on a social group. It is interesting to
   note that the friends and relatives of dying people in Puritan
   New England usually gathered around the deathbed with the

express expectation that the dying person would have unusually profound religious insights to impart.

It appears that different types of trauma tend to lead to different types of psychological disturbances. Single or few traumas usually lead to problems like transient depersonalization syndrome. The chronic depersonalization syndromes more typically result from persistent or recurrent trauma. Noyes et al. (1977) found important differences between the depersonalization experiences of normal persons exposed to danger and those of psychiatric outpatients. The psychiatric patients reported more experiences of mental clouding, whereas the accident victims were fully alert to their circumstances at the time that they experienced depersonalization. This difference may be related to the prolonged nature of the traumas experienced by the psychiatric subjects as opposed to the relatively instantaneous impact of an accident. A heightened state of arousal may not serve the organism well when it is helplessly subjected to chronic physical and sexual abuse, in many cases over several years. Noyes et al. (1977) write,

> The mental clouding factor seemed to represent a more severe form of depersonalization which, by its very nature, excluded awareness of effects included in the detachment factor. Accident victims seemed to experience it when danger was most extreme and when rescue efforts were deemed impossible. (p. 406)

Childhood trauma resulting in the more severe, "mental clouding" type of depersonalization may thus be considered a prolonged, inescapable "accident." The range of human responses to trauma may represent a spectrum of helplessness associated with the overwhelming experience(s). At each point along the continuum there is some mixture of both arousal and numbing. Arousal, however, may predominate in reactions to transient, escapable traumata (such as brief life-threatening episodes), whereas numbing (dissociation from affect and identity) may be more pronounced in reactions to chronic, high-helplessness traumata (such as child sexual abuse lasting for years). Briere (1992) has described detachment and intellectualization as forms of depersonalization in survivors of chronic childhood abuse:

> When it occurs more acutely, detachment may present as a sudden loss of reactivity to internal or external events that otherwise would produce distress or dysphoria. Although not usually considered as such, it is likely that intellectualization—a defense involving excessive, analytic preoccupation with the nonemotional characteristics of threatening events—is a form of dissociative detachment. (p. 38)

In addition, it is possible that people may respond to accidents caused by mechanical problems or other impersonal factors (e.g., weather, natural disasters) with a higher degree of arousal than they do when the traumas are inflicted intentionally by other human beings. A child who suffers abuse at the hands of a relative or other emotionally significant adult may find "mental clouding" a more adaptive response than hyperarousal. Langer's (1991) account of Holocaust survivors indicates that the mental and emotional numbing that people experienced in the death camps was connected to their knowledge that they were victims of human malice and cruelty, not natural disasters or other "acts of God."

■ The Spectrum of Depersonalization

Depersonalization can manifest across a broad continuum of severity, ranging from absence of the symptom to persistent or severe depersonalization (Steinberg 1991; Steinberg 1994b). An isolated episode of depersonalization is a nonspecific symptom and is not pathognomonic of any particular clinical disorder (Brauer et al. 1970; Fleiss et al. 1975). Brief episodes of mild depersonalization are quite common and occur under a variety of circumstances in the normal population (Dixon 1963; Myers and Grant 1972; Roberts 1960; Trueman 1984b). Depersonalization can be induced in normal subjects by several precipitating factors, such as sleep and sensory deprivation, stress, drugs, alcohol, meditation, and fatigue. For instance, brief episodes of depersonalization have been noted to occur in 8.5%–46% of college students (Dixon 1963; Myers and Grant 1972; Trueman 1984b).

In one study by Steinberg et al. (1990), control subjects were compared with psychiatric patients, using the SCID-D's standards of measurement. Control subjects reported none to isolated depersonalization episodes, which were usually brief and associated with stress. Patients with dissociative disorders, on the other hand, tended to experience recurrent to persistent depersonalization and experienced it in the absence of any single concrete psychosocial trauma or mind-altering precipitants, as described previously. SCID-D research indicates quantitative and qualitative differences regarding depersonalization in individuals with dissociative disorder and posttraumatic stress disorder (PTSD), as compared with people with other psychiatric disorders and the general population.

One patient with DID described the high frequency of her depersonalization experiences:

Interviewer: Have you ever felt as if parts of your body or your whole being was unreal?

Patient: Yes.

Interviewer: What's that like?

Patient: It's frightening because it feels as though you could leave and just never, ever come back. Or like you aren't really there. Like it could be invisible. So it's like I want to make sure that somebody sees me. Even if the rest of the world doesn't, make sure that you know, even if you can't see me, that I'm here.

Interviewer: How often have you had the experience of feeling that your whole being is unreal?

Patient: Always—in greater or lesser degree. Sometimes more than others. (SCID-D interview, unpublished transcript)

In depersonalization experiences, the person often feels as if part of him or her has retreated into the role of an observer passively witnessing the behavior of another part, the active, participatory self. In dissociative disorders, this split between participant and observer can take extreme forms. One of the patients in the SCID-D field study described recurrent episodes of "watching" herself from a distance.

> **Interviewer:** Have you ever felt that you were able to observe yourself from a point outside of your body as if you were observing yourself from a distance?
>
> **Patient:** All the time.
>
> **Interviewer:** Can you describe what that experience is like?
>
> **Patient:** Oh yeah. Well, we . . . you know, I watch . . . particularly, I used to . . . like I would decide who should go do something, which of the personalities would be best dealing with a different, specific situation, and I'd watch them do it. I mean I've always, all my life I have watched someone doing something. That's the problem I'm having now, to be involved myself. That's a whole new world. (SCID-D interview, unpublished transcript)

The SCID-D's capacity to elicit additional information about symptomatology was evident later on in this patient's interview, in which she returned to the theme of depersonalized "watching" in response to a question regarding identity disturbance. In this section of the interview, the patient clearly describes herself as a passive observer of situations that she feels powerless to affect or influence:

> **Interviewer:** Have you ever felt your behavior was not in your control?
>
> **Patient:** Oh yes [laughs].
>
> **Interviewer:** Can you describe what that experience is like?
>
> **Patient:** Well, again, it's like the watching business, but it's like . . . as opposed to watching something that you have some control over, it's like watching something and you know that what that person is doing is stupid, but there's not anything you can do. You've got to sit there and watch them make a jerk of themselves.

Interviewer: Who were you referring to?

Patient: Different parts of me. (SCID-D interview, unpublished transcript)

Another key distinguishing feature of depersonalization in the dissociative disorders is that the symptom can manifest in interactive dialogues between the observing and the participating self, as the following excerpt indicates:

> I start to argue with somebody that's in the chair, but I see that person in the chair and I see it's me. I see that person and he's looking at me and he's laughing at me, and he's calling me on to fight him, and fight him, and fight him, and I don't want to fight him . . . I see me outside of myself, in other words, and he's laughing at me, calling out, saying, "Come on punk, fight me, come on punk, fight me." (SCID-D interview, unpublished transcript)

In normal subjects, when depersonalization is accompanied by dialogue, it is not of a personified nature and tends to be experienced as a "metaphorical dialogue" (i.e., a weighing of the pros and cons of a decision). Actual dialogues may be remembered by normal subjects but usually in the form of memories of conversations, not as hallucinations. Nondissociative dialogues take the form of simulations of anticipated interactions and reviewing of past dialogues, usually in the form of fantasized situations and/or reality-based problem-solving. For example, someone getting ready for a date may rehearse possible conversational "openers," or a student preparing for an oral examination may pose and answer a series of likely questions. By contrast, the dialogues that may accompany depersonalization in the dissociative disorders involve distinct personifications and lack the purposeful quality of internal dialogues in normal subjects. In addition to the differential "quality" of depersonalization, the "quantity" of depersonalization is greater in those with dissociative disorders than in the non-psychiatric population. Depersonalization episodes in patients with dissociative disorders tend to last longer and occur more frequently. Thus the severity or pathognomy of the symptoms increases across a spectrum from low intensity and frequency to high intensity and frequency. Here, *intensity* is defined by the degree of interference with social relationships and self-satisfaction as well as the salience of the depersonalization and the personification of the dissociated selves. The lower end of the spectrum tends to manifest in the normal population, the median in mixed psychiatric patients, and the upper end in patients with dissociative disorders and PTSD. DID is assumed to represent the apex of the spectrum. It should be kept in mind, however, that within the population of DID patients, there may be variations in the severity of dissociative symptoms within the range already specified (i.e., the high range of intensity).

In sum, normal subjects usually report mild and episodic experiences of depersonalization that are usually precipitated by stress, fatigue, ingestion of mood-altering substances, or life-threatening danger. Those with dissociative disorders, on the other hand, experience recurrent or persistent episodes that are of high frequency, long duration, high salience (e.g., with interactive dialogues, interfering with daily life), or some combination of these.

■ Differential Diagnosis

The differential diagnosis of patients who experience recurrent or persistent depersonalization should include the dissociative disorders, a variety of other psychiatric disorders, and possible organic etiology. Because depersonalization is rarely the chief or presenting complaint, depersonalization disorder may go undetected (Edwards and Angus 1972). The difficulty in assessing depersonalization may also lead to misdiagnosis supported by a secondary, but highly visible, symptom. Common initial diagnoses include depression due to characteristic lack of affect (Ackner 1954; Lower 1972; Roth 1960) and panic and anxiety disorders due to the frequent coexistence of panic and anxiety (Ambrosino 1973; Cassano et al. 1989; Roth 1959). Accurate differential diagnosis and appropriate treatment depend on systematic assessment to determine the primary symptom and its context.

Anxiety Disorders

Anxiety and panic often accompany symptoms of depersonalization (Ambrosino 1973; Roth 1960). Cassano et al. (1989) found depersonalization to occur in 34% of 150 patients with panic disorder/agoraphobia during the panic attacks. A number of researchers have proposed that, in terms of causation, anxiety exhibits both primary and secondary roles with respect to depersonalization (Cassano et al. 1989; Nemiah 1989a). Primary anxiety, such as is produced by panic attacks, may result in an episode of depersonalization. Depersonalization, as stated by Nemiah (1989a), "is often accompanied by considerable secondary anxiety, and frequently patients fear that their symptoms are a sign that they are going insane" (p. 1042).

This anxiety-depersonalization-anxiety cycle may become semiautonomous because the patient's dissociative reaction to excessive anxiety triggers further fears of loss of control and being labeled by others as dysfunctional. These fears may in turn feed back into the cycle as primary anxiety, thus setting off another episode of depersonalization (Trueman 1984b). One of the patients in the SCID-D study described this cyclical pattern of anxiety and depersonalization quite clearly:

> **Interviewer:** Do you have frequent episodes of anxiety or panic attacks?
>
> **Patient:** Occasionally.
>
> **Interviewer:** Occasional panic attack or occasional anxiety?
>
> **Patient:** I guess both. Um, well, yeah, I guess you'd call it panic attack.
>
> **Interviewer:** What do you experience?
>
> **Patient:** Um . . . very nervous. The heart starts racing.
>
> **Interviewer:** And how often does that occur?
>
> **Patient:** Um, it's hard to say [pauses]. Not a whole lot. Well, it's kind of . . . if someone's talking to me, and I can't understand what they're saying, or I'm just not thinking clearly, then it's

kind of a panic that they're going to notice that. Or if I'm driving. Sometimes I'd have problems driving for awhile.

Interviewer: Is the anxiety and the panic kind of feeling related to your feelings of being unreal and being in a daze?

Patient: Oh yeah.

Interviewer: How are they related and what comes first? That might be a hard question.

Patient: Well, because if something seems so unreal and you're afraid that you don't have control of the situation or something, that kind of makes you panic.

Interviewer: OK. How often would you say they are related? Is it occasionally, or frequently, or most of the time?

Patient: It's always. (SCID-D interview, unpublished transcript)

The frequent coexistence of phobic anxiety, panic attacks, and depersonalization has led some authors to describe a phobic anxiety-depersonalization syndrome (Ambrosino 1973; Roth 1959) that is thought to be relatively common. Patients in this category experience a collection of symptoms, including panic attacks, phobic anxiety, anticipatory anxiety, depersonalization, derealization, somatic preoccupation, and reactive depression (Ambrosino 1973). Depersonalization surfaces most often in the early and acute phases of the syndrome, fading as the disorder becomes chronic (Roth and Argyle 1988). Phobic anxiety-depersonalization syndrome seems to be more common in women, with typical age at onset in the late 20s. Precipitants include severe emotional trauma, pregnancy, and childbirth. Proper establishment of the etiology and assessment of this syndrome requires further research (Linton and Estock 1977), particularly in regard to the possibility that it exists within the context of a dissociative disorder.

The SCID-D field study included one patient with obsessive-compulsive disorder, diagnosed on the SCID-D as having dissociative disorder not otherwise specified (DDNOS), who reported significant instances of depersonalization:

It's happening all the time. It's happening now, of, an observer. A witness. Of me being outside of myself, taking global stock in what I've done in my life . . . I have the illness, and yet I have a witness who's very healthy, and very alive, and can see people my age going on, getting good jobs, buying their first house, when I haven't. . . . Even though I can communicate with [my doctor] in English, I can't communicate feelings, and what it's been like moment to moment, day to day, and the problems that it's caused in my personal life, in my professional life. And the saddest thing is that this witness knows that I'm a very good person, and that a bad thing is happening to this very good person. It makes me very sad. I feel like I've lost time that I can't make up. I don't feel as though I can blame myself for it, yet I still feel like somebody has to be accountable for it. (SCID-D interview, unpublished transcript)

Detachment from feeling may signify an adaptive function of dissociation—that is, distancing from anxiety in order to function, even though the patient's functioning is far from optimal.

Depression

Depression is the most common misdiagnosis attached to patients who have severe depersonalization and phobic anxiety (Roth 1960). Clinicians should note that any of the following are possibilities: depersonalization may 1) mimic the symptoms of depression (Roth 1960), 2) coexist with depression or be a feature of depression in later life (Anderson 1936), or 3) be triggered by depression. Accurate differential diagnosis and appropriate treatment depend on systematic assessment to determine which symptom is primary. One of the patients in the SCID-D study, diagnosed as having DID, indicated that one of her alter personalities was depressed. However, she described the depression from the perspective of a depersonalized observer:

Interviewer: Have you ever felt as if your emotions were not in your control?

Patient: Oh yeah.

Interviewer: If so, can you give an example of what that experience is like?

Patient: I don't know. It's such a common thing. Again it's like, it's like intellectually I will feel that I should be upset or I shouldn't be upset. Intellectually there's no reason to be upset; I understand what they're doing and everything, but I'm furious at the same time . . . it's getting better, but I've had trouble getting the intellect to kind of calm the hysterics down or the depression, real severe depressions, and intellectually I can rationalize the whole bit, but I can't pull the person out of the depression.

Interviewer: When you say, you can't pull the person out of the depression, you're referring to yourself?

Patient: Yeah. Yeah. I do that a lot. (SCID-D interview, unpublished transcript)

The emotional numbing that is a concomitant of depersonalization may cause the symptom to appear like depression to the untrained eye. Lower (1972) reported that "in many [cases of depersonalization] the sense of emotional numbness, of being dead or detached from life around them, was the primary complaint and the disturbance in the sense of self [specifically feeling unreal, or as if an observer of oneself] was uncovered only on questioning" (p. 569). Typical descriptions of the affective detachment of depersonalization that can be mistaken for depression include

I "I'm doing things, but it's as though I'm standing off from things, not involved—as though I'm not real."
I "It's like watching a not very interesting mildly amusing movie. It's not painful; it's just an absence of all feelings."
I "It makes me feel frozen and numb." (SCID-D interview, unpublished transcript)

One of Pessoa's (1991) diary entries reflects an emotional constriction that could easily be read as depression: "I've lived without thinking. Today, suddenly, I returned to the person I am or dream I

am. It was a moment of great fatigue, after an unrelieved labor. . . .
I immediately felt the uselessness of life" (p. 120).

Schizophrenia

Depersonalization was once thought to be a predominant symptom of schizophrenia (Galdston 1947). However, more recent studies have challenged an overly simplistic view of the relationship between the two. Although people with schizophrenia commonly experience episodes of depersonalization (Blackmore 1986; Sedman and Kenna 1963), the phenomenology of depersonalization as associated with schizophrenia is qualitatively different from the type found in depersonalization disorder and DID (Steinberg 1993b). The chief qualitative difference is the loss of reality testing in schizophrenia.

The maintenance of reality testing in depersonalization in the dissociative disorders is a clear line of demarcation between dissociative disorders and the psychoses. The other chapters of this manual will demonstrate that this criterion applies to all the dissociative symptoms as a boundary between schizophrenia and the dissociative disorders. For example, the depersonalization that is characteristic of DID is typically described in "as if" terminology. Many descriptions by patients with DID of their depersonalization experiences are metaphorical. The experience almost always remains incredible to the patient (Ackner 1954). Patients usually differentiate between what they feel is going on within their selves and what is (or might be) observable to others around them.

In contrast to depersonalization in the dissociative disorders, depersonalization experiences in people with schizophrenia manifest poor reality testing. A schizophrenic patient's answer to one of the depersonalization questions on the SCID-D reflects this particular feature:

Interviewer: Have you ever heard yourself talking and felt that you were not the one choosing the words?

Patient: Yes.

Interviewer: Can you describe that for me?

Patient: I felt that what I was thinking was coming out of the top of my head and that other people could read, could hear what I was thinking, and they could put words back and they were talking into my brain. (SCID-D interview, unpublished transcript)

The same patient was later asked, "Have you ever felt as if your behavior was not in your control?" She answered as follows:

I felt that others were controlling me again through food and when they talked about the food, and when I ate it, it did certain things to me—it made me aware of other things, when in fact, I was very delusional. (SCID-D interview, unpublished transcript)

What differentiates patients with schizophrenia from patients with DID is that patients with schizophrenia experience delusions, psychotic episodes, and have poor reality testing, whereas patients with DID have intact reality testing and are not chronically psychotic. Furthermore, both groups may experience hallucinations, but the hallucinations of the patient with DID are usually experienced as being "internal" (i.e., internal personalities debating, as opposed to the patient's thinking that they are communicating with a real, famous person).

Horowitz (1975) defined hallucination as "an image experience in which there is a discrepancy between subjective experience and actual reality." In other words, the person who is hallucinating perceives internal sensations as external, or *ego-alien*. In DID, by contrast, the patient perceives the "hallucinations" as being internal. Thus some of the severe symptoms of depersonalization that can occur in DID can be termed *parahallucinatory*, because the experiences involve distortions in the perception of the self rather than distortions of "actual reality." Moreover, the alterations in identity that characterize DID are "real," whereas a patient harboring a delusion that he or she has been transformed into another existing person (e.g., the Pope) is not in touch with reality. In other words, when Suzy states that she is now "Beth,"—that is, that one of her alters has emerged—at that moment she *is* Beth. On the other hand, when Margaret says she's "Princess Diana," she is *not* Princess Diana. In extreme cases, however, the boundary between inner and outer is both tenuous and complex. For example, a patient with DID may believe that she is talking to another "him" or "her" across the room, or that she is seeing herself sitting in a chair while another "her" is floating near the ceiling, looking down on the patient. Instances of this sort are relatively unusual. In most cases, the patient with DID recognizes that only he or she can perceive the existence of the duplicate person.

Borderline Personality Disorder

As with schizophrenia, borderline personality disorder has also been associated with experiences of depersonalization. In one study, Chopra and Beatson (1986) noted that depersonalization occurred in 11 of 13 patients with borderline personality disorder who had experienced transient psychotic episodes. Severe dissociative experiences, including depersonalization and derealization, have been thought to be particularly common and discriminating of borderline personality and are given added weight in the Diagnostic Interview for Borderline Patients (Gunderson et al. 1981). These studies of patients with borderline personality disorder, however, do not include a group of patients with dissociative disorders in the patient sample. As a result, they are inadequate to establish the efficacy of the Diagnostic Interview for Borderline Patients to distinguish between patients with borderline personality and patients with dissociative disorders. Pope et al. (1985) noted that this inadequacy may have led their study to overlook the presence of dissociative disorders in some of their subjects. Thus previous studies of borderline personality disorder may not have recognized the coexistence of depersonalization disorder and the other dissociative disorders.

Substance Use Disorders

Acute intoxication or withdrawal from a variety of drugs or alcohol can result in symptoms of depersonalization that are indistinguishable from those characteristic of depersonalization disorder

(Good 1989). Depersonalization has been most commonly reported in association with marijuana (Moran 1986; Szymanski 1981), hallucinogens such as LSD (Ludwig 1966; Waltzer 1972), and mescaline (Guttmann and Maclay 1936). It may also occur with the use of alcohol, cocaine, phencyclidine, narcotics, sedatives, and stimulants (Good 1989). Acute intoxication with these drugs may also intensify preexisting feelings of depersonalization. In addition, prolonged episodes of depersonalization (occurring months after only a few occasions of marijuana use) have been reported to occur in conjunction with mood-altering substances, especially when the patient resorted to using them under stress. Such patients were diagnosed as meeting DSM-III criteria for a variety of psychiatric disorders, including depersonalization disorder (Keshaven and Lishman 1986; Szymanski 1981). In addition, recurrent depersonalization that had been initially connected with marijuana use has been associated with the development of agoraphobia. This phenomenon may be understood as a manifestation of a "fear of 'uncontrolled' depersonalization" (Moran 1986, p. 187).

A history of drug and alcohol use and of the temporal history of depersonalization is essential for accurate diagnosis. The patient who mentions experiences of alcohol- or drug-induced depersonalization should be evaluated for these symptoms when he or she is not using drugs or alcohol. Because coexisting psychiatric disorders are common in individuals who abuse drugs or alcohol, the presence of an underlying psychiatric disorder, of which depersonalization is a symptom, should be ruled out. Szymanski (1981) reported that although depersonalization may initially be understood as a pharmacologic effect of marijuana, "after the patients had experienced depersonalization, external stressors and intrapsychic factors may have contributed to its continued use as a defense mechanism."

Seizure Disorders

Depersonalization, along with a variety of other psychiatric symptoms, may be observed in patients with seizure disorders, particularly temporal lobe epilepsy (Bear and Fedio 1977; Flor-Henry

1976; Slater et al. 1963). A variety of dissociative phenomena, including dissociative fugue, dissociative amnesia, depersonalization, and derealization, have been reported to occur in the seizure disorders (Bear and Fedio 1977; Flor-Henry 1976; Slater et al. 1963). These phenomena may be seen during preictal, interictal, or postictal states, and have been most commonly associated with temporal lobe epilepsy. An investigation using the Dissociative Experiences Scale (DES; Bernstein and Putnam 1986) noted that there was a 20% overlap in DES scores of seizure disorders and DID, indicating that one in five patients with epilepsy had significant dissociative experiences (Devinsky et al. 1989). On the other hand, the most comprehensive study to date (Bowman, personal communication) found that there was little overlap of dissociative symptoms between a population of seizure disorder patients and a population of dissociative disorder patients, as measured by the SCID-D. In one study (Roth and Harper 1962), depersonalization occurred in 11 of 30 patients with temporal lobe epilepsy and in 17 of 30 patients with phobic anxiety depersonalization syndrome. Derealization occurred only in the psychiatric group. Age at onset for epileptic patients was commonly under the age of 20, whereas age at onset of the phobic anxiety depersonalization group was over the age of 20. The authors also noted that patients with temporal lobe epilepsy were likely 1) to have had earlier age at onset, 2) to be male, 3) to have automatic stereotypic behavior, and 4) to have loss of consciousness during seizures. These hallmarks were not characteristic of the patients who had presented with phobic anxiety depersonalization syndrome (Harper and Roth 1962). The appearance of dissociative disorders in individuals with seizures was reported in two case studies (Mesulam 1981; Schenck and Bear 1981). At present, researchers have not established whether these associations are coincidental or causal. Other investigations have noted the misdiagnosis of epilepsy in patients whose psychiatric disorders manifest dissociative symptoms (Roth and Harper 1962).

Standard clinical practice currently relies on an index of suspicion based on a history suggestive of seizure disorder. An electroencephalogram (EEG) is then performed to rule out the presence of a seizure disorder. Although depersonalization may occur in the seizure disorders, it may be differentiated from depersonalization as it occurs in the major psychiatric disorders and normal control subjects. The depersonalization present in patients with psychiatric disorders (particularly the dissociative disorders) may be quite complex and elaborate. For example, a patient may report watching herself from a distance and engaging in a dialogue with herself, and the episode may last for hours to days (Steinberg 1991). Depersonalization in the seizure disorders, however, is usually brief (lasting from seconds to minutes), with stereotypic and repetitive content that is rarely elaborated. Although automatic behavior and speech may occur with depersonalization within the psychiatric disorders, it is typically complex and elaborate, purposeful, and well organized (Harper and Roth 1962). In the seizure disorders, there is also perceived automatic behavior and automatic speech, but they are typically purposeless and repetitive (e.g., lip smacking). Similarly, seizure disorders often manifest speech automatisms in which the "patient utters a mixture of words and sentences which may be linguistically correct but bear no appropriate relation to the present situation" (Bingley 1958). Such inappropriateness is not a salient feature of depersonalization in psychiatric patients (see Table 5–1).

Organic Illnesses

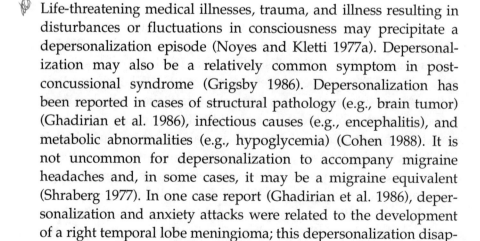

Life-threatening medical illnesses, trauma, and illness resulting in disturbances or fluctuations in consciousness may precipitate a depersonalization episode (Noyes and Kletti 1977a). Depersonalization may also be a relatively common symptom in post-concussional syndrome (Grigsby 1986). Depersonalization has been reported in cases of structural pathology (e.g., brain tumor) (Ghadirian et al. 1986), infectious causes (e.g., encephalitis), and metabolic abnormalities (e.g., hypoglycemia) (Cohen 1988). It is not uncommon for depersonalization to accompany migraine headaches and, in some cases, it may be a migraine equivalent (Shraberg 1977). In one case report (Ghadirian et al. 1986), depersonalization and anxiety attacks were related to the development of a right temporal lobe meningioma; this depersonalization disap-

Table 5–1. Depersonalization in patients with dissociative disorders versus those with epilepsy

	Dissociative disorders	Epilepsy
Duration	Variable (seconds–ongoing)	Brief (seconds–minutes)
Content	Elaborate descriptions and internal dialogues	Repetitive content
Speech	Elaborate, lucid speech	Speech automatisms (mixture of words)
Behavior	Complex and purposeful	Repetitive and purposeless
EEG	Normal	Abnormal

peared following removal of the tumor. Depersonalization has also been noted to accompany complaints of vertigo, presumably because of vestibular dysfunction, and has been reported in association with two cases of Ménière's disease, a disorder characterized by episodic vertigo, progressive hearing loss, and fullness in the ear usually associated with tinnitus (Grigsby and Johnston 1989). Similarly, depersonalization may occur in cases of acute and chronic organic syndromes, such as cerebral arteriopathy and Korsakoff's psychosis (Kenna and Sedman 1965).

Medication Side Effects

Case reports have noted depersonalization as a side effect of a variety of medications, including the neuroleptic haloperidol (Lukianowicz 1967), the anti-inflammatory agent indomethacin (Schwartz and Moura 1983), alpha-methyldopa (Lukianowicz 1967), and the amphetamine-like agent fenfluramine (Imlah 1970). Drug-induced depersonalization is usually transient and commonly disappears upon discontinuation of the medication. However, these case reports did not systematically evaluate the baseline level of depersonalization prior to the initiation of medication therapy. Therefore, it is unclear whether these medications prompted new episodes of depersonalization or exacerbated preexisting depersonalization, or whether the association is coincidental.

CHAPTER 6

Assessment of Depersonalization

By its very nature, depersonalization is an elusive symptom that is difficult for most patients to put into words. As Fewtrell (1986) describes it,

> [Depersonalization] involves a strange absence of feeling and an apparent reduction of vividness and reality. It is therefore difficult for many people to articulate. Whereas most subjects can readily describe an anxiety bout or feelings of morbid depression, a curious state of non-being is much more difficult to put into words. (p. 264)

Depersonalization can easily go unnoticed because it is difficult for the subject to express this intangible experience (Fewtrell 1986; Torch 1987). This ineffability largely stems from the associated features of unreality and numbed affect. Description may also be difficult for the patient because symptoms of depersonalization are often experienced as being "strange" (Cattell and Cattell 1974) or uncanny. During the SCID-D interview (Steinberg 1993b), one patient with DID described an episode of depersonalization in these words:

> It's like everything is not real. It's hard to describe. Because I don't think there are words, that someone that has not felt it, can understand. Because it doesn't make a whole lot of sense. You just become unreal. There's this gap between you and reality. Either by becoming invisible or by stepping back and watching yourself, or just existing in sort of an unreal world. (SCID-D interview, unpublished transcript)

Another patient with DID had difficulty describing feelings of depersonalization compounded by anxiety:

Interviewer: Have you ever felt like a stranger to yourself, as if you didn't know yourself any better than someone who was a stranger?

Patient: Sometimes.

Interviewer: What's that like?

Patient: It's actually very fearful [sic] because I, you know, I have to wonder what's real and what isn't, and it's hard for me sometimes to distinguish it. (SCID-D interview, unpublished transcript)

On the other hand, subjects with depersonalization may not be markedly distressed by its symptoms. Chronic depersonalization, moreover, is often accompanied with little distress, if the patient has become habituated to it. Sometimes depersonalization is accompanied by comfort (Ackner 1954) and may consequently go underreported. For these reasons, depersonalization may not be a presenting report (Ackner 1954; Mayer-Gross 1935; Shimizu and Sakamoto 1986).

Another reason why patients may be reluctant to disclose symptoms of depersonalization is the fear of being labeled "crazy" by friends, employers, or doctors (Ackner 1954; Fewtrell 1986). Fear of stigmatization provides a serious motive for the concealment of symptoms when people understandably prefer to maintain jobs, friendships, and family ties without disruption. In addition, a person's recognition of the symptoms of depersonalization in him- or herself may elicit fears of loss of control or of psychological inadequacy. This reluctance to disclose evidence of depersonalization may be present even when the patient is experiencing chronic depersonalization (Ackner 1954; Edwards and Angus 1972; Shorvon et al. 1946). One patient with DID in the SCID-D study spoke quite candidly about the stress created by chronic feelings of depersonalization as well as her feelings of hurt about having been labeled "crazy" by her family:

Interviewer: ... when you do see yourself from a point outside of your body, is that experience by itself stressful to you or is that a calming experience?

Patient: Well, it's becoming increasingly stressful as I'm aware of it. It used to be just the way I was, and now that I know what I'm doing and, you know, I'm into the integration process, it's becoming real stressful that I can't make connections when I want to.

Interviewer: While you were experiencing these feelings of being disconnected, were you under treatment for any other psychiatric problems?

Patient: Oh yeah. Yeah, I went through the usual, um, you know, in and out of various therapists since I was in college. Actually, I was called crazy when I was a very young child by my family, um, and, uh, they tried various labels on me and stuff. (SCID-D interview, unpublished transcript)

Because of these problems in presentation, clinicians have regarded depersonalization as a rare symptom until very recently. Yet numerous investigators have found that episodes of depersonalization are quite common in the psychiatric population and are as commonly misdiagnosed. Depersonalization is the third most frequent reported problem among psychiatric patients, after anxiety and depression (Cattell and Cattell 1974).

However, clinicians have also contributed to the misdiagnosis of depersonalization. Reasons for misdiagnosis by the clinician include skepticism regarding the patient's sincerity and lack of awareness of dissociative symptoms. For example, patients are often more likely to present secondary symptoms such as depression and anxiety, and clinicians may not be prepared to investigate further. A psychiatrist simply may not expect to discover feelings of depersonalization behind reports of depression or anxiety. The skepticism of the clinician, as well as his or her difficulty with what the untrained might consider "bizarre" symptomatology (e.g., out-of-body and possession experiences), may predispose the clinician to interpret the patient's dissociative symptoms as evidence of schizophrenia or psychosis, when the correct diagnosis may be one of the dissociative disorders such as depersonalization disorder or dissociative identity disorder (DID).

Realistically, the misdiagnosis of depersonalization can be attributed to the interaction between a clinician's faulty assessment and masked presentation. For instance, the common lack of overt impairment in social functioning associated with depersonalization (Levy and Wachtel 1978) may act synergistically with a clinician's reluctance to consider depersonalization as a diagnosis. Changes in consciousness are more difficult to detect than changes in behavior; as a result, clinicians who have been primed to focus mainly on behavior (and, more specifically, behaviors that they recognize) may overlook the indications of changes in consciousness brought about by depersonalization.

■ The Many Facets of Depersonalization

The SCID-D's assessment of depersonalization opens with straightforward questions, such as question 38: "Have you ever felt that you were watching yourself from a point outside of your body, as if you were seeing yourself from a distance (or watching a movie of yourself)?"; question 40: "Have you ever had the feeling that you were a stranger to yourself?"; and question 41: "Have you ever felt as if part of your body was foreign to you?" If the answer is "yes," the interviewer may follow up with, "What was that experience like?" The specific symptom of depersonalization can present in many forms. It can be experienced as an out-of-body experience, loss of feeling in parts of the body, a sense of detachment from emotions and sense of self, an impression of watching a movie of oneself, and many other variations. Although all of these symptoms represent some kind of detachment from the self, or from an aspect of the self, these symptoms could go unnoticed if the interview failed to cover all the relevant considerations. For instance, one subject was diagnosed by his referring clinician as suffering from "alcohol abuse." However, when questioned by a SCID-D interviewer, he presented a different picture. For example, when the subject was asked question 38: "Have you ever felt that you were watching yourself from a point outside your body, as if you were seeing yourself from a distance?" he gave a negative response. However, question 40 yielded this exchange just a few moments later in the interview:

Interviewer: Have you ever felt as if a part of your body or your whole being was foreign to you?

Patient: Yeah, I *have* had that.

Interviewer: Tell me about it.

Patient: I experienced and I continue to experience times when all of a sudden I can't feel my hands, or I can't feel my feet. Everything just seems very unreal. Like I'll be driving in my car, and all of a sudden I'll feel like I'm not driving the car. It's like I'll have to reassure myself that I can feel my hands. I'll wiggle my toes—pinch myself—to make sure that I'm all there. It's a little unnerving. (SCID-D interview, unpublished transcript)

Correct diagnosis requires an interview that investigates the many aspects of depersonalization. In this case, the patient's positive response to this question about depersonalization was one of the many clues that led to the diagnosis of dissociative disorder not otherwise specified (DDNOS).

Feeling "Dead" or Invisible

One common manifestation of depersonalization is the sense of being "dead" or invisible. Two patients with DID put it this way:

Sometimes I think I'm dead. That I'm not really here. That nobody can see me and stuff. I'm just walking, just walking, but nobody—just invisible. I guess like invisible. (SCID-D interview, unpublished transcript)

Interviewer: Have you ever felt as if part of your body or your whole body disappeared?

Patient: No. [Pause.] Well, yes, because I felt invisible. I didn't think of that.

Interviewer: Do you feel that at those times that you felt that your whole body disappeared?

Patient: Yes. I've been invisible ever since I was a child.

Interviewer: What do you mean?

Patient: That the only part of me that existed was my eyes—that the rest of me was not there. That happens very frequently. That is something that has happened to me many, many times. It can be just on an average stressful day or on an unaverage stressful day, that I just become invisible. (SCID-D interview, unpublished transcript)

Out-of-Body Experiences

In some cases, the depersonalization is experienced in the form of an out-of-body experience. The precise nature of the experience may vary with each patient. One patient with DID used the word *hover* to describe her experiences:

Interviewer: Have you ever felt that you were watching yourself from a point outside of your body, as if you were seeing yourself from a distance?

Patient: One of these [alternate personalities] can fly, and I believe that she could, even though I say that's not possible. There's my dilemma. You see? That's not possible. I say to myself, that's not possible. But I *know* she could—when I say fly—she could hover above the ground, and I know when and where she learned how to do it. I remember that. I remember that.

Interviewer: How did she learn how to do it?

Patient: Same way a plane does, she'd taxi down the runway.

Interviewer: How often have you had that experience?

Patient: A lot. I don't reach the heights she reaches. . . . Although I tend to think that I don't hover off the ground as high as she did, that I can't get the height that she had. She could go 6 feet off the ground—10 feet off the ground. I never seem to get higher than 3 feet. (SCID-D interview, unpublished transcript)

Out-of-body experiences result from a dissociation of consciousness from the body. This detachment from the body can range from a sense of strangeness (e.g., "This is not my face"), to a sense of physical detachment from the body (e.g., "Where is my face?"), to hallucination-like distortions in body perception (e.g., "My face is getting bigger"). A patient with severe depersonalization may describe feeling as if his or her head, limbs, or entire body has become foreign or disconnected, as in the following excerpt:

> I felt like I do not belong in this body. I, I'm in the wrong body. I don't know how to explain that. . . . I feel that I was not supposed to have been born into this body. Which body it is, I don't know. It was not this body. . . . I always felt I had the wrong face. (SCID-D interview, unpublished transcript)

Changes in Perception of Body Size/Integrity

One associated manifestation of depersonalization involves perceived changes in the sizes of one's limbs, as in the following excerpt:

> **Interviewer:** Have you ever felt that your arms or legs were bigger or smaller than usual?
>
> **Patient:** Sometimes I look in the mirror—my arms would seem bigger. But then I'd look again, and then they'd look smaller. . . . Then I'd look again, and then they'd look normal size to me again. (SCID-D interview, unpublished transcript)

One woman patient saw herself as shrinking in overall size:

> **Interviewer:** Have you ever felt that your arms or legs were bigger or smaller than usual, or you were changing size?
>
> **Patient:** Um, a few times, just recently.
>
> **Interviewer:** What's that like?
>
> **Patient:** Oh, just a sense of, you know, you're smaller.
>
> **Interviewer:** That you felt your size was smaller?

Patient: Smaller. Yes, I felt very little. (SCID-D interview, unpublished transcript)

Some patients experience these changes in self-perception as frightening, as in the following excerpt:

Interviewer: Have you ever had the feeling that part of your body was disconnected from the rest of you?

Patient: Yes, sometimes my legs, even my arms feel as though they are not connected. Most of the time I am in a trance when all of this happens, you have to know that.

Interviewer: OK, and have you ever felt as if part of your body, your whole body had disappeared?

Patient: No, not too much, my whole body no.

Interviewer: Or part of your body?

Patient: Sometimes part of me. But I would be able to see myself, I mean I would never lose my ability. . . .

Interviewer: What part of your body felt as if it might have disappeared?

Patient: I guess my legs, sometimes my arms, but I would never just see my head. I think that would do me in.

Interviewer: Sounds like a frightening experience.

Patient: Ah, it is real frightening. (SCID-D interview, unpublished transcript)

Clinicians using the SCID-D may occasionally find that patients may give sex-specific answers to questions regarding changes in apparent body size. Because women in our society are acculturated to be more concerned about their physical appearance, specifically about slenderness, women subjects may endorse questions about their body size with answers reflecting these cultural preoccupations, or with remarks having to do with fluid retention during the menstrual cycle. One interview subject replied in the following way:

Interviewer: Have you ever felt that you were changing in size or your arms or legs were getting bigger or smaller?

Patient: Actually, I did yesterday. I felt my ankles were really getting fat, and my hands, but I do have water retention. It was something I was thinking of. It just seemed that the more I looked at my ankles the bigger they were getting, when actually they weren't getting that much bigger. (SCID-D interview, unpublished transcript)

Another woman spoke of changes in her self-perception that seem to represent a combination of feelings of depersonalization and self-dislike related to apparent weight gain:

Interviewer: Have you ever felt that parts of your body were unreal?

Patient: Unreal, yeah. I don't feel that this is my body. You know I know it is.

Interviewer: Can you describe what that feels like to you?

Patient: Well, I look in a mirror and I look at myself again and I see this heavy . . . you know, I feel like I'm really a big blimp, and I don't feel . . . see, it's like I don't see myself . . . it's like another person. The person I want to be is where I was. I was thin and I looked good, and like that, and you know, when I got heavy I just all of a sudden looked at myself and I was heavier. . . . When I go to buy clothes, it's like I buy bigger sizes and . . . you know, it's like I don't know who I'm putting them on. I know they're going on me, but it doesn't feel like I'm putting them on me. (SCID-D interview, unpublished transcript)

Perception of Loss of Self-Control

Another facet of depersonalization to be investigated are the features of self-control that make up a person's sense of identity. In depersonalization, an individual may often feel distant from his or her self in situations in which he or she experiences loss of control over actions, thoughts, or emotions. The SCID-D asks if subjects experience periods of time when their activity seems to evade their control:

Interviewer: Have you ever heard yourself talking and felt that you were not the one choosing the words?

Patient: Yes. Yes.

Interviewer: What is that like?

Patient: That's a weird feeling. I'll give you a "for instance." I was asking a friend how his Mom was doing, because his Mom's got emphysema. And I says, "Yo. How's your fuckin' mother doing, Joe?" And then I realized what I said. [I said,] "Joe, I'm so sorry. I didn't mean to say it that way." But that's right. A voice came out of my mouth and I realized I shouldn't have said it . . . and it wasn't me that wanted to say it. I wanted to say, "Gee Joe, how's your Mom doing, Joe?" But it came out, "Joe, how's your fuckin' mother's emphysema, man?" (SCID-D interview, unpublished transcript)

Another patient described how an episode of depersonalization overcame him during a tennis game:

It wasn't really me. It was me watching me . . . I was playing tennis with a guy about 20 years younger than me, and I really didn't feel comfortable playing. And he made the remark, after he beat me, 6–3, he said, "I didn't even work up a sweat." So I said, "Let's play one more time." And I beat him 6–love. I whipped his ass something terrible. It was like it really wasn't me. It was like I almost let someone else, within me, take over so I could rest, 'cause I was worried about my heart—this guy wasn't. And I'll never forget how fierce that guy beat him. And how I just focused on that imaginary person—it was very real— and the tennis ball. I didn't see him, I didn't care where the shots went. I just listened to the sound of the racket and knew that he couldn't possibly return it. (SCID-D interview, unpublished transcript)

It should be noted that some clinicians have recommended specific self-support techniques for patients who are disturbed by frequent episodes of depersonalization. Briere (1992) has remarked that such patients are often helped by being taught to *ground* or locate themselves as a way of recovering a sense of personal identity and self-control, together with contact with the here-and-now. *Grounding* consists of repeating one's name and location to oneself (e.g., "I'm John, I'm in the Orange Street coffee shop, I'm safe, I'm here, I'm real"), touching or visually focusing on objects in the immediate environment, or pressing one's feet against the floor or one's body against one's chair.

At the other extreme, there are patients who experience depersonalization as a phenomenon under their control that they can induce at will, rather than as a disturbing indication that they are out of control. One woman in the SCID-D study, diagnosed as having DDNOS, described her ability to "change" the apparent size or location of her limbs:

Interviewer: Have you ever felt as if part of your body was foreign to you or was disconnected from you?

Patient: [Pauses.] No. You mean like a physical part of my body is disconnected? I can make that happen if I want to.

Interviewer: Can you describe what you mean by that?

Patient: I think I could make that happen. I think I could just sit there and feel like the arm is not attached. . . . I could do that. I don't like to. You know, I could do it, but I don't like to do it. . . . The energy comes all out of your hands, and I can see it, the white energy. I see my hand getting white, all white, and it gets thin and light. It's my hand, but it's like almost starting to detach.

Interviewer: I see. How often would you say that occurs?

Patient: That, I can make occur.

Interviewer: What do you do to make that occur?

Patient: I see a lot of . . . I don't know if you see it, but I see a lot of white dots all the time, little, little, like, um, little tiny little dots. Maybe nobody sees clear, I don't know this. You look through something . . . I look at that wall . . . that wall has got . . . that white wall has tons of gold dots on it, little tiny ones. So at nighttime it's very simple to do that. . . .

Interviewer: And it feels as if your hand is growing in size.

Patient: Yeah, you can see it. Actually it's like the white coming; it's like the energy coming out and you could feel it. If I put my hand here, I can actually feel it here on this side. I can feel it here, and it can grow longer and longer and it's just like a lot of energy. (SCID-D interview, unpublished transcript)

Recurrent Interactive Dialogues

SCID-D research indicates that depersonalization in patients with dissociative disorders is often accompanied by ongoing, recurrent interactive dialogues between the observing and the participating self, as opposed to mere thinking or reminiscing (Steinberg 1991; 1994b). A question about depersonalization that is answered with accounts of continuous interpersonal dialogues (with one's self) is characteristic of subjects who have either DID or DDNOS.

The following excerpt from a SCID-D interview is an example of depersonalization accompanied with internal dialogue. This particular patient reported having "temper outbursts." He also had a long history of alcohol abuse.

Interviewer: Have you ever felt that part of your body was disconnected from the rest of you?

Patient: Yes. Yes. Like I told you. Seeing myself sitting in that chair and laughing at me . . . He just keeps asking me, "Let me out, let me out." And I tell him, "Get out. Nobody's stopping you. Go do what you got to do." And he starts laughing at me. . . . If you know how to get rid of him tell me, I'll go along, 'cause I don't know how to get rid of him. . . . A lot of times I feel there is almost two people inside of me or what it might be. But I actually see this person. This lasts, like I say, seconds. He'll sit there. He's staring at me. With big green eyes and jet black hair, and this guy's big. He's very big. And he sits there and he'll say to me, "When are you gonna let me out, man?" I go, "What are you talking about?" [He says,] "Let me out." I'll say, "Let yourself out, asshole, don't break my fucking stones! You know how to get out." [He says,] "Let me out." And I don't know how to let this guy out. And I tell him, "Leave! Nobody's holding you, you don't even pay rent any-

ways." But, it's confusing. I find myself in an argument with
him, and it's weird, very weird. But it only lasts a few seconds,
and it is gone. (SCID-D, unpublished transcripts)

Another example that was reported by the same patient
demonstrates a dialogue with himself regarding the outcome of a
baseball game:

> Well, like I'll be talking about watching a baseball game, and I'll
> say, "Now this guy is going to hit a home run," and then I'll
> hear, "This guy is not going to hit a home run. This guy is going
> to strike out." And I'll turn around and look in the chair and
> say, "I'm telling you—watch it. I'll bet you 10 dollars he's going
> to hit a home run." And the person sitting there, which is me,
> will turn around and say, "He's going to strike out, and the 10
> dollars is up." "Well, put the money up," I tell him. Those kinds
> of conversations. (SCID-D interview, unpublished transcript.)

Behavioral manifestations of depersonalization may include a
trancelike appearance, lack of affect, disavowal of behaviors and
talents (due to estrangement from oneself), and impaired relationships with others. Difficulties in relationships may occur in both
directions, as it were: a patient experiencing episodic depersonalization may be criticized or rejected by others on account of his or
her odd or apparently inexplicable behavior, particularly if the patient cannot verbalize it effectively.

In other cases, the individual may refrain from trying to establish relationships with others because he or she feels so ill at ease
due to the feelings of depersonalization. The poet Pessoa (1991)
recorded his inability to start a courtship by addressing some notes
in his diary to the woman he admired from a distance, in terms
suggesting dissociative experiences:

> I wouldn't know how to prepare my soul to bring my body to
> possess yours. Even thinking about it, within myself, I fall over
> obstacles I don't see, I entangle myself in cobwebs without
> knowing what they are. How many more things would happen
> to me if I really wanted to possess you? (p. 203)

Spontaneous Elaboration

When taking a history of dissociative symptoms, the interviewer should note spontaneous elaboration—that is, a voluntary description of symptomatology not directly related to the given question. These often provide additional information in support of a tentative diagnosis and confirm the validity of the subject's reported symptoms. In the following interchange, note that the second question on depersonalization elicits the subject's spontaneous elaboration about interactive dialogues between two parts of the self:

> **Interviewer:** Have you ever felt that you were watching yourself from a point outside of your body, as if you were seeing yourself from a distance?
>
> **Patient:** Absolutely.
>
> **Interviewer:** What is that experience like?
>
> **Patient:** It's . . . I want to say crazy. The feeling is so strange. I could be sitting here, and I could be sitting there. Or I could be sitting there, and I could be sitting over there. And I can carry on a conversation. You know, like having a friend in the room? That feels very strange . . . I was lying on the floor, unconscious, and I was on the ceiling looking at myself. And I was saying, "What's the matter now? Why don't you get up? There's nothing wrong with you." Sometimes I would be a mirror of myself. Other times I would be slouched in a chair. This person was yelling at me, or saying things that were hurting me. And I wouldn't be able to speak up. Sometimes I would get angry and speak at me. . . . That's really what it's like. (SCID-D interview, unpublished transcript)

Indeed, it may be unrealistic to expect subjects to answer each interview question in a cut-and-dried fashion, without giving somewhat larger scope to their symptomatology. The clinician should expect related features of dissociation (e.g., inner dialogue with out-of-body experience) to be presented in tandem. In this way, each question is an individual piece of the puzzle but also a microcosm of the disorder in itself: a miniature mirror that reflects the entire object to the viewer.

Distress and Dysfunction

To decide if a subject meets the criteria for a diagnosis of a dissociative disorder, the interviewer must obtain information about the severity of depersonalization and whether distress and/or impairment occur as results of the depersonalization (see Figure 6–1). It is therefore necessary to include questions about the duration of the depersonalization episodes, mode of onset, age at onset, and associated dysphoria such as anxiety or distress. Impairment in social relationships and employment is one of the most important aspects to consider when assessing the severity of the symptoms. Dysfunctionality is common among patients with DID and may occur in the absence of emotional distress. One patient reported a dreamlike quality to her life as a result of her depersonalization episodes:

> It's the way I've been living lately, in this dream. It's like, uh, I just go from thing to thing, from here to here. I mean I go to work. I do whatever the stuff is I do. . . . I don't even want to do what I'm doing. I don't want to be bothered doing this. So I just go and do it. . . . So I just do it and then I may be going home

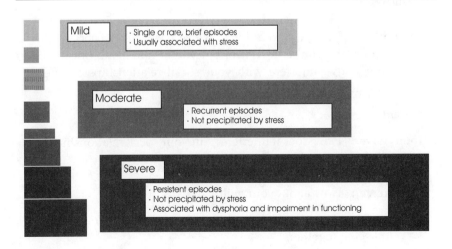

Figure 6–1. Severity range of depersonalization.

and I sleep, or if I just don't feel like going home I go to a friend's . . . sometimes I pick my daughter up from school and take her to work. So it's like I just go off and I just lose track and then sometimes I just kind of lost this track, and all of a sudden I'm not sure what I'm doing or where I'm doing or why I'm doing it, if I have a day like that. (SCID-D interview, unpublished transcript)

On the other hand, the following patient experienced a great deal of anxiety during her episodes of depersonalization:

When it gets really bad, if it doesn't go away, I'm in a panic. And I get extremely dizzy and the room begins to sway or the sidewalk begins to do this [flails arms] and I actually begin to lose my sense of balance, and I feel as though I'm losing consciousness. I have that sense, a lot. I don't ever faint. Ever. But I feel like I'm losing . . . and I'll get so dizzy. You know I'll go into the ladies' room and I'll look at the water, but I'll never faint. I frequently feel dizzy. (SCID-D interview, unpublished transcript)

Another patient exhibited both distress and social dysfunction in association with her episodes of depersonalization. She reported the following:

Interviewer: Do any of the things we've been talking about—the feeling like you're in control but you're not, being outside of your body—interfere with your social relationships or affect your ability to work?

Patient: Yes.

Interviewer: How does it interfere with your social relationships?

Patient: Because I then start not being around people.

Interviewer: How about your ability to work?

Patient: Then I can't work because I'm spending all my time trying to keep it together.

Interviewer: Are these experiences . . . associated with stress?

Patient: Yes.

Interviewer: Does it cause you discomfort or distress?

Patient: Yes. (SCID-D interview, unpublished transcript)

For the following patient, the distress of her depersonalization was so intolerable that she injured herself to relieve the feelings. After seeing a play in New York with her fiancé, she reported the following:

> We were driving up Park Avenue, and then all of a sudden I realized that everything was unreal. It was like a stage set. And I struggled to get things back, but I couldn't. Things were not working out well. . . . This thing about being unreal kept on. And I went into the bathroom and I found a razor blade and I cut my wrist, and then things came back together again. Then things were real again. But I found that if things are unreal or if I start fragmenting, if I cut then I bring things back together again. And then I'm whole again. (SCID-D interview, unpublished transcript)

▌ Conclusion

Depersonalization is a universal experience that can range in severity from hypnagogic consciousness to waking intrapersonal dialogue and out-of-body experiences. Depersonalization manifests in a variety of ways, parallel to the varied ways we experience the self. One can experience perceptual depersonalization (body perception distortion, seeing oneself from a distance), kinesthetic depersonalization (a sense that the body is not familiar or even absent), emotional depersonalization (a sense that emotions are unfamiliar or unaccountable), and even behavioral depersonalization (a feeling that actions are not under control). Most often, these manifestations occur simultaneously. For instance, in out-of-body experiences one can see oneself sitting in a chair while another part of the self is hovering on the ceiling, and at the same time, see the person in the chair talking while the seat of consciousness is in the ceiling-person at the time. As another example, one subject interviewed by the SCID-D researchers reported drowning two cats and then weeping, not knowing why he had done it. There was a split between the part that had drowned the cats and another part that had observed what was happening. In this case, there was no perceptual depersonalization but there was significant emotional and behavioral depersonalization.

In normal subjects, depersonalization is transient, mild, and is precipitated by stress. In dissociative disorders, depersonalization tends to be recurrent and persistent, and is associated with distress and/or dysfunctionality (see Figure 6–1 and Tables 6–1 and 6–2). SCID-D indicates that the distinguishing diagnostic feature of depersonalization in subjects with dissociative disorders is the ongoing interactive dialogues (Steinberg 1994b). In nondissociative psychiatric disorders, depersonalization manifests differently. In schizophrenia, detachment from the self is associated with lack of reality testing and delusional beliefs. Other disorders may involve episodic depersonalization, such as organic illnesses, depression, and borderline personality disorder. However, in these other disor-

Table 6–1. The spectrum of depersonalization in the SCID-D

	No psychiatric disorder	**Nondissociative and personality disorders**	**DID and DDNOS**
Patient description	No spontaneous elaboration	No spontaneous elaboration	Depersonalization questions elicit descriptions of identity confusion and alteration
Presence of interactive dialogues	No interactive dialogues	No interactive dialogues	Interactive dialogues
Frequency	None–few episodes	None–few episodes	Recurrent– persistent episodes

Note. SCID-D = Structured Clinical Interview for DSM-IV Dissociative Disorders; DID = dissociative identity disorder; DDNOS = dissociative disorder not otherwise specified.

Table 6–2. Distinguishing between normal and pathological depersonalization

Common mild depersonalization	Transient depersonalization	Pathological depersonalization
Context Occurs as an isolated symptom	Occurs as an isolated symptom	Occurs within a constellation of other dissociative or nondissociative symptoms or with ongoing interactive dialogues
Frequency One or few episodes	One episode that is transient	Persistent or recurrent depersonalization
Duration Depersonalization episode is brief; lasts seconds to minutes	Depersonalization of limited duration (minutes to weeks)	Chronic and habitual depersonalization lasting up to many years
Precipitating factors ■ Extreme fatigue ■ Sensory deprivation ■ Hypnagogic and hypnopompic states ■ Drug or alcohol intoxication ■ Sleep deprivation ■ Medical illness/toxic states ■ Severe psychosocial stress	■ Life-threatening danger; this is a syndrome noted to occur in 33% of individuals immediately following exposure to life-threatening danger, such as near-death experiences and auto accidents (Noyes et al. 1977) ■ Single, severe psychological trauma	■ Not associated with precipitating factors in column 1 ■ May be precipitated by a traumatic memory ■ May be precipitated by a stressful event but occurs even when there is no identifiable stress ■ Occurs in the absence of a single, immediate, severe psychosocial trauma

Source. Reprinted with permission from Steinberg M: *Interviewer's Guide to the Structured Clinical Interview for the DSM-IV Dissociative Disorders (SCID-D), Revised.* Washington, DC, American Psychiatric Press, 1994. Copyright 1994, Marlene Steinberg, M.D.

ders, the patient does not report or construct interactive dialogues.

Systematic assessment of depersonalization requires careful investigation of a complicated phenomenon in all its complexity. Depersonalization is a disturbance at the core of the human being: our very sense of personal integrity and stability.

CHAPTER 7

Derealization

The Unreal World

But alas, not even the bedroom was stable—it was the old bedroom of
my lost childhood! Like a fog, it drifted away, it materially penetrated
the white walls of my real room, which emerged clear and smaller from
the shadow . . .

—**Fernando Pessoa,** *The Book of Disquiet*

In the epigraph above, the poet Fernando Pessoa is essentially
describing an episode of derealization. Derealization is a dissociative symptom consisting of a feeling that one's home, workplace, or other customary environment is unknown or unfamiliar,
or a sense that friends or relatives are strange, unfamiliar, or unreal. In some instances derealization may include changes in the
visual perception of the environment; for example, a person may
think that buildings, furniture, or other objects are changing in
size or shape, or that colors are becoming more or less intense.
Derealization is a commonplace occurrence in the dissociative disorders as well as in other psychiatric disorders (Fleiss et al. 1975;
Steinberg 1994a). However, derealization has some different features in dissociative disorders and occurs with greater frequency.

There have been very few systematic investigations of derealization in the literature because of a lack of diagnostic tools. Most
research has involved case studies with spontaneous descriptions
of derealization that emerged in the course of the patient's therapy,
or has involved controlled studies using questionnaires that concentrated on the symptom of depersonalization. In contrast, the
SCID-D (Steinberg 1993b) focuses on five dissociative symptoms,
one of which is derealization. The SCID-D has thus allowed for
detailed investigations into derealization even though it does not
focus on derealization exclusively. The body of current literature

on derealization is so small, in fact, that the SCID-D field-study transcripts of 130 patients constitute the largest primary resource for further investigation. SCID-D research indicates, for example, that recurrent derealization frequently coexists with amnesia. Whereas some researchers classify derealization as a disturbance of recognition (e.g., Reed 1988), the absence of a familiar affect usually associated with a particular object or person may well be the salient factor (Siomopoulos 1972). A person with derealization may feel that his or her friends or environment are unreal or unfamiliar, or may find it difficult to recognize family members, yet is usually aware of his or her actual identity and history. One patient with dissociative identity disorder (DID) in the SCID-D field study felt that in some indefinable way her entire surroundings were rendered suddenly unreal:

> **Interviewer:** Have you ever felt puzzled as to what's real and what's unreal in your surroundings?
>
> **Patient:** A lot.
>
> **Interviewer:** Can you describe what that experience is like?
>
> **Patient:** Well, it's part of being real disconnected and everything around me and me seeming very, very unreal. It's sort of a part of a whole. (SCID-D interview, unpublished transcript)

Depersonalization and derealization commonly occur together; that is, they are often experienced simultaneously, although the individual is often unaware of one or the other at first. Derealization more commonly occurs with depersonalization than it does alone. In fact, a number of patients in the SCID-D field study endorsed experiences of derealization when asked questions regarding depersonalization. One patient with dissociative disorder not otherwise specified (DDNOS) described an episode of derealization that occurred during a final exam in a European university:

> I was doing a paper . . . and I don't know whether it was the material I was writing about . . . but, I thought I was going to pass out, and I actually was able to get up . . . and walk out . . . and go outside . . . and everything, um, things have happened

with me in terms of like color . . . [laughs] . . . like that particular time it was blue . . . that was my first real sensation of things being very unreal. And I had a strong, strong sense of not knowing what was going on. I almost felt like I was from another planet. I felt that disconnected. But I did go back in and finish the exam. And I don't even know how I did that. (SCID-D interview, unpublished transcript)

This coexistence has led many to conclude that the derealization and depersonalization are one and the same (e.g., Hollander 1989) or that derealization is merely a subcategory of depersonalization (e.g., psychoanalytic theories). Those who do not consider derealization only an aspect of depersonalization often use the term *depersonalization–derealization* (e.g., Christodoulou 1986) to connote the range of alterations in consciousness from self to environment. However, many other researchers (e.g., Krizek 1989; Mayer-Gross 1935) have made an effort to separate the two as independent systems of experience. Nemiah (1989a) has argued that derealization can be seen as being *wider* in scope than depersonalization, in which only the self is derealized. Current opinion favors separating the two symptoms, at least in principle. The potential occurrence of one symptom without the other is widely accepted, as can be seen in the DSM-IV (American Psychiatric Association 1994) dissociative disorder classification "derealization unaccompanied by depersonalization," a variant of DDNOS (p. 490).

Depersonalization, as Chapter 6 indicates, may be defined as an alteration in the experience of the self. It involves a sense of unreality and estrangement from the self, a feeling of detachment as if one were an external observer of one's own mental or physical processes. Patients often describe it as a dreamlike state, a sense of watching a movie of themselves, or feeling like a robot. Depersonalization can also be experienced as a feeling of numbness or absence of feeling. SCID-D research indicates that another dimension of contrast between the two symptoms concerns patients' subjective sense of normality. As has been mentioned in earlier chapters, persons who become habituated to chronic depersonalization tend to consider it normal until informed otherwise. By contrast, people almost always experience derealization as an abnormal state of consciousness, even though they may have different emotional responses to its abnormality.

In both depersonalization and derealization, perceptual disturbances are common. In depersonalization, these disturbances include autoscopy (i.e., having a hallucination of one's own body—sometimes described as an out-of-body experience) and proprioceptive hallucinations (e.g., feeling as if one's body is floating or nonexistent). By contrast, perceptual disturbances during an episode of derealization include seeing changes in the size, shape, or color of objects. The patient may also experience difficulties with vision or hearing, or may have an altered sense of the passage of time—more specifically, that it is moving very slowly or has stopped altogether (see Figure 7–1).

Lastly, the patient may experience other people as "dead," mechanical, or robot-like. One woman in the SCID-D study diagnosed with DDNOS described her episodes of depersonalization in the following way:

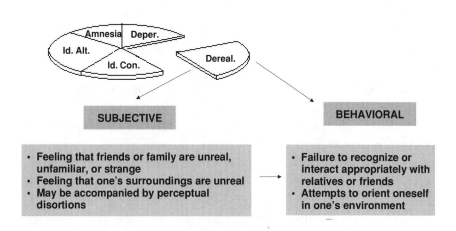

Figure 7–1. Manifestations of derealization.

Interviewer: Have you ever felt as if familiar surroundings or people seemed unfamiliar or unreal?

Patient: Yes.

Interviewer: What happened?

Patient: When I had my ... my reality, is, um ... I feel like I'm dead, and I just feel like the people around me, the people and places and you know ... things are just not living. Everyone is just dead. I can touch myself, but that doesn't prove a lot.

Interviewer: How often does that happen?

Patient: I don't know. I talk to my therapist about it sometimes, but not all the time. (SCID-D interview, unpublished transcript)

■ Clinical Manifestations of Derealization

Derealization is most commonly a dissociative disturbance of adults, although some researchers have reported instances of childhood derealization (Fast and Chethik 1976). This apparent difference may have more to do with the lack of systematic evaluation of dissociative symptomatology in children than with a difference in actual incidence. Derealization is most pronounced in the dissociative disorders; however, it can also appear in other disorders.

■ Derealization in the Nondissociative Disorders

The nondissociative psychiatric symptoms most often associated with derealization are anxiety, depression, and psychosis. Derealization has been observed as a response to a variety of traumas, including near-death experiences (Noyes and Kletti 1977a; Putnam 1985), combat, and the loss of a loved one.

Derealization in Anxiety

From a psychodynamic standpoint, anxiety is a common trigger of derealization episodes (Fast and Chethik 1976); however, the current state of research is lacking in systematic investigations of the causal connection between derealization and anxiety. It is not yet clear whether anxiety precipitates the derealization or whether derealization produces the anxiety. Studies of *phobic anxiety-depersonalization syndrome* have included derealization as a component of this particular syndrome (Ambrosino 1973) in which anxiety and depersonalization/derealization cyclically reinforce each other. Several patients in the SCID-D study mentioned a connection between episodes of derealization and panic attacks, although they gave a variety of answers as to which symptom triggered the other. A female subject, diagnosed with depersonalization disorder, regarded her derealization experiences as setting off the anxiety attacks rather than the reverse:

> **Interviewer:** Is the anxiety and the panic kind of feeling related to your feelings of being unreal?
>
> **Patient:** Oh yeah.
>
> **Interviewer:** How are they related and what comes first? That might be a hard question.
>
> **Patient:** Well, because if something seems so unreal and you're afraid that you don't have control of the situation or something, that kind of makes you panic.
>
> **Interviewer:** OK. How often would you say they are related?
>
> **Patient:** It's always [related]. (SCID-D interview, unpublished transcript)

Patients with high levels of anxiety have been found to experience more severe derealization, and patients with high levels of derealization have been found to experience more severe anxiety (Cassano et al. 1989; Trueman 1984a). Patients with diagnoses of anxiety disorder have also been found to experience more derealization than other patients. It seems likely that patients with high levels of anxiety have a stronger need for some form of dissociative defense. Cassano et al. (1989) found that panic disorder patients who experienced derealization were more severely anxious, obsessive, and depressed and had earlier onset of panic disorder. Thus the presence of derealization may reflect higher levels of psychopathology and perceived intrapsychic danger as well as a problematic configuration of other psychiatric symptoms. However, further research is necessary to clarify the relationship between derealization and anxiety. Moreover, clinicians should systematically assess patients with anxiety disorders for the presence of underlying dissociative disorders. As the preceding transcript excerpts indicate, the SCID-D is a highly effective instrument for the study of anxiety and depersonalization as well as for the detection of previously unsuspected dissociative disorders coexisting with anxiety.

Derealization in Schizophrenia

Derealization has also been observed in connection with schizophrenia and other psychotic disorders (Christodoulou 1986), which is not surprising because these syndromes typically include severe distortions in reality testing. However, when a person with a dissociative disorder has an episode of derealization, reality testing is typically maintained.

There are few studies that have investigated the prevalence of derealization symptoms in schizophrenic subjects. A field study of the SCID-D involving schizophrenic subjects found them to have none or few derealization episodes, whereas patients with dissociative disorders experienced recurrent or persistent episodes (Steinberg et al. 1994). Typically, the schizophrenic subjects misunderstood the SCID-D items concerning derealization or interpreted them idiosyncratically. For example, one male subject interpreted a question on derealization in terms of other people behaving in uncharacteristic ways:

> **Interviewer:** Did you experience any of your relatives as being unfamiliar?

Patient: Now if it's unfamiliar, like also with my cousin, how she handled herself when I was sick, and I never . . . and also how she handled herself about money, how hard-nosed she is at times, I've known my cousin for 45 years, and I'd never realized how hard-nosed she can be about money. But she's also generous on the other side.

Interviewer: So it sounds like sometimes familiar people . . . sometimes they behave in ways which are surprising to you. But you never lose the sense of who they are.

Patient: Right. (SCID-D interview, unpublished transcript)

Derealization in the Dissociative Disorders and Posttraumatic Stress Disorder

Derealization is a prominent feature in patients with posttraumatic stress disorder (PTSD) (Spiegel and Cardeña 1991; Steinberg et al. 1989–1992; Steinberg et al. 1990) as well as in patients with dissociative disorders. A common context in which derealization occurs is the *flashback*, which is experienced by many patients who have dissociative disorders. The flashback is accompanied by age regression, or "reliving the past as though it were occurring in the present, with age-appropriate vocabulary, mental content, and affect" (Spiegel 1984, p. 522). The superimposition of a past reality onto the present results in a sense that current events are strange and unreal. For example, Pessoa's (1991) experience of his bedroom in Lisbon in the 1930s being suddenly transformed into the bedroom in which he slept as a child made him feel disoriented, as if he were in a "fog." Flashbacks consist of two SCID-D dissociative symptoms known as identity alteration (i.e., age regression) and derealization. Investigations using the SCID-D indicated that patients diagnosed with PTSD described episodes of derealization in terms identical to those used by patients with dissociative disorders (Steinberg et al. 1989–1992; Steinberg 1994b).

Investigations using the SCID-D have found that patients with dissociative disorders have higher levels of derealization than patients with other psychiatric disorders (Steinberg 1993b; Steinberg et al. 1990).

Derealization in Other Disorders

Derealization is also a frequent concomitant of borderline personality disorder and eating disorders (Gunderson et al. 1981; Torem 1986). However, further research is necessary to evaluate whether the derealization is a symptom of an undiagnosed dissociative disorder in these two patient populations.

❚ Theories of Derealization

Psychophysiological Theories

Few researchers have investigated the mechanisms in the brain that are the immediate causes of derealization experiences. One study by Timsit-Berthier et al. (1987) induced dissociative symptoms by administering nitrous oxide. Although the experiment was amusing or enjoyable for the subjects who participated, the results were not conclusive. The nitrous oxide caused distortions in vision, time, proprioception, and hearing, which as a whole were considered by the researchers to be highly similar to states of depersonalization and derealization. Through various physiological measures, Timsit-Berthier et al. concluded that they had found a brain state they called "dissonant" that other researchers correlated with states of helplessness and inability to find relations between response and response-outcome. Although it is useful in correlating states of derealization to other dysfunctional states, the dissonance theory is too simplistic to fully explain the symptom of derealization, even on the biological level.

Perceptual and Affective Theories of Derealization

Some theories attempt to explain derealization by appealing to processes of perception connected to emotion. Siomopoulos (1972) proposed a perceptual-affective system, whose holistic nature is disrupted during derealization. Normally, perceptual wholes (e.g., visual recognition of a person) and their affective counterparts (e.g., emotions reflecting a particular style of relationship with the person) combine to form larger *object-affect wholes*. This structure is disturbed in derealization. The feeling that "*x* is not real" may reflect a person's awareness that a familiar affect was lacking in the normal experience of the other individual. Siomopoulos sharply differentiates derealization from anomalies of recognition, stressing that derealization is a disturbance in *affective memory*, in which intellectual acknowledgment of the presence of the derealized object or person is maintained but the affect is withdrawn. Siomopoulos also differentiates derealization from repression, as psychoanalysis often interprets the term. *Repression* as classically defined involves the loss of awareness of an idea. Derealization involves the loss of a familiar affect and also an *awareness* of the missing relationship between the affect and the perception.

However, other patients in the SCID-D field study mentioned episodes of derealization that involved various forms of heightened positive affect. One patient thought of her derealization episodes as a source of artistic creativity or inspiration:

Patient: It's not something that I can't pull out of.

Interviewer: Right.

Patient: OK. And it's not unpleasant.

Interviewer: Mmhmm.

Patient: In fact, some really vivid and wonderful [emphatic] things have happened from that place. It's like being super-real [gestures dramatically]. (SCID-D interview, unpublished transcript)

In short, although Siomopoulos' hypothesis accounts for a significant range, perhaps the majority, of dissociative patients' experiences of derealization, it is inadequate to explain the responses of artistic or intellectually curious subjects for whom the symptom represents an expansion of consciousness. Further research is needed in this area.

Cognitive Theories of Derealization

Derealization has been associated with a variety of unusual cognitive phenomena such as déjà vu, delusional mood, Capgras' syndrome, and the agnosias (Christodoulou 1986; Reed 1988; Siomopoulos 1972).

Reed (1988) considers derealization to represent a "breakdown of automatization." He compares the experience of derealization to any routinized or automatized behavior, such as driving a car. Normally, one is not conscious of the many different actions, judgments, and reflexes that are necessary for operating a vehicle safely. However, when hand-eye coordination is complicated by factors such as the emotional stress of nearly having an accident, extreme fatigue, or being in training, the driver becomes conscious of many different specific operations, such as the need to focus on shifting gears or switching on a turn signal. In derealization, normal automatized consciousness is broken up, and the person becomes aware of the feeling of reality, which is normally an unconscious subcomponent of experience. Reed calls all such experiences "attentional reemphases related to shifts in hierarchical organization" (p. 131), in which "hierarchical" refers to the habitualization of the subcomponents under a governing integrator. It is possible that Reed's theory may have affinities with the reports of subjects in the SCID-D field study who indicated that they thought they could control experiences of derealization or bring them on at will. The last patient cited in the previous section described derealization as something that she could "pull out of." Another woman, who experienced derealization as "feeling like a robot," nonetheless maintained, "I could do it when I want to do it" (SCID-D interview, unpublished transcript). Although clinicians should keep in mind that patients' claims regarding intentional control over dissociative symptoms are by no means infallible, nonetheless their perception of voluntary control offers some support to Reed's hypothesis.

Cognitive restructuring, in the sense in which Reed defines it, is most often triggered by emergency situations. The traumas that cause dissociative symptomatology could have this effect by disrupting the normal flow of experience. As an effect of childhood abuse, for instance, consciousness can break down and the child may become aware of previously "behind-the-scenes" elements of consciousness. Reed's view has received support from some researchers. For instance, Coleman (1933) coined the concept of *cenesthesia*, or "the feeling of the function of life of the organism" (from Christodoulou 1986). Cenesthesia is a part of normal experience, although the individual is not normally aware of it. Like Siomopoulos, Coleman emphasizes that derealization is the awareness of a *loss* of a normal part of experience. The theory of cenesthesia is interesting; however, it is difficult to conceptualize the notion of an element of experience that remains unconscious, and the hypothesis awaits further refinement and corroborative research.

With regard to flashbacks in particular, the derealization that accompanies them could be explained by the patient's experience of conflicting cues to reality. Researchers found that flashbacks in both posttraumatic and drug intoxication conditions involve a triggering of contextual information that is stored together with memories (McGee 1984). During a flashback, this contextual information may conflict with other contextual information that emanates from the present environment, resulting in the patient's confusion as to which set of contextual information represents "reality."

The term *jamais vu* has been defined as "an inappropriate absence of familiarity" (Sno and Linzen 1990). This definition is identical to cognitive descriptions of derealization. Although there has been little research on this phenomenon, the experience of déjà vu has been described as being related to derealization (Siomopoulos 1972; Sno and Linzen 1990). Descriptions of déjà vu were not uncommon patient responses to SCID-D questions about derealization, indicating that both déjà vu and derealization may involve a disturbance in the perception of familiarity.

Psychoanalytic Theories

Most psychoanalytic theories consider derealization to be an ego defense mechanism directed against anxiety that cannot be mastered. Arlow (1966), for instance, posited that the ego guards against an intrapsychic danger (e.g., a particularly abhorrent aggressive or sexual wish) by displacing it onto perceptions of reality.

As a result, the outside world is repudiated and thus feels foreign to the patient. Arlow saw derealization as a splitting phenomenon, resulting in an experience of division between an observing self and a participating self. The participating self, as well as its context, are repudiated by the patient as being unreal and not part of the real self. Object-relations theorists, on the other hand (e.g., Jacobson 1959), describe an imbalance and disorganization between various identifications of the ego. Derealization would then represent the patient's subjective experience of this disorganization. Psychoeconomic theories (e.g., Sarlin 1962) suggest that derealization involves a withdrawal of cathexis (i.e., personal or emotional investment) from one's "object representations," resulting in feelings of nonidentification with aspects of the outside world. (This is in contrast to decathexis from *self*-representations, which results in depersonalization.) Derealization, according to a psychoeconomic definition, involves the loss of an internalized object whose function normally is the validation of experience.

Derealization has also been discussed by developmental psychoanalysts. Their models point to disturbances in the stages of the individual's psychosexual development as precursors of derealization. For example, Arlow (1966) suggested that experiences during the anal stage, for instance, predispose a child to repudiate either a part of him- or herself or a part of the environment. Psychoanalytic theories often focus on *object loss*, rather than on the more severe and intrusive traumas that are considered to be more common antecedents of dissociative symptoms. Theorists in this tradition sometimes consider *fantasy* and *narcissism* to be more powerful than objectively verifiable external events. Collective denial of the frequency and significance of child abuse on the part of professionals is a legacy that was handed down from Freud's era and sadly continues to this day (see Miller 1984).

■ The Traumatic Origins of Derealization

Dissociative symptoms commonly result from severe physical and/or sexual abuse in childhood (Coons et al. 1988; Fine 1990;

Spiegel 1991; Terr 1991). Specifically, child abuse has been linked to derealization by at least one study (Ogata et al. 1990). Derealization (rather than depersonalization, masochism, or promiscuity) was found to be the number one predictor of childhood sexual abuse in patients with borderline personality disorder. One subject in the SCID-D study spontaneously described having been molested at the age of 8 in the context of explaining changes in visual perception: "Colors just popped out" (SCID-D interview, unpublished transcript).

However adaptive derealization may be as a childhood coping strategy, it becomes maladaptive in later life, causing difficulties with relationships, work, and inner serenity (Gelinas 1983). Derealization in its severe form, as with all dissociative responses, causes dysfunction and/or distress in all aspects of a person's life and functioning.

❚ Conclusion

Derealization is a dissociative symptom that severs a person's consciousness from familiar perceptions of the outside world. Derealization is similar to depersonalization and often occurs together with it. However, derealization can also occur independently of depersonalization.

Derealization may result from altered states of consciousness within the normal range, such as exhaustion, hypnagogic states, and alcohol or drug intoxication. Derealization can also occur in organic brain syndromes and a variety of psychiatric illnesses such as schizophrenia, affective disorders, and anxiety disorders. Derealization, as it occurs in dissociative disorders, is distinguished by the maintenance of reality testing, recurrent frequency, and the frequent concurrence of other dissociative symptoms such as depersonalization and amnesia.

Derealization is a posttraumatic symptom and, in the dissociative disorders, is a predictable by-product of persistent and recurrent child abuse. Derealization is often experienced in connection with the perpetrator of the abuse, such as a parent or sibling, or in connection with a person who serves as a carrier for projected memories of past abuse, such as the patient's boyfriend or girlfriend.

CHAPTER 8

Assessment of Derealization

Derealization is the third of the five dissociative symptoms assessed by the SCID-D (Steinberg 1993b). Its main characteristics include feelings of estrangement from the environment, feelings of detachment from the world, a sense that one's immediate environment is not real, or a sense that events are not really happening. The parts of the environment that seem unreal typically include friends, family, the workplace, or the home. Derealization may also manifest in more general or vague respects; for example, it may affect the patient's sense of his or her general surroundings or the passage of time. Derealization is often associated with subjective feelings of fear and anxiety.

Derealization frequently coexists with depersonalization and only rarely occurs alone. Like depersonalization, it is often associated with a variety of perceptual distortions. These can include a feeling that objects are changing in size, changes in the appearance of objects and people, and changes in the perception of time. Behavioral manifestations of derealization may include failure to interact appropriately with family or close friends, and attempts to orient oneself in one's environment by, for instance, identifying personal belongings. As was mentioned earlier, patients may describe episodes of derealization when questioned about depersonalization; in addition, questions about derealization may yield spontaneous references to identity confusion or alteration.

The SCID-D investigates derealization by a number of direct questions, such as question 79: "Have you ever felt as if familiar surroundings or people you knew seemed unfamiliar or unreal?" and question 84: "Have you ever felt puzzled as to what is real and what is unreal in your surroundings?" Patients with severe derealization describe recurrent feelings that close relatives, particularly their parents, are unreal and that their own home is foreign to them. Often, these feelings are associated with traumatic memories of childhood events, which patients may spontaneously share when describing intense derealization experiences.

Derealization involves a sense of loss of familiarity from something or someone previously invested with that familiarity. Patients experiencing derealization feel that the people around them, people that they should know very well, suddenly seem strange or alien to them. This type of derealization is commonly experienced for familiar places, as is shown in the following excerpt of a patient with newly detected DID:

> **Interviewer:** Besides your mother, did you ever have trouble recognizing close friends, relatives or your own home?
>
> **Patient:** A few times I had a hard time finding my house. I mean I'd have to really get in touch with my house, you know, to figure out where it was. (SCID-D interview, unpublished transcript)

The following woman with newly detected DID described her derealization for both her family and for her home:

> **Interviewer:** Has there ever been a time when familiar people or places seemed unfamiliar or unreal?
>
> **Patient:** Yes.
>
> **Interviewer:** Can you describe when that occurred?
>
> **Patient:** My room. My room seems unreal, um, unfamiliar. My closet. Uh, my family. A lot of times it doesn't seem like I'm part of the family, like they're a family and I'm off to the side somehow . . . I don't drive, and people, you know, friends drive me places, or going home, saying they've never been to my house before, and I can't find it. You know, it's like, you stall and drive around for a little while. (SCID-D interview, unpublished transcript)

Many SCID-D questions inquire about factors that assist the clinician in assessing the level of severity of the derealization.

These include question 86: "What is the longest period of time that [the derealization] ever lasted?" and question 91: "When you experienced [the derealization], did it ever interfere with your social relationships or affect your ability to work? Question 94 asks if the patient experienced the derealization together with depersonalization. This question may provide additional information to rule out the DSM-IV DDNOS category *derealization unaccompanied by depersonalization* (American Psychiatric Association 1994, p. 490). The final set of questions in this section of the SCID-D inquire about exclusionary factors such as head injury or substance abuse to rule out an organic etiology.

■ Derealization as Loss of Familiarity

Episodes of derealization that affect the patient's perception of people can involve any person that was previously familiar, but the most common type of derealization is connected to perception of family members, particularly one or both parents. When asked which person of their acquaintance has a tendency to seem most unfamiliar to them, patients typically indicate the mother or the father, as in the following excerpt from an interview with a patient with DID:

Interviewer: Have you ever felt as if familiar surroundings or people you knew seemed unfamiliar or unreal?

Patient: Probably unreal.

Interviewer: Who seemed unreal?

Patient: People that I should know. People that I looked at and I kept thinking, "I know those people, why am I scared to death?" That type of thing. My parents. Especially my mother. (SCID-D Interview, unpublished transcript)

The predominance of parents as objects of derealization is not surprising because of the posttraumatic nature of dissociative symptoms and disorders. The symptom of derealization makes sense when understood as a response to the traumas inflicted on such patients when they were children or teenagers. It is natural that a person who has been abused by his or her mother or father would feel as if the parent were alien to them. This symptom was (and unfortunately still is) a way for them to integrate the experiences of the parent as caretaker and at the same time as a source of severe pain, neglect, or deprivation. On the other hand, patients may endorse experiences of derealization with a friend or relative who has not abused them but may partially resemble the abuser or trigger memories of the abuse.

Several patients with DID and DDNOS in the SCID-D field trials mentioned employers or office colleagues rather than relatives in the context of derealization episodes. The most likely explanation for this would be either that the employer or co-worker resembles a previous abuser, or that the patient transfers feelings originating in childhood to authority figures in general. One patient with DID discussed the impact of her experiences of derealization on her workplace environment:

> **Interviewer:** Have you ever felt as if familiar surroundings or people you knew seemed unfamiliar or unreal?
>
> **Patient:** Unfamiliar.
>
> **Interviewer:** What's that experience like?
>
> **Patient:** Weird. It's strange. It's . . . um, you're scared to death sometimes that you're going to get caught. I mean it's like, it's usually, it can happen sometimes up at work, when I'm talking to someone and they'll feel unfamiliar, different. It's like I can hear us talking, you know, telling, "OK, guys, come on, let's get your act together, we've got to get through this." And then it's like we all come together and start working, and then everything will start calming down. But it can be very scary because, again, you've got this job you've got to carry out.
>
> **Interviewer:** What kinds of experiences have you had, or what has seemed unfamiliar to you in your surroundings or people you know?
>
> **Patient:** People, um, just their behavior, their, uh, just them [sic] themselves might seem unfamiliar.

Interviewer: And these are people that you really should have been familiar with?

Patient: I work with them on a daily basis. (SCID-D interview, unpublished transcript)

Although episodes of derealization triggered by the patient's workplace or supervisor may be less common than those connected with family members, clinicians should not underestimate their potential seriousness. As this book has emphasized, the dissociative disorders often have major consequences for patients' employment. Episodes of derealization at work may be connected with amnesia or identity alteration, either of which can affect a person's work performance in a number of ways.

Occasionally, subjects will endorse a general loss of familiarity for objects in the environment. One patient described "an alienated feeling. I'll look at a chair or something [and say,] 'What the hell's that?' Sometimes things do seem more real than others" (SCID-D interview, unpublished transcript).

Derealization commonly occurs for close friends and sometimes acquaintances. In patients with DID, relationships with friends can become complex when the patient has created several independent social networks (i.e., one personality is amnestic for relationships maintained by another personality). Such patients may experience derealization when approached by people who have become friends of one of their alter personalities, as was noted by the following patient with DID:

Interviewer: Have you ever been unable to recognize close friends, relatives, or your own home?

Patient: Yes.

Interviewer: OK, can you describe what occurred?

Patient: Walking down the street towards a group of friends and not recognizing them until they stop and, not corner me, but you know, they'd all start talking to me and then I realize that, oh, maybe I know these people, and then after a little while I do. (SCID-D interview, unpublished transcript)

Many patients are quite vocal about the unpleasantness of derealization. One male DID patient mentioned a strong desire to leave the situation when he had a derealization episode:

> **Interviewer:** Have you ever felt as if close friends, relatives, or your home seemed strange or foreign?
>
> **Patient:** [Thinks for about 15 seconds] Yes.
>
> **Interviewer:** What is that like?
>
> **Patient:** Well, the person, you sort of want to get away from them. You know who they are, whether friends or acquaintances, but you . . . at this particular moment in time, they're neither of that.
>
> **Interviewer:** Mmhmm.
>
> **Patient:** And your home . . . it's a question I ask myself: "What the hell am I doing here?" And I get an urge to flee. "Why am I here?"
>
> **Interviewer:** Mmhmm. How long does that feeling last?
>
> **Patient:** Sometimes for days. For as long as 3 months. (SCID-D interview, unpublished transcript)

∎ Derealization as Subjective Confusion

Derealization typically results in a subjective sense of confusion because it involves an internal contradiction: the patient has lost the sense of reality or familiarity of something that was previously experienced as familiar. It is thus common to feel incongruent feelings or perceptions about familiar people, such as was described by the following woman with DID:

> I would think to myself, "Who is this person, it isn't my mother." I would hear myself thinking, "This person isn't my mother. Who is this person? She's not my mother." (SCID-D interview, unpublished transcript)

One patient with DID experienced considerable distress resulting from her subjective confusion:

Interviewer: Have you ever felt as if close friends, relatives, or your own home seemed strange or foreign?

Patient: Yeah.

Interviewer: What was that experience like?

Patient: Again, it's scary. Because you're . . . faced with . . . you know that this is reality . . . but . . . you don't know who they are. Yet they're here, and you're in this house, and you're living with these people, obviously, and . . . you wake up. And, you know, this lady's serving you breakfast and you don't even know who she is. It's your mother, y'know.

Interviewer: Have you ever felt puzzled as to what is real and unreal in your surroundings?

Patient: Yeah.

Interviewer: What is that experience like?

Patient: You feel like you've been dumped in the Twilight Zone. (SCID-D interview, unpublished transcript)

This feeling of confusion regarding what is real and familiar is one of the primary sources of fear and distress in these patients. It also causes dysfunctionality, because it becomes difficult for them to relate normally to a close friend or family member who is suddenly perceived—and treated—as if they were a stranger.

Derealization in patients who have dissociative disorders is accompanied by intact reality testing as well as the ability to cognitively recognize a "derealized" person or thing. For example, one subject who endorsed episodes of derealization concerning people in general, as opposed to family or friends, was well aware that his subjective perceptions were a distortion of reality:

Interviewer: Have you ever felt as if familiar surroundings or people were unfamiliar or unreal?

Patient: [Chuckles] Yeah, in a way, surroundings, places I've been, I've felt like, y'know, these people ain't for real, they can't be for real, y'know. I found like they're staring at me. But they're not really staring at me. (SCID-D interview, unpublished transcript)

In the same way, derealization experiences can be distinguished from amnestic episodes, in which the patient in the previous excerpt would be asking simply, "Who is this person?" Derealization *can* occur in tandem with amnesia, such as we saw in one of the previous examples. If the woman with the "unfamiliar friends" had had amnesia at that moment, she would have been unable to recognize the person near her, rather than being oppressed by a feeling that "this is not my mother." Some information was telling her that it is her mother (i.e., the family setting), whereas her feelings indicated that her mother was a stranger. A patient experiencing derealization has an intellectual connection or understanding that this person, for instance, is his or her mother. But emotionally there is dissociation of the affect about who this individual is, which may be an adaptive way of coping with an abusive figure who should be familiar.

The following example describes this point with respect to an experience of derealization involving a patient's father:

> **Interviewer:** Is there anyone in particular in your family who seems the most unfamiliar or unreal?
>
> **Patient:** My father.
>
> **Interviewer:** When you feel that he is unfamiliar, do you have a sense that he may be someone else who is not your father, or what do you think?
>
> **Patient:** No, I think he's my father, I'm pretty sure he's my father. No, I know he's Mr. Jones and I'm his daughter, which makes it even stranger because I know that this is where I am, and why am I feeling this way? (SCID-D interview, unpublished transcript)

▌ Derealization and Perceptual Disturbances

As was noted previously, experiences of derealization, as with depersonalization, sometimes involve perceptual disturbances. Whereas in depersonalization a person often loses the perception of part of the self or body, or sees an image of the body where it does not exist, derealization can involve a loss of perception of one's surroundings or a change in the normal appearance of the environment. For instance, there can be an "Alice in Wonderland" kind of phenomenon, in which, for example, people can seem as if they are increasing or decreasing in size. The room can seem as if it is getting larger or smaller; the chair that the person is sitting on can seem as if it is shrinking. Other perceptual disturbances include colors seeming more vivid, the visual field appearing fuzzy, auras surrounding objects, and a narrowing of the visual field. One patient reported experiences in which he "got out" as if he were escaping through a tunnel: "There is always a light somewhere, you have to find it to get out of there. That is the way I get out. Somewhere there is a light. I could slide down the tunnel and I get out. I slide toward the light and I am out" (SCID-D interview, unpublished transcript).

People experiencing derealization often become aware of a slowing or cessation of time, and often feel as if time has stopped. The stoppage of time is often associated with flashbacks, in which, as we will see, past events become superimposed on the present.

One of the questions in the derealization section of the SCID-D, which appears in the following excerpt, addresses perceptual disturbances directly. However, all of the questions in this section elicit spontaneous reports of perceptual disturbances. The following patient describes a perceptual distortion in her vision and hearing during the episode:

Interviewer: Have you ever felt as if your surroundings or other people were fading away?

Patient: You mean like in loss of vision? I have a distancing thing that happens where I lose ... it's like I get very narrow like this [places palms next to each other] ... this is all I can see. And then, and then I lose vision altogether. ... My eyes close and at the same time it's like a roaring sound. I thought everybody had it. (SCID-D Interview, unpublished transcript)

Another subject mentioned a combination of sharper visual focus and selective awareness of specific colors:

Patient: I've had this happen, say in a bookstore, with a book I picked up. And I was reading something, and I think it triggered something. And the friend I was with . . . I mean . . . and the bookstore became . . . it almost takes on an unreal look and feel to it.

Interviewer: How so? What does it look like?

Patient: It's like as if I'm in a dream [pauses]. I feel a bit strange also. It's that . . . now I don't panic with it. I just let it be there. It's almost like being totally out of focus, or something, and then it comes back into focus.

Interviewer: Flatter? Sharper?

Patient: Very much sharper. Like in the bookstore . . . it was [the color] red at that time too. Everything in the bookstore that was red just popped out. I've done it in Claire's office too. Claire is my therapist. It's happened there that everything that's yellow will just pop out. It becomes really highly vivid. And other things just fade into the background, including my therapist. I can hear her voice, but she just fades. (SCID-D interview, unpublished transcript)

One patient, who found a certain measure of artistic inspiration in her experiences of derealization, was very specific with the interviewer about her understanding of question 84:

Interviewer: Have you ever felt puzzled as to what is real and what is unreal in your surroundings?

Patient: Not in terms of being tangible, no.

Interviewer: But of strangeness? Or . . .

Patient: [Pauses] That's hard to answer. I . . . you know, um . . . because I hear it two ways. I hear it as being like a little crazy. But I know that, again . . . you know, I can pull back [gestures]. And that is a very strange thing. Spatial relationships become different. And apartments become different. And, you know, colors take on special things. So, I mean, it's almost like an intensifying. And an abstraction, which gives it an unreal quality. I'm very aware. It's a sofa, there, sitting in front of a fireplace, and there's this strange mauve color, with the canary yellow curtains and all that. But there's one way of looking at it up front, and there's another way of drawing back and seeing it differently. So I'm not sure. (SCID-D interview, unpublished transcript)

No matter how bizarre the symptoms, patients will often feel that their dissociative symptoms are normal, because they have been living with them for most of their lives. One patient, when asked whether he was ever puzzled as to what was real or unreal in his surroundings, replied, "Not puzzled, no. I've just accepted it" (SCID-D interview, unpublished transcript). This is also true, unfortunately, because the diagnosis of a dissociative disorder, as well as acknowledgment of child abuse, often takes years, if ever.

As we will now explore, perhaps the most common perceptual disturbances associated with derealization occur during flashbacks, a type of experience that occurs frequently in people with dissociative disorders, as well as in patients who have posttraumatic stress disorder (PTSD).

■ Derealization and Flashbacks

When questioned about derealization during a SCID-D interview, patients with severe dissociative symptomatology may describe flashbacks and age-regressed states that were accompanied by derealization. When a person is reliving memories as if they are occurring today, he or she is feeling as if things around him or her in the present are very unreal. The symptom of derealization is thus occurring simultaneously with the flashbacks.

The following patient described this phenomenon well:

Interviewer: Have you ever felt puzzled as to what is real and what's unreal in your surroundings?

Patient: Yes, yes . . . It's closely associated with the flashbacks. . . . Flashbacks are not like snapshots that you can put in your album, and put them in the back of the closet, and remember. It's like you're feeling the sensations that you would have felt then *now*. (SCID-D interview, unpublished transcript)

What contributes to the intensity of the derealization experienced during flashbacks is that the remembered event is much more than a memory. The intense realism of the experience sometimes leads to a patient's strong conviction that the traumatic experience actually re-occurred. Sometimes it takes the input of another person to point out the discrepancy in the patient's perception of reality.

A common derealization experience associated with flashbacks is superimposing one familiar face onto another person known to the patient, usually a friend or loved one. The superimposition has the effect of making the second person appear unfamiliar. Thus patients can experience seeing a person who does not look like the person they were talking to a minute ago, as in the following excerpt:

> **Interviewer:** Have you ever felt as if familiar surroundings or people you knew seemed unfamiliar or unreal?
>
> **Patient:** Sometimes when I look at my doctor, I see the face of my father or my ex-husband, and I tell him about it right away. It's usually because I'm afraid he'll do the same thing to me that they will, even though there's no reason not to trust him and he's a very, very wonderful person, and he would never hurt me. . . . And, when I was married, sometimes I'd look at my ex-husband and see my father's face. (SCID-D interview, unpublished transcript)

As commonly occurs in descriptions of flashbacks, the patient in the previous excerpt *spontaneously* offered information about abusive actions inflicted on her by her parent or other person. Flashbacks that occur in dissociative disorders typically involve a vivid memory of a past traumatic event, be that a person's face or the whole event. In another case, a woman while on a date experienced a flashback of the face of a man who had abused her and became very frightened:

> **Interviewer:** Have you ever felt puzzled as to what is real and what's unreal in your surroundings?
>
> **Patient:** Yes. When I have flashbacks. That's what I call them. It's like I'd be out on a date with a boyfriend and see a totally

> different guy. It's like really weird. That's happened where it's a flashback of one of the guys that raped me. You know, I'd be with him, and then, oh my God, I'd run out of the theater or something. (SCID-D interview, unpublished transcript)

The SCID-D does not make an effort to compel or elicit specific memories of physical or sexual abuse; it doesn't ask direct questions about particular traumatic experiences. However, in exploring dissociative symptoms, the SCID-D interviewer is eliciting information about how patients with severe dissociative symptoms have survived traumatic experiences. When patients describe their coping mechanisms, their accounts sometimes flow naturally into descriptions of painful experiences that had to be survived and incorporated somehow into their lives. For this patient population, dissociating from their own consciousness (e.g., experiencing derealization) was the only means to get away from past traumatic experiences from which physical escape was impossible.

▍ The Spectrum of Derealization

Derealization occurs in people from all groups in all degrees of severity (see Table 8–1). The SCID-D's severity rating definitions outline specific criteria that designate episodes of derealization according to several levels of severity.

Mild derealization is common in the general population and consists of a few episodes that are brief and are usually not unpleasant. Normal, mild derealization is typically brought on by stress, fatigue, hypnagogic states, alcohol use, or drug use. Mild derealization generally occurs in people without psychiatric illnesses.

Derealization is assessed as moderate if the episodes are recurrent (i.e., more than 4 times). These may be either brief or prolonged. Derealization may also be considered moderate if a person experiences one or a few episodes in which there is no dysfunctionality or dysphoria, the derealization is not precipitated by stress, or the episodes last more than 4 hours. Moderate derealization can occur in patients with nondissociative disorders (e.g., borderline personality disorder) and in some dissociative disorders, such as DDNOS.

Finally, severe derealization entails persistent episodes of over 24 hours or recurrent episodes that occur daily or weekly. In addition, episodes that produce significant impairment in functioning, that are not precipitated by stress, or that are associated with dysphoria are also considered severe. Severe derealization commonly occurs in patients with DID and PTSD (see Figure 8–1).

Table 8–1.   The spectrum of derealization in the SCID-D

	No psychiatric disorder	Nondissociative and personality disorders	DID and DDNOS
Nature of episode	Brief episodes linked to stress	Rarely occurs for family and home	Occurs with respect to parents, home, friends
Associated w/amnesia and identity alteration	No	No	Yes
Associated w/flashbacks and age regression	No	No	Yes
Disturbances in perceiving environment	No	May experience disturbances	Yes
Frequency of episodes	None–few episodes	Few episodes	Recurrent episodes

Note.   SCID-D = Structured Clinical Interview for DSM-IV Dissociative Disorders; DID = dissociative identity disorder; DDNOS = dissociative disorder not otherwise specified.

episodes

· Recurrent episodes
· Not precipitated by stress

nt, persistent episodes (24 hours or longer)
ecipitated by stress
ated with dysphoria and impairment in functioning

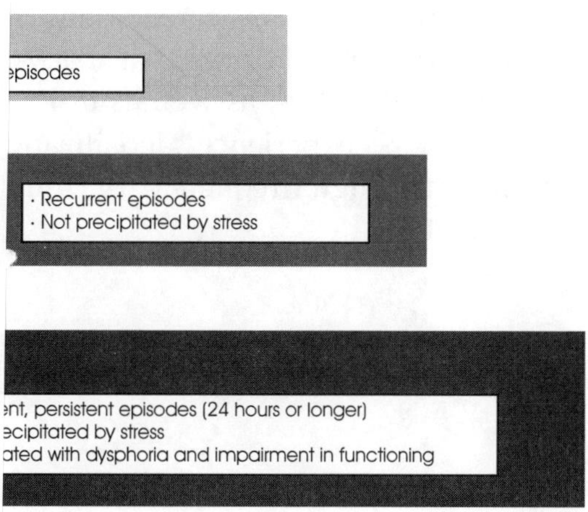

Figure 8–1. Severity range of derealization.

In patients diagnosed with dissociative disorders, derealization occurs less frequently than the other dissociative symptoms (i.e., amnesia, depersonalization, identity confusion, and identity alteration). Patients with DID may not endorse as many episodes of derealization as of the other symptoms, but as with all the dissociative symptoms, the dysphoria, duration, frequency, or nature of the symptom (e.g., not recognizing parents) will indicate a high level of severity.

The only syndrome that is characterized by a *predominance* of derealization is *derealization unaccompanied by depersonalization*, one of the variants of DDNOS. Patients with DID commonly experience severe derealization, particularly in the context of flashbacks.

■ Conclusion

Derealization is a common dissociative symptom experienced by patients with dissociative disorders. Derealization may occur by itself or together with depersonalization. During an episode of derealization, a person may lose a familiar feeling associated with another person or with a place. This often occurs in association with romantic partners, parents, and the home. Derealization is typically experienced during flashbacks, which are common in the dissociative disorders, as well as in PTSD. Patients with dissociative disorders experience derealization at a severe level, as indicated by high frequency or duration, dysphoria, or dysfunctionality.

CHAPTER 9

Identity

Theoretical Perspectives on the Self

Who is to carry the research beyond this point? Who can understand the truth of the matter? O Lord, I am working hard in this field, and the field of my labours is my own self. I have become a problem to myself, like land which a farmer works only with difficulty and at the cost of much sweat.

—St. Augustine, *Confessions*

I sculpted my life like a statue made of material different from my being. Sometimes I do not recognize myself, so external am I to myself. . . . Who am I behind this unreality? I don't know. I must be someone.

—Fernando Pessoa, *The Book of Disquiet*

Identity is a primary concept in understanding and treating the dissociative disorders, in that the dissociative disorders not only directly involve the symptoms of identity confusion and identity alteration, but they also affect the patient's sense of identity. In Chapter 9, I overview theoretical questions concerning identity as they relate to dissociative disorders. (Chapter 10 deals with the clinical assessment of identity disturbance.)

■ Identity as a Contemporary Sociocultural Problem

From a social science perspective, the recent increase in incidences of dissociative disorders could be regarded as a reflection of the increasing fragmentation, political and cultural, of the larger society. Commentators such as Charles Taylor (1989) have spoken eloquently about the loss of a common shared framework in contemporary society: "No framework is shared by everyone, can be taken for granted as *the* framework tout court, can sink to the phenomenological status of unquestioned fact" (p. 28). Although there are, of course, persons or families for whom traditional religion, certain political convictions, or other strongly held ideals still provide structure, all such persons are still very much aware that their ideals or values would be questioned by others. Personal identity, in sum, must be constructed and maintained nowadays apart from, sometimes in opposition to, a confused and seemingly indifferent society.

One of the genuinely painful paradoxes of modern life, at least in the United States, is that the consolidation of a strong personal identity has become simultaneously a social duty, incumbent on every mature adult yet more difficult to attain than ever. Whether we begin with the intrapsychic or the interpersonal components of identity, we find that contemporary society insists on the importance of personal integration and independence while multiplying obstacles to its achievement. If, in this context, we reconsider the five core symptoms of dissociation as consisting of three *dimensions* of identity dissolution (see Figure 9–1), we can better understand them as reflections of identity disturbance on both the intrapsychic and interpersonal planes—that is, as symptoms of disordered social relationships as well as evidence of loss of internal structure and orientation. DSM-III-R (American Psychiatric Association 1987) defines *identity* as "the sense of self, providing a unity of personality over time" (p. 399). *Amnesia*, which has already been described as the fundamental dissociative symptom in relation to the other four, can be thought of as a rupture of the sense of temporal continuity of personal identity. When a person is amnestic for large blocks of time, his or her sense of identity as a continuous life story, with a narrative "shape" and coherence over time, is compromised or lost. *Derealization* and *identity alteration* can be defined as disturbances of the external and spatial dimension of personal identity. Taylor (1989) cites Heinz Kohut to the effect that identity disturbances are not infrequently experienced by patients as spatial disorientation as well as a generalized sense of emotional crisis: "Uncertainty about where one stands as a person seems to spill over into a loss of grip on one's stance in physical space" (qtd. in Taylor 1989, p. 28). The frequency of fugue episodes in dissociative identity disorder (DID) or dissociative fugue can be regarded from this angle as a spatial expression of identity disturbance; by traveling to another city or country in a state of dissociation, the patient is acting out his or her "loss of grip on [his or her] stance in physical space" (Taylor 1989, p. 28) In identity alteration, the person's identity disturbance is manifest in behaviors that affect others or are visible to them. Lastly, *depersonalization* and *identity confusion* can be thought of as the loss of the person's subjective sense of internal coherence and structure. Figure 9–1 provides a schematic dimensional representation of the five core symptoms.

The cultural pressures within North American society that combine to make individuality a major desideratum should not be minimized. Although it is still the case that other cultures, in the Third World and elsewhere, subordinate the individual's identity to that of the family or clan, clinicians working with patients in the United States who have dissociative disorders are dealing with a population that generally values individual rights and privileges over those of larger social units. Sociologists such as Robert Bellah and colleagues have studied the results of America's highly personal interpretation of the right to life, liberty, and the pursuit of happiness (Bellah et al. 1985). The paradox of the current situation is that this ideal of the highly differentiated individual is basically a collective value; that is, it is articulated and enforced by the society as a whole.

Macrosocial Pressures on Personal Identity

It may be helpful at this point to provide a brief review of pressures in the larger society that make personal identity increasingly problematic for growing numbers of people:

Freedom of Choice

Generally speaking, most middle-class people in American society assume that one's personal identity is a composite or sum total of a number of conscious choices made during adolescence and early adulthood: one goes to a particular college; selects a major; chooses a vocational path; finds, woos, and weds a specific mate; and so on. In a book regarded as a classic study of adolescent identity problems, Erik Erikson (1968) observed that the choices that society requires young people to make during their teenage years are a source of pressure and, for some, precipitate a crisis: "With dire urgency [new identifications] force the young individual into choices and decisions which will, with increasing immediacy, lead to commitments 'for life'" (p. 155). Most of us cannot imagine, except by the most strenuous efforts of historical reconstruction, a society in which men and women had everything from their ruler, to their religion, to their place of residence, occupation, and future spouse "chosen" for them by the accident of birth. Yet this was precisely the lot of most Western Europeans between the collapse of the Roman Empire and the coming of the Industrial Revolution. The assumption that personal identity is the end result of a series of free choices is a comparatively recent historical development. Moreover, the extent and variety of available choice has expanded

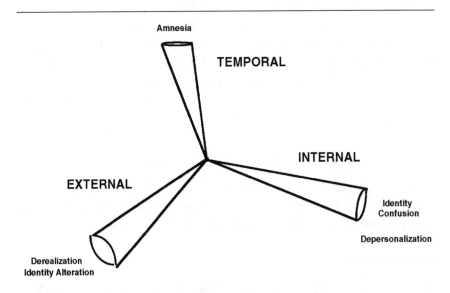

Figure 9–1. Three dimensions of identity disturbance.

and accelerated since Erikson published his book in 1968. In the quarter-century since then, the temporal duration of people's commitments to institutions or vocations has been abbreviated while the number of options continues to grow. In 1968, college students who transferred from one institution to another were in the minority; today, transfer students, students who interrupt their education for several years, and students who change majors frequently are no longer unusual. In 1968, it was unusual for people in midlife to change professions; nowadays, some professional schools have a sizable enrollment of students over 40. In 1968, monogamous marriage was still considered the normative middle-class lifestyle; 25 years later, people may not only opt for "alternative lifestyles," but move in and out of a variety of family and cohabitation patterns. For example, the sociologist Kenneth Gergen (1991) lists some situations he has encountered in the past several months: 1) a neurologist married to one woman, who visits a second woman by whom he has a child on Tuesday and Thursday nights; 2) a male lawyer who marries a female lawyer and invites both partners' former lovers to the wedding—all of these former lovers are women; 3) a woman who has switched careers four times in the past 15 years, from working as a drama teacher to becoming a fundraiser, then a stockbroker, then manager of her own antique business. Gergen (1991) summarizes the pressures placed on a person's sense of identity by the contemporary "cafeteria mentality": "The postmodern sensibility questions the concept of a 'true' or 'basic' self, and the concomitant need for personal coherence or consistency. Why, the postmodern asks, must one be bound by any traditional marker of identity—profession, gender, ethnicity, nationality, and so on?" (p. 178). The net effect of this emphasis on choice is a mild case of identity confusion in many people in the general population and a more severe degree of it in those who are particularly vulnerable by reason of growing up in troubled families.

Technological Change

Changes in technology are related to pressures on personal identity on several different levels. First of all, technological advances in transportation have increased people's mobility, both in terms of relocation because of employment and extensive daily travel as a part of one's employment. It is not only no longer unusual for people in managerial or professional positions to relocate themselves and their families every several years, but in addition many of them travel frequently as a matter of routine. To use only one example, that of a professor, Pierre Janet made one trip to the United States in the course of his professional career as a psychologist and traveled to Berlin or London by rail or sea once or twice a year on the average to attend congresses and other academic meetings. Today's academic may fly thousands of miles every few weeks to keep up with his or her discipline. As a result, it is increasingly difficult for many people to have a firm sense of geographical "place" or position. In its own way, DSM-IV (American Psychiatric Association 1994) has recognized the impact of this particular form of contemporary stress by including the category of *adjustment disorder* to account for patients who are reacting to the strain of relocation and comparable stressors.

Second, changes in communications technology affect personal identity both in terms of the speed of communications and the sheer number of people with whom one may have contact in the course of the day. Gergen's (1991) book opens with an account of the surprising number of letters, faxes, phone messages, electronic mail, and telegrams that piled up on his desk during a 2-day absence. When a person has to communicate with more people in an average day than his or her grandparents did in a month, a sense of one's own personal center sometimes wears thin.

Third, technological change affects people's sense of identity by the simple fact of making them more aware more frequently of the range of choices mentioned earlier. The mass media, ranging from movies, to tabloid newspapers, to MTV, to talk radio, to inexpensive paperback books, to videos and compact disc recordings, constantly bombard the public with dramatic portrayals of different lifestyles, information about different cultures around the world, different experts' opinions on a vast range of topics, and so on.

Lastly, the unending flow of random stimuli can sometimes generate a sense of "systems overload" in people. Some stress management experts have noted an increasing tendency in people to function in a "polyphasic" manner—that is, to divide their conscious attention among several different activities simultaneously. For example, a person's job as an administrative aide may require her to deal with people face to face, answer phones, respond to an intercom, and operate a word processor, all more or less at the same time. Or an air traffic controller may have to monitor several different radar screens, microphones, and computer terminals. Moreover, even during their free time, people who are habituated to polyphasic splitting of attention may "relax" by doing a number of things simultaneously (e.g., driving while conducting a conversation with a friend, listening to a tape, and mentally planning an upcoming social event). Although this complex and multilayered form of functioning may seem far removed from dissociative disorders, there is some evidence that modern technology is teaching the population as a whole to become accustomed to split or divided attentiveness as normal. It has been hypothesized that polyphasic functioning can, over the course of time, affect a person's sense of identity by increasing the difficulty of distinguishing between events or stimuli that concern core elements of his or her personhood (e.g., fundamental beliefs or moral convictions, close relationships) and those that affect only peripheral matters (e.g., where to eat lunch on a particular day) (Karasek and Theorell 1990). Moreover, to the extent that polyphasic thinking or functioning is required by a person's occupation, it will be increasingly difficult for someone presently affected by a dissociative disorder to feel adequate to the demands of his or her job. This book has already mentioned the impact of amnesia on people's general sense of competence and functioning. It is easy to understand how such amnestic episodes would upset or frighten someone whose work requires simultaneous attention to many different tasks or communications devices.

Conflicts in Definitions of Identity

Another factor complicating a clear sense of personal identity is the potential conflict between previous cultural definitions of categories or groups of people and the group's own newly forged sense of identity. For generations of Western professionals, it was assumed that educated white men could satisfactorily define, analyze, or speak for other groups or classes of people. Within recent years, racial and ethnic minorities, women, and gay people have challenged the cultural stereotypes about them and have claimed the right to define their own identities. As a result of greater social sensitivity to issues of self-definition on the part of groups or individuals, many individuals do often feel a sense of internal dissonance or momentary identity confusion when they are in situations in which their own self-definition is at odds with someone else's perception of them. Real-life examples are not difficult to find:

1. An Episcopal priest finishing a doctoral degree at an Eastern university puts on his running gear one evening and goes out for a jog. As he approaches a pedestrian on the sidewalk, she flinches and assumes a general attitude of wariness. He has gotten used to the fact that many women in urban areas are uneasy around men that they do not know personally.
2. A physician driving along a highway notices that an accident has happened around the next curve in the road. She pulls onto the shoulder to give assistance and is motioned away by a state trooper who says, "Move on, lady—we need a doctor here" (Shainess 1984, p. 224).

Although some advertisers and other people in media are making an effort to break down stereotypes—one recent airlines ad depicts a female executive being served a meal by a male flight attendant—the persistence of stereotypes still affects people's sense of internal coherence.

Microsocial Pressures on Personal Identity

Moving from the level of mass culture and technology to the level of the family, we note that there are a number of factors present in many nuclear families that have negative effects on identity formation in children. Because a child's basic sense of identity depends on identification and interactions with family members, dysfunctional relationships in early life can leave a young person at risk for identity disturbances in adolescence and early adulthood. Mounting evidence that DID in particular is the consequence of abuse in childhood suggests the importance of taking a careful family history as part of the assessment of dissociative disorders (Hornstein and Tyson 1991). (A more detailed account of identity formation as the result of parent-child interactions follows in a later section of this chapter; our immediate concern is with family dysfunction in relation to later identity disturbances in individual members.)

Child Abuse and Parental Projections

There is a consensus in the literature that dissociative disorders result from the patient's having been abused in childhood. Most writers distinguish between physical, sexual, and emotional abuse, while acknowledging that most dysfunctional families manifest a combination of these forms. With regard to physical abuse, many therapists assume the correctness of Kluft's (1984b) four-factor theory of the etiology of DID, which posits a biological substratum or capacity to dissociate as the first factor in defense against abuse. However, as Confer and Ables (1983) have observed,

> Little information is provided [in the literature on DID] as to how the formation of multiple personalities occurs in response to trauma, other than suggesting that the person is overwhelmed by an affective state associated with specific traumatic events which is responded to by repression of feelings and development of alternate states. (p. 26)

This hypothesis was outlined by Wilbur (1984a) as the child's response to the discovery that rage resulting from abuse "is unacceptable and must not even be 'felt.'" Van der Kolk's (1989) research suggests that humans have biological responses to trauma, such that they become habituated to chronic hyperarousal and manifest a decreased ability to modulate strong affect states. However, it is not clear at the present time how these biological responses to abuse cause alterations in the person's sense of basic identity.

With respect to the interpersonal dimension, the abuse is itself often an expression of the parent's delusional views of the child. Some abusive parents simply have poor impulse control and are accustomed to lashing out physically when they feel angered or frustrated by the child's needs or demands. Others, however, react to the child with physical violence because they momentarily identify the child with a hated or feared parent or older sibling. Henry Kempe (1962), one of the first researchers in the field of child abuse, reported that many of the abusive parents that he studied "heard" the voice of their own authoritarian parents in their child's cries or whining. This delusional identification seemed to be the source of their belief that the child deliberately tried to annoy them, was intentionally bothersome or burdensome, or generally "asked for it." In some instances, abusive parents may "read" the child's facial expressions as a justification for abuse; as Gil (1988) remarks, "The abuser may interpret the look as defiance, pleasure, fear, or anger—any of which may elicit further abuse" (p. 22). It is understandable how a child who is not only maltreated but verbally invalidated and accused of provoking or deserving the maltreatment would eventually experience a form of identity confusion.

Societal Emphasis on the Rights and Privileges of Adults

A number of commentators have pointed to the contemporary cultural preoccupation with the rights of adults to experiment with "self-fulfillment" and "self-gratification" as one source of mistreatment of children within the family. This problem has a number of different dimensions. One has to do with the impact of the cafeteria mentality mentioned previously on the stability and continuity of the nuclear family. Many children have had their lives disrupted when their parents divorce, remarry, or decide to live with a same-sex partner. Some researchers believe that the high incidence of incestuous abuse in the United States is in part a by-product of divorce and remarriage; stepparents are less likely than biological parents to be inhibited by traditional incest taboos. There are cases reported of men marrying into a single-parent family in order to have access to the new wife's daughters (Russell 1986). But even when a parent's new partner does not become sexually involved with a child, the child's exposure to the complications of adult sexual permissiveness can affect normal development. As Wilbur (1984a) has observed, "Chronic exposure to sexual displays and sexual acts during infancy and early childhood is abusive" (p. 3). The problem is that many adults do not wish to allow their children's needs for relational stability and predictability to interfere with their own interpersonal options or geographical mobility (Hewlett 1991). One obvious consequence is that children in these situations grow up with an unstable internal sense of self as well as a high level of anxiety regarding relationships with others.

Another dimension of the problem is the widespread assumption that children exist to gratify their parents' needs—for a sense of importance, of belonging, of power, or for nurture and comfort. This attitude, which is all the more powerful in our society because it is often not explicitly articulated, is a comparatively recent historical development. Prior to the Industrial Revolution, children were an economic asset to families, and parents' authority over their children was counterbalanced by cultural injunctions regarding responsibility to them. For example, in medieval Europe, parents were reminded at their child's baptism that they would be required to account for their parenting at the Last Judgment. However, with the breakdown of extended families in the nineteenth century and socioeconomic changes that turned children into financial liabilities, a pattern of role reversal gradually developed in which children have come to be considered extensions of their parents' egos. In some families, parental pressure on children takes the form of emphasis on social prestige or other measurable achievements; the parent is gratified when the child becomes an athletic star, wins beauty contests, marries into a family in the Social Register, or is admitted to a good college. In other families, the child is expected to live up to certain moral standards, accept a particular political or religious ideology, or exemplify the parents' notion of good citizenship. If these pressures are severe enough, the child may well feel some identity conflict because he or she may be confused about the extent to which personal and professional goals or standards are their own, and the extent to which these have been imposed by the parents.

More visible forms of abuse also involve this assumption that children should meet parents' needs. Kempe's (1962) early studies indicated that many physically abusive parents felt justified in hitting or beating their children for failing to meet the parents' standards of behavior or accomplishment. Because many of these adults did not understand the normal human developmental timetable, they often had unrealistic expectations of children's readiness for toilet training, self-feeding, and the like. As the child grows older, abusive parents are likely to continue burdening the child with excessive and premature responsibilities. Putnam (1989a) found that many DID patients reported family patterns like those in alcoholic families; these children were often expected to cook, clean house, and take care of younger siblings when they were only 5 or 6. On a fundamental level, the person who develops DID has been deprived of their childhood (Putnam 1989a). By way of summary, Fontana has grouped parents who abuse out of the general belief that children "owe them" under five headings: 1) emotionally immature parents, 2) neurotic or psychotic parents, 3) uneducated/uninformed parents, 4) parents who are ideological disciplinarians, 5) parents addicted to alcohol or drugs (Fontana 1992). Whatever the specific root of the parent's self-centeredness may be, the child acquires a painful sense of having no rights, only the obligation to subserve the parent's needs or wishes. Briere (1992) has observed that abuse survivors frequently manifest "impaired self-reference," in that he or she cannot "perceive or experience his or her own internal states independent of the reactions or demands of others" (pp. 45–46).

With regard to incestuous sexual abuse, the notion that parents are entitled to act as they please recurs frequently in the accounts of perpetrators. Herman (1981) notes that many incestuous fathers justify their approaches to their daughters by claiming that their wives are sexually cold and withholding: "They apparently assume without question that a wife is required to service her husband on demand, and that if she fails to provide complete satisfaction, the husband is entitled to whatever replacement might be most convenient" (p. 43). Although the incidence of father-daughter incest is admittedly affected by a general cultural attitude that regards sexual access to all women as a male "right" or prerogative, nonetheless the sex dynamic rests upon a still more basic underlying assumption that children are the property of their parents (Kelly 1988).

The last form of adult exploitation of children, which is no less damaging even though it is not physical, is parental violation of the child's psychological boundaries. With the rising divorce rate, many children in single-parent families are drafted into the role of confidant or amateur therapist. It is not uncommon for a stressed and lonely parent to confide in a child or teenager matters that are beyond the young person's level of psychosocial or intellectual maturity. Hewlett (1991) recounts a case history of a middle-class teenager whose divorced mother used her as a "best friend": the young woman commented that she "never thought that my mother could protect me—in fact, even as a little kid, I felt all kinds of pressure to protect *her!*" (pp. 9–10). Again, it is predictable that a young person forced to comfort or counsel a parent about adult problems, in short, to experience a reversal of the roles of parent and child, is at risk for identity confusion. To the extent that healthy maturation requires identification with a parent prior to separation and individuation, a child compelled to identify with a parent who demonstrates self-centeredness or a general lack of maturity has an additional obstacle to overcome in forging his or her own sense of personhood.

Loss of Self in Relationships

The third factor on the microsocial level that exerts a negative influence on identity development is the pressure that abused children and, more generally, most females experience toward second-guessing the moods and possible behavior of others. The hypervigilance that characterizes abused children results from their need to learn how to "read" their abusive caretakers as quickly and accurately as possible to avoid trouble. Goodwin and Briere have identified hyperalertness as a common posttraumatic symptom in adult incest survivors (Briere 1992; Goodwin 1990). The contribution of the abused child's concentration on the behavioral signals of others to identity disturbance is that such children have little opportunity to define, explore, or gratify their own interests or desires. A clear sense of one's personal center derives in part from knowledge and acceptance of one's gifts and interests. By contrast, a boy or girl who is driven by fear of abusive family members to continually scan the interpersonal environment for signals of impending violence has little energy left for investment in positive activities of his or her own choosing. In addition, the fact that many abusive adults act as if they expect others to be able to read their minds adds to the child's predicament. "If you loved me you'd *know* what I want" is an attitude frequently met with in dysfunctional families. Thus many children in such households grow up not only in fear of the consequences of failure in clairvoyance, they believe that it is a reasonable expectation in human relationships. At the same time, they cannot name or define who they are, what they want from life, or what they believe in any profound or coherent fashion. Their sense of identity is more closely connected to avoidance of pain or other negative stimuli than to attraction to interesting, pleasurable, or positively instructive pursuits. Gil (1988) has found that avoidant behavior is a common self-protective response adopted by adult survivors of abuse. Unfortunately, avoidance as a coping style hinders identity formation because the survivor deprives him- or herself of opportunities for corrective experiences and relationships that can help him or her overcome the cognitive distortions that result from growing up in an abusive family.

Female children are doubly at risk for loss of self in relationships because of the pervasive cultural assumption that women exist to meet the psychological and physical wishes of others. Some researchers have commented on the impact of women's "deselfing" even in relatively healthy families; Lerner noted such manifestations as 1) inability to finish graduate or professional training, 2) anxiety related to promotion or success, and 3) general difficulties establishing a clear sense of identity and a "life plan" (Lerner 1988). This process of teaching women to put the demands of others first begins early in life. Orbach and Eichenbaum found in their patient sample that mothers begin depriving daughters of food, comfort, and nurture in infancy as a way of training them to accept deprivation and focus on gratifying others. The result is an adult female with a deep sense of unmet needs, anxiety about having those needs met, and a general lack of a healthy sense of entitlement (Eichenbaum and Orbach 1983). Chernin (1985) and others have hypothesized that the recent epidemic of eating disorders among American and Western European women is directly related to women's difficulties with selfhood and identity. In the last several years, Brown and Gilligan (1992) have studied female adolescents' "difficulties in speaking, the feeling of not being listened to or heard or responded to empathically, the feeling of not being able to convey or even believe in one's own experience" as indexes of women's general sense of invalidation and invisibility (p. 5). With regard to women's experiences of sexual violence within their families of origin and in later life, Kelly (1988) found that one dimension of her subjects' difficulties with abusive behavior is that women have not been allowed to name their own experiences until very recently. The majority of her respondents felt a need to redefine sexual violence in terms of women's experiential reality rather than according to traditional cultural minimizations of it as something that women either deserve, do not mind, or positively enjoy. Furthermore, Kelly's subjects testified to the impact of the notion that women must "place the needs of others before their own" as a factor in their vulnerability to boundary violation (p. 112). Although the present sex ratio imbalance (9 females:1 male; Putnam et al. 1986) in the incidence of the dissociative disorders doubtless has manifold and complex causes, societal pressures on women to have "negotiable" identities and weak personal boundaries are unquestionably part of the problem. As Briere (1992) has stated, "The same social dynamics that support exploitation and victimization of children teach women to be passive, relationship-oriented, and reluctant to express anger or personal needs directly" (p. 72).

Discussion

The material in this section was included to help clinicians situate their patients' identity disturbances in a larger social context. Although patients may not always verbalize their suffering in these terms, those with DID and other forms of identity disturbance must live with their affliction in a society in which "self" and "identity" are considered both positive goods and measures of a person's general competence. Many people with DID feel stigmatized by their disorder, and cultural norms that equate one's basic worth with the ability to achieve self-integration, self-definition, or self-direction exacerbate these feelings of embarrassment or inadequacy. Both Putnam (1989a) and an anthology of first-person accounts of DID (Cohen et al. 1991) mention teasing (e.g., trying to provoke particular alters to come out), criticism, and exploitation by significant others as common responses to the patient's diagnosis. Clinicians who are sensitive to the wider issues posed by the dissociative disorders will be in a better position to help their patients wrestle with questions of personal identity.

▌ Identity in the Psychological and Psychotherapeutic Literature

If we turn from the current social setting of identity issues to the classical psychological and medical literature on identity, we discover that the question of dissociated identity was first posed during a period of rapid historical change, namely the nineteenth century. The earliest recorded case of what we would now call DID dates from 1789 to 1791, when a German physician named Eberhardt Gmelin reported an instance of what he termed *umgetauschte Persoenlichkeit*, or *exchanged personality*. Gmelin's patient was a 20-year-old German provincial woman whose alter spoke upper-class French. Greaves (1993), in his discussion of the case, suggests the name *Gmelin's syndrome* as a replacement for *multiple personality disorder*. In his discussion of the historical precedent set by Gmelin's young patient, Greaves (1993) remarks,

> It would be strange, indeed, were we to surmise that in humankind's vast history, what we now know as multiple personality disorder (MPD) should not have existed prior to 1789. . . . But from an epistemological viewpoint, no knowledge can properly be said to exist before it is conceptualized. (p. 356)

However, Greaves goes no further than to note that Gmelin's patient marks the beginning of discussion of human identity problems as the "secularization" of what earlier centuries would have termed *possession*. Kenny's (1986) study of nineteenth-century instances of DID in the United States interprets them as, in effect, a psychiatric by-product of the breakdown of social consensus. Nineteenth-century Americans were divided over a number of new issues: religious pluralism, changing roles for women, the shift from an agrarian to a manufacturing economy, the growth of large urban centers, changing immigration patterns, and the like. Kenny therefore views his cases as people manifesting "a given idiom of distress that has been seen to answer to the needs of individuals in marginal, ambiguous, contradictory, or transitional personal situations." (p. 185) The same rapid course of cultural transition affected Europe during the same period. Ellenberger (1970), in his classic account of the evolution of dynamic psychiatry, devotes a considerable amount of space to chronicling the changes in the political map of Europe, the growth of nationalistic feelings, the rise of new trends in the arts and philosophy, and changes in relations between the sexes, in order to provide an explanatory backdrop for his analysis of the work of Janet and Freud. These two pioneers were conducting their research and publishing their case histories in a society that contained a growing number of "individuals in marginal, ambiguous, contradictory, or transitional personal situations" (p. 369). For example, one of Janet's patients was a man who came from a family whose Catholicism was tinged with superstitiousness, living in a large city in which anticlerical opinions were published in the newspapers. The man's symptoms of possession began after he violated his own moral code by being unfaithful to his wife during a business trip. To turn to Freud, one of his best-known case histories, that of "Anna O.," involved a young woman caught in the conflict between her advanced education and her monotonous home life, and between her identity as a Jewish woman and the ambiguous social situation of Jews in the Austro-Hungarian Empire of that period.

In addition to the broad-based historical changes that increased the population's vulnerability to dissociative disorders, the nineteenth century saw the rise of different theories or approaches to the therapy of these disorders. Put slightly differently, the period not only saw an increase in the number of people with identity disturbances, it also saw a proliferation of diverse, and often contradictory, answers to the question of personal identity. The one generalization that can be made is that none of these theorists, practitioners, or schools of therapy understood human identity to be a unitary or monolithic given; all of them proceeded from the assumption that identity is a construct, built up by the individual from a set of different elements, experiences, capacities, or components. Two major questions were involved in the nineteenth-century debates and to some extent are still present in discussions of identity:

1. The relationship between the human soul and the human body or, more generally, between spirit and matter
2. The relationship between the various layers or components *within* the human mind

The Mind-Matter Question

Most traditional theories of Western medicine and, within the Church, pastoral care assumed both a distinction and a connection between the soul and the body. In Greco-Roman medical practice, both Hippocrates and Galen indicated that certain diseases of the body were affected in their progress by the patient's state of mind and, conversely, that self-indulgence in emotional excesses increased the body's vulnerability to disease. The major Greek philosophical schools combined techniques of mental hygiene, intended to enable the person to control his or her passions, with physical discipline (i.e., dietary and exercise regimens). The ideal of classical culture was *sophrosyne,* or moderation and balance in all things. The Roman poet Juvenal's capsule advice that a wise person will strive for "a healthy mind in a healthy body" summarized classical antiquity's definition of the underlying basis of functional human identity. What we would term *personality* or *individuality,* was to the Greek or Roman mind a secondary derivative of universal characteristics that all humans have in common. Thus personal identity was to be sought through harmony with the natural and civic order, rather than in distinction from it or opposition to it. And this condition of harmony presupposed respect for both the spiritual and physical components of one's being.

In early Christianity, a major point of objection to Gnosticism, one of the first major heresies, was that the Gnostics taught a radical dualism between soul and body, such that the connection between the two was dissolved. As a result, some Gnostics subjected themselves to destructively ascetical practices to destroy the despised material elements comprising their bodies, whereas others indulged in all kinds of physical excesses out of the belief that gluttony or sexual promiscuity could not affect the soul. In reaction, mainstream Christianity generally followed classical thought in upholding a doctrine of the unity of soul and body within the human subject, although the distinction between spirit and matter was simultaneously maintained. This concept of distinction-within-unity was applied to a number of theological questions, such as how the material elements of the sacraments could confer spiritual grace, or how the resurrection of the body could be understood. However, it had obvious relevance to both pastoral care and medieval medicine. As Ellenberger (1970) has observed, not only the practice of exorcism within the Roman Catholic Church but also pastoral counseling within the Churches of the Reformation has proceeded from the assumption that spiritual disorders affect the body as well as the mind. Whether the precise spiritual disorder was understood to be demonic possession or unconfessed sins, Christians in any of the major traditions generally understood that any human illness, whether of mental or physical functioning, derived from a disordered relationship to God and other persons. In the Judaeo-Christian worldview, *personal identity* could be defined as the sum total of the physical, mental, and spiritual dimensions of a human being in right relationship to his or her creator and his or her fellow humans.

However, with the challenges posed to traditional Judaism and Christianity by the scientific discoveries and philosophical developments of the nineteenth century, this view of the soul-body or spirit-matter question was no longer unchallenged. Some Victorian intellectuals adopted a thoroughgoing materialism, such that they regarded mental or spiritual activity in humans as mere epiphenomena of biological processes. Many of the early studies of brain-damaged patients were undertaken to prove or disprove materialist arguments. Other thinkers in this period became panpsychists; that is, they interpreted all reality as essentially psychic or mental. To the panpsychist, matter is simply a dense form of thought. Although Crabtree does not use the term *panpsychism*, it is obvious that this school of thought is still alive and well in the form of various occult or "New Age" groups and associations. Crabtree's (1985) discussion of the notion that some form of mentation is present even in inert matter and that humans can generate "thought-forms" that affect physical reality as well as interpersonal relationships is a description of common panpsychic beliefs. The contemporary practice of *creative visualization*, which is recommended in a number of self-help books for abuse survivors and addicts in recovery, is a modified version of panpsychism. (Creative visualization in this restricted sense is not to be confused with the more general practice of visualization as a therapeutic practice or relaxation technique.) The third response that developed in the nineteenth century to the mind-body question was spiritualism. The question of the relationship between soul and body has a temporal aspect in that the body's physical disintegration after death raises issues of the soul's survival, permanence, or location. Some nineteenth-century spiritualists believed in the survival of disembodied spirits and attempted to communicate with them through mediums or other forms of séance. In 1882, the Society for Psychical Research was founded in England (with an American branch) to conduct empirical research into paranormal phenomena. Another group of spiritualists adopted a belief in reincarnation (i.e., that souls enter a new body after death rather than continuing to exist in a disembodied state). In any case, it will be evident to the reader that a certain range of inquiries regarding personal identity derive from the more general philosophical problem of the relationship between spirit and matter.

Multiplicity Within the Mind

The late eighteenth and early nineteenth centuries also saw the breakdown of the notion that the human mind is a unified monad. Although it is true that previous generations of philosophers and medical practitioners had generally accepted the model of a so-called faculty psychology (i.e., the notion that the mind can be divided into faculties of reason, emotion, will, appetition, and so on), nonetheless most people still thought of consciousness as basically unified. In other words, one might be aware of a conflict between one's emotions at a particular moment and what one's reason defined as the wise or prudent course of action, but both of these responses to the situation were considered part of consciousness. The same would hold true of moral conflicts; it was assumed that a will divided between the dictates of conscience and the impulse to break the law or violate moral sanctions still had access to all the aspects of the person's consciousness. Prior to Mesmer and the early nineteenth century French hypnotists, no major intellectual authority thought of the human mind as composed of different layers or dimensions of consciousness. Dreams, hallucinations, and other aspects of what we would now call the subconscious were generally assumed to enter the mind from the outside, either by possession or some form of communication with nonhuman entities. Because a sense of personal identity consists in part of a sense of consciousness or self-awareness, the first explorations into hypnosis set in motion a series of changes in the understanding of consciousness as a component of personal identity.

Franz Anton Mesmer (1734–1815) was a German physician who accidentally discovered the technique of hypnosis in the course of treating a patient in 1774. Although Mesmer's underlying theory— he assumed that the curative factor was something he termed *ani-*

mal magnetism—was incorrect, his technique had undeniable therapeutic results. Moreover, Mesmer's conviction that the hypnotist must establish a personal rapport with the patient is still accepted as a fundamental principle of good practice by contemporary hypnotists. Mesmer was followed by Puységur, Braid (who first gave the name *hypnosis* to the technique), Victor, Liebault, Azam, and Charcot. Many of the early cases of multiple personality recorded in French medical literature were treated by these practitioners, such as Azam's patient "Félida." As Ellenberger has observed, it was experimentation with hypnosis in the first half of the nineteenth century that led to two different schools of thought regarding the constitution of the human mind. On the one hand, there were the *dipsychists*, theoreticians who believed that the human mind had two levels of consciousness. One of these, Dessoir, wrote a book in 1890 called *The Double Ego* in which he maintained that each person's mind has two layers, an *Oberbewusstsein (upper consciousness)* and an *Unterbewusstsein (lower consciousness).* According to Dessoir, hypnotism is nothing but a calling forth of this secondary ego or lower consciousness, and dual personality amounts to the lower consciousness's acquiring sufficient strength to compete with the primary personality. The polypsychists, on the other hand, conceived of the mind as a population of subegos subordinate to an "ego-in-chief," which represented our ordinary waking consciousness. The importance of these two schools of thought lies in their contributions to Janet's and Freud's early professional education and first ventures into independent research. Janet drew his concept of the subconscious from the dipsychist model; Freud and Jung began with dipsychist theories and evolved in the direction of a polypsychist model of the mind (Ellenberger 1970).

Since the nineteenth century, experimental studies in a number of different fields of medicine and psychology have been used to advance or defend various models or paradigms of the multiplicity of the human mind. These include the following:

1. **Studies of patients whose cerebral commissures have been cut as a surgical treatment for epilepsy.** These so-called *split-brain studies* have been controversial insofar as research-

ers disagree about the degree of extrapolation to the normal population that is possible from the divided consciousness that characterizes these patients (Glover 1988). Some researchers (e.g., Parfit 1983) have argued that the two separate streams of consciousness experienced by commissurotomy patients are simply synchronized in people who have not had the operation. When the corpus callosum is severed, the synchronized stream of consciousness that is assumed to be unified in normal identity breaks into its basic dual components. Others (Reed 1988) concede that the left and right cerebral hemispheres house different mental specializations, abstract analysis and logical thought being carried out in the left brain and intuitive, artistic, and musical capacities in the right. However, Reed maintains that these specializations do not constitute separate consciousnesses.

2. **Studies of other brain-damaged patients.** With the rise of interest in neuroanatomy in the nineteenth century, clinicians often recorded case histories of unusual instances of trauma. One case was that of "F," the Sergeant of Bazeilles, a French soldier wounded in 1874 by a pistol ball in the left parietal region of his brain. The sergeant survived but was left with sensory disturbances and a tendency to react automatically to idiosyncratically interpreted stimuli. Because his behaviors were interpreted by some observers as a form of DID, researchers such as Ribot were led to theorize that disturbances of identity were secondary to organic trauma or irregularities of body chemistry (Sutcliffe and Jones 1988). Again, however, researchers have disagreed as to the relevance of cases such as these to the incidence of dissociative symptomatology and disorders in the general population.

3. **Research in the areas of time perception, memory, and attention allocation.** Many of these studies have shown that ordinary subjects drawn from the general population experience conditions of divided attentiveness, selective perception, and distorted memory. As has been discussed in earlier sections of this book, the SCID-D (Steinberg 1993b) has been designed to allow interviewers to distinguish between the normal range of

these phenomena (e.g., "highway hypnosis"; going on "automatic pilot" during boring routine activities) and the five core dissociative symptoms.

4. **Sociological studies in role construction, perception, and transition.** With the establishment of sociology as a separate field of scholarship at the close of the nineteenth century, many researchers began to investigate the ways in which social institutions affect an individual's sense of identity. In recent years, these studies have included research into role socialization as part of identity formation in childhood and the impact of role transition or role loss on disturbances of identity. For example, DSM-IV now includes categories for "Additional Conditions That May Be a Focus of Clinical Attention" that include difficulties brought about by role loss (e.g., "Phase of Life Problem," "Identity Problem," and "Acculturation Problem") Again, the sections in the SCID-D related to identity confusion and identity alteration are intended to distinguish between endorsements of commonplace role conflicts (e.g., a woman who feels conflicted between behaviors demanded of her in the workplace and traditional definitions of "femininity") and endorsements of dissociative experiences.

5. **Ongoing investigation of hypnosis.** Because hypnosis is a common therapeutic technique used in treatment of posttraumatic and dissociative disorders, its implications for discussions of personal identity are still significant. Janet's experiments in the mid-1880s with one of his DID patients led him to conclude that the hypnotic trance elicited two distinct sets of responses from the patient, one being role-playing on the subject's part to please or comply with the hypnotist and the other being the unknown personality (Ellenberger 1970). Spiegel (1990) has discussed hypnosis as a phenomenon that "seems possible to change the boundaries between conscious and unconscious experience" (p. 248). For Spiegel, hypnosis bears a resemblance to dissociation in that "dissociation can be conceptualized as a complementary aspect of absorption . . . . The more intensely one focuses on one aspect of experi-

ence, the more the remaining peripheral awareness is dissociated and unconscious. During hypnosis there is less connection among various aspects of experience. Events are dissociated" (p. 248). Frischholz (1985) has also described hypnosis as "a form of dissociation" because it is associated "with changes in awareness, memory and volition" (p. 109). Others have described hypnosis as a technique that can blur the usual participant-observer dichotomy within the mind such that a person can perform actions and observe them as if he or she were not the agent. Milton Erickson (1965) conducted an experiment with Aldous Huxley in which, in response to Erickson's suggestion that he see his wife in front of him, Huxley hallucinated an image of his wife complete with voice, emotion, and intelligence. In addition, the link between hypnosis and identity disturbances in the dissociative disorders has been formulated in terms of the theory that DID represents a form of self-hypnosis on the patient's part (Bliss 1984). Lastly, the hypothesis that multiple personality is an artifact of the interpersonal relationship between hypnotist and patient rather than an intrapsychic disturbance of the patient's own identity has been much discussed in the literature (Frischholz 1985).

In response to evidence accumulating in and across a number of disciplines, various theoreticians constructed metaphorical models for describing the multiplicity of the human mind. These can be grouped roughly as follows: 1) social models, 2) architectural models, 3) astronomical models, and 4) artistic or self-creationist models.

Social Models

Social models include theories of the multiplicity of normal identity that compare the psyche to a group or organization of people, or to a microcosm of society. The nineteenth-century polypsychist notion of an ego-in-chief surrounded by subegos would fit into this category. More recently, Minsky (1980) has rehabilitated this model; he envisions the mind as "composed of many partially autonomous 'agents'—as a 'Society' of smaller minds.... In fact, we'll suppose that it works much like any human administrative organization" (pp. 118–119). The relevance of the social model to DID is that many patients with the disorder spontaneously describe their alters as a group, a horde, or an army. The reader will note several instances of such self-description in excerpts from SCID-D interviews in the chapters that follow.

Architectural Models

Architectural models include theories of personality organization that compare the psyche to a building or similar structure. Masterson and Kernberg, who speak of *personality substructures* and *configurations*, fit under this heading. Again, this model appears in the spontaneous self-descriptions of DID patients, who compare their psyches to a house with a different room for each alter.

Astronomical Models

In astronomical models, the most important figure is C. G. Jung, who introduced what he termed a *polycentric* notion of the psyche—that is, that personal identity consists of a "multiplicity of partial consciousnesses" (Watkins 1986). Jung compared mental processes to a system of constellations of stars and planets. The constellations are *complexes* that may appear as imaginary persons in dreams and fantasies.

Artistic or Self-Creationist Models

Artistic or self-creationist models are the most recent and could fairly be termed *postmodernist*. These models would include the theories of the French deconstructionists, who view a person's identity as a fluid self-creation, a work of idiosyncratic art assembled on an individual basis from the flotsam and jetsam of thought systems that have broken up in the general chaos of contemporary culture. Also included in this category would be what Kenneth Gergen (1991) has termed the *pastiche personality*—that is, a sense of identity cut and pasted together with little sense of a core essence.

As Gergen (1991) has stated, "The pastiche personality is a social chameleon, constantly borrowing bits and pieces of identity from whatever sources are available and constructing them as useful or desirable in a given situation" (p. 150). The difference between this model and the previous three is important in its potential implications for therapy. Whereas the social, architectural, and astronomical models presuppose a kind of basic organization or coherence to the self, the "artistic" postmodernist model assumes that the multiplicity of the self has neither rhyme nor reason. It is on this account that Glass (1993) has attacked the influence of deconstructionism on psychotherapy. In his opinion, this view of personal multiplicity as essentially chaotic leads to an irresponsible glorification of DID as creative liberation from oppressive social constructs, when in fact it results from trauma and inflicts intense suffering on people. Glass (1993) criticizes deconstructionist philosophers for

> discrediting the psychoanalytic distinction between fragmentation and wholeness, multiplicity and unicity, reality and delusion, truth and nothingness, ontological security and insecurity. To obliterate these distinctions . . . is from a clinical perspective to throw the self into a universe of anguish and disconnection. In reality, what comes after the deconstruction of the self is tragedy. (p. 28)

Although this model of identity as multiplex may seem like an exotic academic fad, unlikely to manifest in the patients at the average clinician's facility, it has potentially wider ramifications. First of all, as Glass has documented, deconstructionist notions have influenced some schools of psychotherapy in Europe. Second, a subpopulation of undiagnosed subjects with DID who are presently in college or graduate school might well describe their dissociative experiences in the jargon or argot of deconstructionist thinkers.

▌ Identity and Developmental Psychology

From one perspective, questions of personal identity as measured by consistency of character across time are not new. A number of classical writers, including Aristotle, Plutarch, and Cicero, discussed this dimension of human personhood in relation to the subject of long-term friendships. They pointed out that friendships formed in childhood or adolescence may collapse as the friends mature because young people are not yet fully formed in character and may change as they grow older. Whereas these observations may seem rudimentary to contemporary researchers, nonetheless they indicate that the historical dimension of personal identity has long been a matter of philosophical reflection and pedagogical concern. St. Augustine, in the fifth century C.A.D., began to ask some surprisingly modern questions about character formation in children and the role of various attitudes in the family of origin as well as formal educational practices in affecting children's self-understanding. For example, St. Augustine (1961) relates his intense fear of being beaten in school for not learning his lessons properly and asks why it is that children must go through "a period of suffering and humiliation" (p. 9) in elementary education. "I was constantly subjected to violent threats and cruel punishments to make me learn," he wrote (p. 14). He also notes the influence of what we would call mixed messages nowadays: the narrative epics that were part of learning Latin and Greek literature in his day were full of stories about the gods' immorality, behaviors that the students were taught to consider wrong for human beings. He wrote, "This traditional education taught me that Jupiter punishes the wicked with his thunderbolts and yet commits adultery himself. The two roles are quite incompatible" (p. 16).

St. Augustine's investigations into his memories of his early life proved to be important for later-century thought on developmental issues in human identity. This influence was not only because the *Confessions* contain some wise insights into children's growth, such as the comment that children "learn better in a spirit of free curiosity than under fear and compulsion" (p. 14), but because Augustine's own personal history was filled with a number of sharp vocational and religious breaks and discontinuities. As such, his is a record, unique in the ancient world, of self-examination with regard to questions of identity and what we would now call a sense of self-continuity. It is not surprising that educational theorists during the Renaissance, such as Erasmus and Roger Ascham, the tutor of Elizabeth I, began with Augustine when they wrote their own books on childhood development and education. The sixteenth century also saw the first handbooks of pediatric medicine and the first guides to baby and child care for parents. These so-called *housefather* books were comparatively short, compared with today's editions of Spock and Brazelton, but they did inform parents of such medicines as were available for routine childhood problems, such as colic or teething, and they contained useful advice about the stages of children's development and the ways in which parents could helpfully influence their children's character. It is, of course, the case that educational theory in this period still aimed at character formation in the sense of teaching young people the basic civic and religious virtues that would help them to be good workers and parents in their turn; for the most part, people were less concerned with the issues of individual selfhood and self-definition that preoccupy moderns.

In the nineteenth century, the new ideas that were affecting general theories of human identity and psychological structure began to infiltrate concepts of child development as well. In particular, the *fin de siècle's* preoccupation with sexuality influenced a good many popular writings of that period concerning human psychological development. Freud was by no means the first practitioner to suggest that infants and small children experience sexual feelings, or that children can be seduced by servants or other adults. Freud's real innovation was the introduction and systematization of ideas and concepts that were scattered in the general literature of the period, and to apply them directly to psychotherapy (Ellenberger 1970). Consequently, the often-repeated statement that Freud's writings on psychosexual development aroused widespread anger at the time of their initial publication is untrue; they were actually quite favorably received (Ellenberger 1970). The primary significance of Freud's theories for the purposes of this book is their repercussions for research into the connection between childhood sexual trauma and later development of a dissociative disorder. Although there is a growing consensus in recent research regarding this connection, Freud's recantation of his early discovery of the frequency of incest in his patients' childhoods was a major factor in the minimization of the incidence and sequelae of sexual trauma until very recently. Herman (1981) has outlined Freud's shift from believing his patients' accounts in 1896, when he published "The Aetiology of Hysteria" (Freud 1896/1962) and *Studies on Hysteria* (Breuer and Freud 1895/1955), to suppressing information about some of his case studies, to repudiating his seduction theory entirely. By 1897, only a year later, he wrote to his friend Fliess that "it was hardly credible that perverted acts against children were so general." As Herman (1981) summarizes the aftereffects, "The legacy of Freud's inquiry into the subject of incest was a tenacious prejudice, still shared by professionals and laymen alike, that children lie about sexual abuse" (p. 10). Recent studies in the dissociative disorders indicate that, with respect to a sexually abused child's sense of identity, confusion about one's primary sexual identity or orientation is a frequent result. In the case of DID patients, development of contrasexual alters or homosexual alters is commonplace.

The twentieth century has seen a vast increase in the literature concerning developmental issues in personal identity. Some of this research has been stimulated by studies (Piaget, Mahler, Winnicott, etc.) of the physical and psychosocial development of children. Other studies have proceeded from the growing recognition that the social conditions outlined in the first section of this chapter have made issues of childhood identity formation more critical than ever. Put slightly differently, ours is a culture in which the technological and personal skills required for the completion of advanced degrees and professional training demand that children develop a coherent sense of self as early as possible. Children who are abused and subsequently develop dissociative symptoms and disorders are thus not only at risk for a series of interpersonal problems but for a lifetime of underachievement and/or underemployment.

Although different theorists of childhood development have postulated different schemata of the successive stages of identity formation, one would expect that a child subjected to persistent or repeated trauma in childhood would have difficulty negotiating the successive stages at their proper time or in their proper sequence. To cite Briere's (1992) summary, the impact of child abuse occurs at three different stages during development: 1) initial reactions to victimization, 2) accommodation to ongoing abuse, and 3) long-term elaboration and secondary accommodation. Abuse survivors are affected in all three stages on both the intrapsychic and the interpersonal levels.

To better understand the impact of abuse on identity formation over time, it will be helpful here to review the literature on normal childhood development. One area of research involves a process called *identification.* Identification is the process by which an individual incorporates attributes from others who have had a significant influence on his or her life. Small children identify primarily with their parents: the parents' beliefs, values, behaviors, and so on. As the child matures, identification extends to siblings, relatives in the extended family, peers, and other significant adults, such as teachers, scout leaders, clergy, neighbors, and friends of the family. Erikson (1968) has pointed out that these identifications undergo a continual process of selection, accentuation, and modification. He stated that "from a genetic point of view, then, the process of identity formation emerges as an evolving configuration—a configuration which is gradually established by successive ego syntheses and resyntheses throughout childhood" (p. 163). For example, at any point, the growing young person may decide to identify with one sibling rather than another or to identify with a particular teacher's gentleness and sense of humor rather than his or her specific area of instruction. In addition, identifications include groups as well as individuals; thus the growing child may choose to identify (or reject identification) with a religion, a nation, an ethnic group, a profession, an age cohort, and so on. As is well known, group identifications are one of the particular marks of adolescent development (Erikson 1968). In sum, *identity formation* can be defined as a process of ongoing dialogue between a child and his or her social surroundings; it consists of interpersonal effects on intrapsychic processes and structures. If all goes well, a child privileged to enjoy a normal course of development will be a child surrounded from infancy by siblings and adults who exemplify a range of positive personality traits, so that the child will have a choice of favorable identifications. The young person's selection and modification of these identifications will not receive undue interference. Environmental feedback will be sufficiently consistent and predictable to allow the child to grow up without cognitive distortions of reality. Interpersonal relationships will be adequately supportive and affectionate to permit the child to move out into the world without the extremes of either timidity or aggressive belligerence.

However, any or all of these aspects of normal identity formation can be sabotaged or derailed altogether by abuse. To begin with primary identifications, a child abused within the family of origin is forced to identify with negative traits or behaviors rather than positive or constructive ones. Moreover, secondary identifications with others outside the family are impaired by the impact of abuse on the child's social persona and skills. Many times abused children develop behavioral responses to maltreatment that make them unattractive to others (Fontana 1992); even in cases in which the child attracts favorable attention and affection from outsiders, he or she may be too afraid of these better role models to identify with them.

With respect to self-selection of identifications, abusive families frequently interfere with a child's growing ability to discriminate between traits that are ego-syntonic and those that are not. Some families force a so-called *negative identity* on a particular child; the child may be singled out as the family scapegoat or repeatedly told that the parents expect him or her to "come to no good end." In addition, the family may actively teach the child to develop antisocial or socially unacceptable attitudes and behaviors; Garbarino et al. (1986) have identified *corrupting* as one of eight items of psychological abuse that may occur in dysfunctional families (in Briere 1992). In other instances a parent's unresolved problems with other family members may result in the parent's interactions with a child being skewed by these projections or anxieties. For example, Erikson (1968) recounts the story of a young man whose mother was afraid that he would recapitulate the life pattern of her alcoholic brother. She selectively responded only to those traits in her son that reminded her of her brother. In still other families, the abusive parents may criticize or invalidate the child's attempts to identify with an admired adult outside the family; for example, a child who has been befriended by a teacher may be told that the teacher does not deserve admiration or that he or she only pretends to like the child.

To some extent, the early stages of DID can be understood as a malformation of the normal process of identification. Many DID patients have alters who are essentially introjects of the original abusers. In addition, researchers who hypothesize that an abused child's imaginary playmate or companion may eventually become an alter personality have observed that these imaginary playmates are frequently modeled after a real-life or fictional person with whom the child identifies (Sanders 1992b). Lastly, Confer and Ables (1983) mention the hypothesis of Horton and Miller (1972), that DID results from the child's forced identification with parents with contradictory personality traits coupled with "a meaningful emotional relationship with a substitute identification figure. The syndrome follows the loss of this relationship" (Confer and Ables 1983, p. 27). The difference between this and the more normal pattern of identification is that the child in the process of developing DID cannot choose among his or her various identifications in order to integrate them because these identifications are the nuclei of alter personalities that may be amnestic for one another. Furthermore, once dissociative symptomatology develops in the child, he or she may begin to manifest behaviors that either provoke additional maltreatment from the original abusers or that make it additionally difficult to attract supportive attention from adults who are better role models. As Kluft (1985b) has pointed out, many children in the early stages of DID find themselves accused of being "bad," "absent-minded," "possessed," or "being a chronic liar" (p. 174). Thus an abused child's resorting to dissociation as a coping mechanism is an example of Briere's second point: it is a form of accommodation to ongoing abuse. By the time an adult survivor manifests the symptoms of full-fledged DID, the level of identity confusion and identity alteration is usually severe.

At present, therapy for DID patients includes addressing issues of identity formation. Kluft (1993a) and Fine (1988) mention specific therapeutic objectives in this direction, including helping the patient to achieve perceptual congruency, addressing and correcting cognitive errors, reducing separateness and conflict among the alters, and modeling an attitude of personal responsibility. Putnam (1989a) has noted that DID patients who have achieved fusion or integration usually need some supportive therapy afterward in order to deal with changes in self-image and "their new identity as 'singles,'" particularly as these changes affect their relationships with others (p. 319). Briere (1992) has outlined a treatment philosophy of *abuse-focused therapy*, which combines self-oriented, cognitive, and trauma-specific approaches that are adapted to fit the patient's specific history and needs. With regard to self-work, Briere summarizes its goal as "help[ing] the survivor build a positive source of identity, so that he or she is able to monitor internal states, call upon inner resources at times of stress, maintain internal coherence in interactions with others, and foster improved affect regulation" (p. 113). Briere acknowledges that one of the difficulties in self-work is precisely "the fact that self-development occurs primarily in childhood, as opposed to later in life . . . thus it is not always clear how to accomplish this task outside the normal developmental sequence" (pp. 112–113). He hypothesizes that a safe and supportive therapeutic environment facilitates self-work in that it reverses the abusive process that caused the patient to become *other-focused* in the first place by "free[ing] the survivor to move attention from the external environment to internal experience" (p. 114). Finally, Watkins and Watkins (1993) propose a model of ego-state therapy, which favors a form of integration that is *not* defined as a fusion of the patient's alters into a single entity. Their work presupposes a model of normal personal identity, which allows for "segmented divisions in personalities" (p. 278).

In any event, whichever model of self-work a clinician favors, he or she can make use of the SCID-D in patient education to provide the patient with a better understanding of the nature, origin, and prognosis of his or her symptoms. Chapter 15 of this book includes a sample SCID-D interview and patient feedback interview in order to provide the reader an example of the instrument's utility in therapy as well as diagnosis and assessment.

■ Identity Confusion and Identity Alteration in the Dissociative Disorders

It has been understood for some time by researchers in the field that identity disturbance is a major component of the dissociative disorders as a group. Whether the disturbance consists of amnestic loss of personal history or information, fugue states, or the development of alter personalities, all persons with any of the dissociative disorders have experienced a compromised sense of personal integrity and coherence. The SCID-D's assessment of five core dissociative symptoms includes two that directly concern identity disturbance: identity confusion and identity alteration. The SCID-D defined specifically the categories of identity confusion and identity alteration in order to assess both the internal and external dimensions of identity disturbance. *Identity confusion,* as defined by the SCID-D, includes subjective feelings of uncertainty, puzzlement, or conflict regarding one's identity (Steinberg 1993a, 1993b; Steinberg et al. 1990). As Figures 9–1 and 9–2 illustrate, identity confusion can be represented as the subjective internal dimension of identity disturbance. Identity confusion consists of two wider subjective affects: difficulty in self-understanding and a sense of dysphoria resulting from internal conflict. Identity alteration, on the other hand, represents the external behavioral manifestations of identity disturbance.

Identity Confusion in the Dissociative Disorders Based on SCID-D Research

The symptom of identity confusion, as with the core symptoms previously discussed, occurs across a spectrum of severity. Persons in the general population, depending on the degree of cultural or familial stressors in their lives, experience mild levels of identity confusion. Persons diagnosed as having nondissociative psychiatric disorders score in the mild-to-moderate range, whereas those with dissociative disorders typically manifest severe levels of identity confusion.

As has been previously noted, mild identity confusion is an unremarkable concomitant of life in so-called postmodern society. It is a frequent sequela of adolescence and other points of transition in the adult life cycle, such as completion of education, marriage, adjustment to aging, and retirement. Moreover, mild identity confusion may either precede or follow an important life decision, such as the choice of a vocation, going public about one's sexual orientation, a decision to marry or divorce, geographical relocation, and the like. These transitions can generate subjective experiences of internal confusion, either because the person desires a stable sense of personal identity or has to decide among conflicting aspects of his or her identity. However, the type of mild identity confusion that clinicians encounter in the general population is ordinarily transient, episodic, and connected to a specific stressor.

Moderate levels of identity confusion are, by contrast, recurrent, not always precipitated by obvious crises or other stressors, and connected with impairment in social or occupational function-

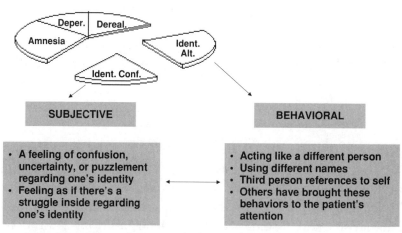

Figure 9–2. Identity confusion and alteration.

ing. For example, a person with a personality disorder might experience ongoing or recurrent doubts about sexual identity that are unconnected to the biological changes of puberty or the climacteric, on the one hand, or to specific events like the break-up of a relationship, on the other. Furthermore, these doubts would manifest in behavior that disrupt normal functioning, such as an inability to complete one's schooling or sustain healthy relationships with others. Lastly, moderate identity confusion is characterized by subjective feelings of dysphoria.

Severe levels of identity confusion are an intensification and prolongation of the characteristics of moderate identity confusion; that is, that the subjective feelings of internal uncertainty or conflict are persistent, that there may be episodes of complete loss of and/or alterations in one's identity, that social and vocational functioning are more extensively affected, and that the patient's feelings of dysphoria are more acute. In patients diagnosed with a dissociative disorder, histories of long periods of unemployment, marital disruption, and hospitalization are common.

❚ Identity Alteration in the Dissociative Disorders Based on SCID-D Research

The SCID-D defines *identity alteration* as a shift in role or persona that is manifested in external behaviors such as voice changes, age regression, clothing styles, and rapid mood switches. Figure 9–1 shows the relationship of identity alteration to the other core dissociative symptoms and to the external dimension of the patient's world.

As with identity confusion, SCID-D research has found that identity alteration manifests along a spectrum of intensity (Steinberg et al. 1990) In the general population, identity alteration occurs at mild levels of severity; in patients with nondissociative psychiatric disorders, it ranges from mild-to-moderate levels. In this latter group, identity alteration may take the form of delusional identifications with celebrities (as in schizophrenia) or of personality changes secondary to drug or alcohol use. The most severe levels of identity alteration are found in patients with dissociative disorders. Identity alteration is the *sine qua non* of DID, in which alter personalities compete with the host personality for executive control of consciousness, behavior, memory, and affect.

Identity alteration at its mildest level is typified by the role playing and role switching that most persons experience in the course of ordinary life, such as the transition between one's "official" or "work" personality and the behaviors characteristic of private relationships and recreation. In these situations, the person is usually conscious of the role performance or switching but feels that it is under his or her control. For example, a flight attendant may be self-consciously aware that her job requires toleration of unpleasant or obstructive behavior from passengers that she would not permit in her household. However, she is usually also conscious of her degree of success in maintaining a proper demeanor and attitudes while on duty, and to take corrective measures, such as a brief break, if her self-control wears thin under stress. Mild levels of identity alteration are usually not associated with amnesia or dysfunction.

Moderate levels of identity alteration are characteristic of non-dissociative psychiatric disorders but also of dissociative disorders such as DDNOS. At this level, the patient may report acting like two (or more) different people; however, it is unclear whether the identity alterations assume executive control of the person's behavior *or* whether these alterations represent complete personalities. In cases of DDNOS, for example, the patient may experience conflicts between his or her usual self and specific fragments of identity. Moreover, a patient exhibiting moderate levels of identity alteration will manifest subtle intra-interview cues, such as variations in vocal pitch or tone, body movements, or general style of response. These intra-interview cues are less pronounced than in cases of severe identity alteration.

In cases of severe identity alteration, the patient experiences distinct loss of executive control to alter personalities. These alters are more clearly defined and distinctive than the personality fragments that characterize moderate levels of identity alteration. In addition, the patient has serious indications of identity alteration, such as the use of several names, consideration or implementation of a sex-change operation, reports from others of complete personality changes, experiences of having one or more people inside who are capable of influencing or controlling external behavior, and spontaneous age regressions. Lastly, intra-interview cues for severe identity alteration include distinct changes in voice, speech patterns, dress styles, body posture and movements, and so on.

CHAPTER 10

Assessment of Identity Confusion

As Chapter 9 indicates, there are many different theories that attempt to define and explain the concepts of human identity and selfhood. This theoretical material is relevant to the clinician in that it provides a context and point of departure for the assessment of dissociative disorders. Disturbances such as identity diffusion (borderline personality) and identity alteration (DID) are more approachable with a better understanding of what comprises identity. However, only recently have diagnostic tools been available to accurately assess the phenomenology of identity disturbances. The two identity disturbances assessed in the SCID-D (Steinberg 1993b) are identity confusion and identity alteration. *Identity confusion* is defined as a subjective feeling of uncertainty, puzzlement, or conflict about one's own identity or sense of self. *Identity alteration,* on the other hand, is defined as a shift in one's social role that is often perceptible to others due to the patient's changed behavior patterns (Steinberg 1993b; Steinberg et al. 1990). Identity alteration may manifest in a variety of behaviors, including the use of different names; the possession of a learned skill, such as the ability to play a musical instrument or to speak a foreign language, for which one cannot account; and the discovery of items in one's possession that one cannot recall having purchased.

The SCID-D contains one section that assesses identity confusion, one section that assesses identity alteration, and a separate section assessing features associated with identity disturbance. The interviewer can tailor or adjust the course of a SCID-D interview to each patient by asking questions contained in a series of follow-up sections at the end of the instrument. These follow-up sections are designed to be administered to patients suspected of having identity disturbances so that the precise content and extent of the identity disturbance may be explored more fully. For example, the interviewer may choose to follow up on rapid mood changes, flashbacks, feelings of possession, and the like, if the patient endorses those symptoms in the course of the fourth and fifth sections of the interview.

∎ Identity Confusion

The clinician may find that the SCID-D format elicits a variety of thematic clues that suggest the presence of identity confusion. To begin with, the theme of an ongoing inner struggle or warfare regarding one's identity is a characteristic feature of identity confusion seen in patients with dissociative identity disorder (DID) and dissociative disorder not otherwise specified (DDNOS). Feelings of disturbances in self-knowledge or an insecure sense of self also frequently appear in identity confusion. Often, the two themes emerge simultaneously. One patient's self-description articulates the two themes quite clearly:

> Recently there's been a lot of struggle. It's been like terrible. It's been like a fight to live. OK, it's like a fight to struggle to get out of this hole I'm in, and it's a fight to get rid of the one who has seizures, the part of me that has seizures; I can't stand it. There's a fight on that. . . . I guess there's a fight to be a good wife and mother and all this. There's a fight to do good in school, a fight to do good in work and a lot of me is, you know, starting to give up. (SCID-D interview, unpublished transcript)

SCID-D questions regarding identity confusion include question 101: "Have you ever felt as if there was a struggle going on inside of you as to who you really are?" and question 105: "Have you ever felt confused as to who you are?" The symptom of identity confusion is often difficult for the patient to put into words.

Here is how one patient with DID described her subjective experiences of identity confusion:

> I know who I am. I know what I am about, I know my thought process. I know what it feels like to be me. And then I have this . . . gosh, it's always been there . . . this sense that I don't know who I really am, and I'm not really . . . there's a physical feeling to it, but I don't know how to describe the physical feeling. . . . There's still these parts of me. I just don't feel together. I don't feel *whole*. That's the word. I just don't feel whole. (SCID-D interview, unpublished transcript)

Another patient with DID referred to different levels of consciousness but then personified them:

> It's as if I have several levels of consciousness and they all have an equal amount of, um, um, an equal amount of, um [pauses] . . . what it takes to be, an equal amount of what it takes to be a human being, bear a name. They argue and they pull and struggle and battle. (SCID-D interview, unpublished transcript)

■ The Spectrum of Identity Confusion

The spectrum of identity confusion ranges from the absent/normal to the severe/pathological (see Figure 10–1). The severity of identity confusion depends on its nature, frequency, and duration; the degree of stress, dysphoria, and dysfunctionality associated with it; and the involvement and extent of sexual identity confusion. Mild identity confusion is transient, nonpathological, and often associated with stress or life transitions (e.g., a death in one's family, graduation, marriage, retirement). By contrast, moderate identity confusion is recurrent, prolonged, and includes dysphoria. Severe identity confusion involves a persistent internal struggle regarding one's identity and recurrent episodes of dysfunctionality accompanied by dysphoria. Severe identity confusion may also include a complete loss of identity or a struggle regarding sexual identity.

Normal adults tend to reply to SCID-D questions about identity confusion either negatively or in terms of a felt need to integrate one's various social roles (e.g., "wife" and "educated professional"). One question for future SCID-D research would be the extent of correlation between this latter form of mild identity confusion and patients' perceptions of conflicts between work and sex roles or between racial/ethnic identity and some other social variable. Patients with nondissociative disorders, including schizophrenia, often verbalize identity confusion in terms of a struggle to find an appropriate role or function in the world and unhappiness with their stigmatized identity as a person labeled "mentally ill." Identity confusion in nondissociative disorders is often less severe than in the dissociative disorders, although clinicians should note the many exceptions to this general rule.

Patients with DID and DDNOS typically describe a persistent and recurrent internal struggle or uncertainty as to their identity (see Table 10–1). These self-descriptions are usually associated with distress and/or dysfunction. Internal conflict between alter personalities—particularly if the patient experiences copresence— and amnesia for past events are major components of the subjective experience of identity confusion.

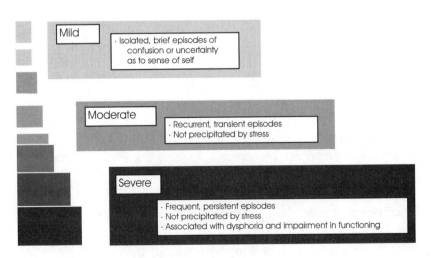

Figure 10–1. Severity range of identity confusion.

▮ Normal Identity Confusion

To consider the spectrum of identity confusion in the general population in more detail, we can start with the lower end of the continuum. One common form of identity confusion is brought on by simple life change, such as the decisions about one's future that middle-class adolescents must make, or the transient sense of disorientation that may result from a person's changing careers or moving to a new city. The SCID-D is designed to allow the interviewer to help the patient distinguish these normal forms of identity confusion from more serious dissociative symptoms. In an early segment of the identity confusion section in the SCID-D, the interviewer has the option of asking how the patient's current sense of identity confusion differs from adolescent identity confusion. Here is the response of one patient with DID:

Table 10–1. The spectrum of identity confusion in the SCID-D

	No psychiatric disorder	Nondissociative and personality disorders	DID and DDNOS
Symptoms	Transient episodes related to stress	Confusion regarding one's roles; struggle among "good" and "bad" parts	Persistent struggle regarding identity
Ongoing dialogues	No	No	Yes
Occurs w/amnesia	No	No	Yes
Severity of episodes	None–mild	Mild–moderate	Recurrent–persistent

Note. SCID-D = Structured Clinical Interview for DSM-IV Dissociative Disorders; DID = dissociative identity disorder; DDNOS = dissociative disorder not otherwise specified.

Interviewer: Adolescents and other individuals may have periods of confusion about their identity. How does your confusion differ, or is it similar?

Patient: No. It's this feeling of being split, like you're not part of your hand. . . . When you go through adolescence and you have an identity crisis, you know you're a whole person. You're just trying to put your values and your sense of self in place. But *this* is a feeling of being split, of not being whole.

Interviewer: Which is different than trying to just struggle with what your values are?

Patient: Oh yeah. Totally different. (SCID-D interview, unpublished transcript)

It should be emphasized that identity confusion in dissociative disorders is an identity *disturbance.* The majority of people with dissociative disorders have experienced persistent or overwhelming trauma throughout childhood. People within the normal range of identity confusion were most likely reared without recurrent episodes of abuse and are responding in a predictable fashion to a moderate and transient period of stress in their lives.

▮ Identity Confusion and Nondissociative Psychiatric Illness (Schizophrenia): Issues of Differential Diagnosis

This section examines schizophrenia as an example of a non-dissociative psychiatric disorder in order to clarify some of the major considerations in differential diagnosis. Schizophrenia lies at a different point on this particular symptomatic spectrum. (See Table 11–2 in Chapter 11, this volume, for a summary statement of the relevant differences between the SCID-D findings for the dissociative disorders and for schizophrenia.) Identity confusion in the psychoses often arises from a general sense of personal instability, dissatisfaction with life, and problems with reality testing. Schizophrenic subjects typically score in the none-to-mild range of severity for the symptom of identity confusion as measured by the

SCID-D. In part, this lower range of severity is because the identity confusion characteristic of schizophrenics is not produced by alter personalities or by amnesia. One schizophrenic patient described his experience of identity confusion in a manner that is typical for this population—not as an encounter with fragmented consciousness but in terms of his illness' effect on his life:

> I am frustrated as to who I am because I wonder what my future is going to hold for me, being on disability or in a limbo. You know, you're kind of a kid, you're not really an adult, you're not really at a job, and you're not really that secure. So, you know, it's up to grabs, what might happen to me. So it's frustrating, it might be painful at times. It might be agonizing. (SCID-D interview, unpublished transcript)

This lower severity of identity confusion in schizophrenic subjects has been demonstrated empirically in field tests of the SCID-D. In one study, 50 subjects (19 with DID, 31 with schizophrenia or schizoaffective disorder) were given the SCID-D. All of the patients with DID showed severe identity confusion, whereas the majority of the schizophrenia and schizoaffective subjects showed mild-to-moderate identity confusion. The exceptions were 3 patients with referring clinician diagnoses of schizophrenia or schozoaffective disorder who were found to have previously undetected DID following administration of the SCID-D (Steinberg et al. 1994).

What *is* distinctive about dissociative symptoms in schizophrenia is their psychotic context. Put slightly differently, the nature, content, and meaning of the symptom of identity confusion differ between schizophrenic patients and patients with DID. A diagnosis of schizophrenia is made when the patient's symptoms occur together with delusions, with hallucinations other than alter personalities, or with identifications with people who are (or were) real people or fictional characters. The following patient's identification with Jesus is typical of the type of identity confusion that occurs in schizophrenia:

> Yes. I thought this arm was Jesus and this arm was me and I would hold my hand like this to take care of Jesus because

I thought he was hurt or something. I would take care of this arm because I felt he was hurt. That happened for about a week and I was sent back to the hospital. (SCID-D interview, unpublished transcript)

To use a hypothetical example, a patient might claim to be the Pope. If the person is schizophrenic, the content and meaning of the statement is shaped by magical thinking; the patient has transformed himself or herself into another real person, thinks he or she is infallible, and assumes that he or she is living in the Vatican. On the other hand, patients endorsing symptoms of identity confusion in the context of a dissociative disorder describe their experiences as having an "as if" quality in that their sense of reality testing remains intact. A patient with DID who identified with the Pope would not believe him- or herself to *be* the Pope, but would assign the title to an alternate personality who was an internal self-helper or who represented the patient's moral or religious convictions. In the following example from the SCID-D field study, the patient responded to one of the interviewer's follow-up questions about identity confusion with the kind of "like" or "as if" wording that characterizes patients with dissociative disorders:

Interviewer: Have you ever felt that words would flow from your mouth as if they were not in your control?

Patient: That's happened.

Interviewer: Can you describe what that experience is like?

Patient: OK. The one time was 15 years ago, I went to the hospital, these words came out of my mouth. I don't know what they were because I . . . I was like unconscious or passed [out] or sitting there, and all I can remember is my girlfriend saying to me, "What are you talking about?" I didn't know what was going on. . . . I mean I didn't tell her that. I said, "Oh, I don't know, I'm just mumbling." But I could feel it . . . my mouth was moving and I could feel the pain from the thought, and then that was it. (SCID-D interview, unpublished transcript)

The other important major diagnostic differential has to do with the nature and significance of auditory hallucinations. In schizophrenic patients, the voices are perceived as emanating from sources outside the patient's head. For example, the person may claim that beings from outer space or CIA agents are "beaming" thoughts into his or her mind or otherwise invading the person's brain from the outside. By contrast, patients with DID perceive the voices of alter personalities as internal phenomena. One patient described the internal character of his voices quite clearly:

Interviewer: Are you having any dialogues now while you are talking to me?

Patient: Inside my head, oh yeah. Somebody is telling me not to tell the truth. It is no fun sometimes, you know. Don't tell the truth. I think it is the half that does not want me to remember. You know.

Interviewer: He'd like to keep the past secret.

Patient: He . . . sometimes it is he or many he's.

Interviewer: When you say "many he's," what do you mean?

Patient: Sometimes there are two people, sometimes 2,000. (SCID-D interview, unpublished transcript)

Other features that may be helpful to the clinician in establishing a differential diagnosis, such as the flat affect or catatonia that characterize schizophrenia, are summarized in Table 11–2 in Chapter 11.

■ Identity Confusion in Patients With DID

We can locate the identity confusion characteristic of DID in the middle-to-upper range of severity. Identity confusion is a significant factor in DID, when an environment created and sustained by one personality conflicts with the expectations of another personality who is not prepared to function in this alternate environment. Although it is certainly the case that most individuals find themselves drawing upon different aspects of their identity at different times during the day and in different situations, DID can precipitate problems that are very different from ordinary role switching. For example, most people have been socialized to keep personal matters separate from their work lives. A person whose job performance begins to suffer because of preoccupation with family difficulties may be criticized or reprimanded by a supervisor; even if that does not happen, the person may be concerned about his or her inability to compartmentalize the strong feelings that he or she may be having. However, temporary inefficiency in role transitions due to stress is well within the normal range of experience. A patient with DID, on the other hand, may have an alter personality completely lacking in the training or skills necessary to perform the dominant personality's work. If this particular alter emerges in the patient's workplace, considerable confusion or misunderstandings may result. The following excerpt is one example of such a patient's subjective experience of confusion with regard to work:

> It's like sometimes you come in [to work] and you don't know what you're supposed to do that day. I've walked into work wondering who the hell am I? Not knowing, OK, what is my job? What is my title? What am I supposed to do? And then when you start asking for help, then all of a sudden you know what to do. (SCID-D Interview, unpublished transcript)

In another instance, a patient who had been praised by her previous employers for the high quality of her work as an executive secretary found herself in a painful situation with a new employer because an alter personality had emerged in the interim who knew nothing about typing, dictation, or an executive secretary's duties.

> Right now I'm learning typing all over again. It's like my brain was damaged, it's gone. . . . I told [the corporation] I had 10 years' experience, but it doesn't look like I had more than a week experience to them. . . . The vice president told me I had absolutely no secretarial ability whatsoever and yet I got straight As and I was told by all [my previous employers] that I had A-#1 performance and I was considered good. . . . This one executive wanted me to come work for him. He said, "I've been

trying for 10 years to get you to work for me." I went to work for him for 1 month. . . . I couldn't perform even like anything. He said, "I can't believe what happened to you," and started yelling at me. (SCID-D interview, unpublished transcript)

As we see in the preceding material, presentations of identity confusion are often accompanied by the more disturbing symptoms of identity alteration. Patients may (perhaps intentionally) present themselves as having only identity confusion, when in fact they have more than one personality. They may delude themselves into thinking that they can control their alter personalities when in fact the alters emerge and act independently of the primary personality. The factors that may affect this delusion of control may include misdiagnosis by a previous therapist, the administration of neuroleptic drugs that temporarily suppress the voices of the secondary personalities, and the patient's fear of being labeled as crazy.

■ Common Themes of Identity Confusion in DID

At this point it may be helpful to review some recurrent themes in patients' descriptions of their experiences with DID. As is summarized in Table 11–2 in Chapter 11, these themes are relevant to accurate clinical diagnosis insofar as they do *not* characterize the schizophrenic population. The latter typically experience identity confusion in terms of a global diffuseness, a lack of a sense of identity, and a lack of a corresponding place in the social order. As will be evident from the material that follows, patients with DID frequently describe identity confusion in distinctive ways.

Puzzlement and Uncertainty

The themes of puzzlement and uncertainty are common in cases of identity confusion. Patients may refer to a disquieting lack of knowledge regarding their "real self," and a corresponding sense that their roles and characteristics are not integrated into a coherent identity. As an example of the kind of spontaneous elaboration encouraged by the SCID-D's format, one patient with DID responded to a question in the depersonalization section with indications of identity confusion:

> **Interviewer:** Have you ever had the feeling that you were a stranger to yourself?
>
> **Patient:** Yeah, all the time. I don't know who I am. I don't know.
>
> **Interviewer:** Can you say some more about that?
>
> **Patient:** I don't know, I guess my Mom named me Janet, but I'm *not* Janet. I don't know who I am. I'm mixed up. I don't know. I wish I did know who I was. I just feel so many different ways. (SCID-D interview, unpublished transcript)

Another patient replied as follows to question 102:

> **Interviewer:** Have you ever felt as if there was a struggle going on inside of you as to who you really are?
>
> **Patient:** Yes, for years, and I still can't find out who the fuck am I, man. Excuse my language, doctor. I don't know who the fuck I am.
>
> **Interviewer:** What do you mean by that?
>
> **Patient:** Who is [A.B.]? Who the fuck am I? I don't know. I don't know who I am. I really don't know who I am. I look at the rest of my family and I say, "I ain't part of this family, man, this can't be. They're all different than me. They also look alike, but they look different to me." (SCID-D interview, unpublished transcript)

As the preceding example indicates, the theme of puzzlement is characteristic of patients at all levels of educational achievement and verbal ability. The clinician should be alert to the presence of this theme in the self-descriptions of all patients endorsing dissociative symptoms, not just in those of patients who completed a college degree or who are accustomed to introspection and self-analysis.

The Theme of Internal Struggle

Severe identity confusion frequently elicits experiential descriptions that incorporate the theme of the internal struggle. The patient is likely to describe the internal struggle as a competition or conflict between incompatible wishes or goals. It is certainly true that most people in the general population experience a sense of inner conflict from time to time; commonplace examples include a dieter's feeling torn between a craving for a calorie-laden treat and the wish to lose weight, or a person's indecision about a major purchase such as a house or car. However, this sense of struggle is qualitatively different in patients with DID insofar as it affects their sense of personal identity and stability, which connects this theme to the theme of uncertainty and puzzlement. The ordinary person who feels tempted to go on a food binge or is weighing the options involved in a purchase does not usually feel as if his or her personal coherence or integrity is at stake. The following excerpt illustrates the intensity of internal struggle as experienced by a patient with DID:

Interviewer: Have you ever felt as if there was a struggle going on inside of you as to who you really are?

Patient: Oh God, yes. That's like daily, hourly. I feel like an amoeba with 15 thousand different ideas about where it wants to go. And it's like literally being pulled in every direction possible until there's nothing left, and it's like split in half. That's a constant battle. (SCID-D interview, unpublished transcript)

People with DID often experience conflicting advice or opinions emanating from their alter personalities. Individual alter personalities may have coherent, consistent identities, but, taken as a group, the incompatible internal personalities generate an atmosphere of conflict as well as incoherence. As one patient described it, "Do you know how hard it is to get a hundred and four minds to come together to a single decision?" The spontaneous elaboration of such identity alteration is common in DID responses to items about identity confusion, as is noted in the following excerpt:

Interviewer: Have you ever felt as if there is a struggle going on inside of you?

Patient: Yes.

Interviewer: What's that like?

Patient: That person that wants to come out. . . . He struggles, struggles with me. And this guy must think I'm nuts, if I'm gonna let him out. If I let him out, I'm never gonna get myself back in. And that's what scares me the most.

Interviewer: What's the struggle like?

Patient: It's like a tug of war. Pulling, pulling the rope, pulling, you keep pulling and pulling, and he pulls you back and you pull it forward, and he pulls you back, and you pull it forward, and you want to say, "Hey, man. Take the damn thing." And I keep pulling that rope, and he keeps pulling it back, and I pull it again [raises voice and sounds very annoyed]. One of these days, he might win. (SCID-D interview, unpublished transcript)

The struggle over identity is often accompanied by a feeling of anxiety related to fears of loss of control over the self. These fears may be associated with depersonalization, in which the person has subjective feelings of losing touch with reality or with his or her identity and a corresponding fear that he or she will never "come back."

The Theme of War or Battle

Extreme manifestations of identity confusion often elicit descriptions of military combat or civil war. The patient may experience the fight as a pitched battle between the self and a hidden other, or may describe it as a full-fledged war, with many participants or even whole armies.

One man described his inner combat as something like a barroom brawl between his dominant self and an internal personality:

Interviewer: What are the dialogues like, that you have with yourself when you see yourself outside?

Patient: Most of the time it's like a war. Anger. He'll look at me, he'll laugh. He'll go, "Ha ha ha ha ha ha. I'm gonna get you, man." I'll say, "You aint gonna get nobody. You can get the fuck out of here, man." 'Cause I'll pick up a board, and I'll go at him. And he'll disappear. (SCID-D interview, unpublished transcript)

Descriptions of the inner battle are often accompanied by distinctive and detailed visual images. The images may go so far as to include the tools or weapons used in the battle and physical descriptions of the combatants. One person with DID described his struggle in the following terms:

Interviewer: Have you ever felt as if there was a struggle going on inside you?

Patient: Yeah, a fight. I do. I feel that a lot of times like somebody's punching somebody out inside of me.

Interviewer: What does that feel like?

Patient: Kind of like a push and a pull. It's a lot of turmoil. It's kind of traumatic actually. It's very traumatic sometimes because that's when I get really scared because I know I can't control that. I see these two little men with gloves on and they're punching each other. (SCID-D interview, unpublished transcript)

In some instances, the patient may experience himself or herself as the battleground or location of the conflict, as this man's comparison of himself to a punching bag indicates:

Interviewer: Have you ever felt as if there was a struggle going on inside you?

Patient: Sometimes.

Interviewer: What is that experience like?

Patient: Sometimes there is half of me that wants to remember; the other half does not. I am not sure, it is a strange feeling inside. You feel like a punching bag after a while, you know. I want to remember; well, I don't. So . . . you get to feel like a punching bag and you start to lose your air and it starts to make you crazy. (SCID-D interview, unpublished transcript)

The following patient's imagery for her inner battle was considerably more elaborate, consisting of "armies of children," organized into groups headed by leaders, with each child a separate alter personality. This patient, who was diagnosed with DID, discussed her "internal army" as consisting of hundreds of faceless children and a guerrilla leader.

Interviewer: Have you ever felt as if there was a struggle going on inside of you as to who you really are?

Patient: As to who is in charge, yes . . . well you think you're in charge. . . . . If there is reason to call up the army then [Lisa, an alter,] will take over and she will command the army because it's a matter of life or death and she will not allow anyone to be killed without putting up one hell of a fight.

Interviewer: Is this struggle [frequent?]

Patient: [Interrupting] Twenty-four hours a day. (SCID-D interview, unpublished transcript)

This quote demonstrates the high severity of this patient's identity confusion in two respects. In the first respect, the patient is wrestling with separate and distinctive identities that are engaged in a battle for control over her mind and body. In the second, the patient mentions her experience of her symptoms of identity confusion as ongoing, "twenty four hours a day." The SCID-D assesses this degree of persistence in identity confusion as severe. Furthermore, the transcript indicates that the patient interrupted the interviewer with her reply, which is an additional indication of the persistence of her symptom and the intensity of her reaction to it. In response to another question in the identity confusion section, the same patient provided a more detailed account of her inner struggle:

Interviewer: Have you ever felt as if there was a struggle going on inside of you?

Patient: Yes . . . a battle. It's just like this humongous battle, this clashing of . . . it's a struggle for survival. It really is. For inner survival.

Interviewer: What are the sides of the struggle?

Patient: I become . . . I can't talk. I lose my ability to talk. Because there is such a battle going on and such a struggle that all the energy is concentrated inside on living this battle. . . . I can give you an example, that is the best way. The meeting a few weeks ago that I needed to attend and I went to go and attend it, and I went to walk into the room and the only chair that was available was between two men. And I remember being in this meeting before and I turned around and walked out. And I didn't turn around and walk out but my body turned around and walked out. And I couldn't talk to save my soul because there was this battle going on about whether or not I should go into the meeting and someone wanting, some memory to come up and someone else suppressing it. . . . I didn't actually get to physically sit in the meeting because I went inside and my body turned around and walked out, although I tried to walk into that meeting but I couldn't do it. (SCID-D Interview, unpublished transcript)

In this description of a stressful situation at work, the patient expresses her identity confusion in terms of a battle over the issue of seating in a conference room. One part of herself that felt vulnerable about having to sit between two males in the meeting— possibly an alter personality—took control of her body and impelled her to perform an action that another part of her resisted. The interdependence of dissociative symptoms that occurs in DID is also evident in this transcript. In this one episode, the patient experienced identity confusion (a struggle over volition), identity alteration ("someone else suppressing it"), depersonalization ("my body walked out"), and amnesia ("suppressing the memory").

Confusion Regarding Sexual Identity

Patients with dissociative disorders frequently experience disturbances in their sexual identity. In some cases the disturbance has to do with sex identity; in others, it may include confusion about sexual orientation. Many patients with DID have alter personalities of the other sex. Thus the patient may not only feel torn by an internal conflict, he or she may experience the conflict as a literal "battle of the sexes." One female patient in the SCID-D field study described a male alter named Joe. In some cases the person may not only have alters of the other sex, these alters may be bisexual or homosexual. For example, a well-known instance of DID involving a man convicted of rape indicated that the personality who "came out" during the actual commission of the rapes was not only female but lesbian (Crabtree 1985). Thus the clinician attempting to assess a patient's descriptions of sexual identity confusion in cases of DID will need to note the orientation as well as the sex of the alter personalities. A dissociative patient's anxiety about his or her basic sexual orientation may be either due to the simple presence of alters of the other sex, to the presence of homosexual alters, or to a combination of both types of presence. Indications of sexual identity confusion cover a range of symptoms, including fluctuations in the patient's sense of primary sex or the expressed desire for a surgical sex change. One patient with DID whose primary personality was a male named Michael described his sexual identity confusion in the following terms:

> I had many periods in which I felt I needed a sex change, debated if I was a homosexual. . . . I have pictures of myself in drag, and I have some vague ideas of what Michelle [female alter] looks like, and probably Michelle has some vague ideas. And I'm not so sure Michelle's happy. She's not happy with my genitalia, and I'm not so sure she's happy with my weight, and with my bone structure and with this and that and the other thing. . . . Michelle has her own agenda. She would like to see me dissolved from this person. . . . She has told me the way she's gonna do that is to have the sex change. And so she's not going to do anything that's gonna endanger her chances of leading a happy life. I keep trying to tell her that if she comes out to my therapist and we work this out we'll be one person, but she doesn't want to be one person with Michael in charge. (SCID-D interview, unpublished transcript)

On the other hand, some patients with DID experience sexual identity confusion as a more diffuse symptom; that is, they may report a general sense of bewilderment about their primary sex rather than specific descriptions of alters of the other sex or of different sexual orientations. For example, one woman described her sexual identity confusion as a generalized state of perplexity, rather than as a sharply defined inner struggle or conflict between different personalities:

> **Interviewer:** When you say that you don't know who you are, what do you mean by that?
>
> **Patient:** I don't know . . . should I tell the truth, doctor?
>
> **Interviewer:** Sure.
>
> **Patient:** I don't know if I'm a man, or I don't know if I'm a woman. I don't know. I'm just mixed up. I don't know, I don't know who I am. My name's Janet I guess, but . . . my mother named me that, but . . . I don't know. I'm just confused. Confused. I don't know what I'm about. (SCID-D interview, unpublished transcript)

The SCID-D's optional follow-up sections include questions related to exploration of this aspect of identity confusion. Clinicians should be aware that sexual identity confusion is a multifaceted problem insofar as it can manifest on any of the different levels that comprise a person's sexual identity. As the *Penguin Dictionary of Psychology* (Reber 1985) indicates, *sex differences* can be defined on at least three different levels that affect personality:

1. **Primary sex characteristics,** which are understood to include genetically determined traits of the organism that are closely related to biological reproduction; in humans, these are the genitalia and internal organs of reproduction.
2. **Secondary sex characteristics,** which are genetically determined traits not closely associated with reproduction; in humans, these include patterns of body hair and musculature, vocal pitch, and so on.

3. **Mental, emotional, and social behavior patterns;** in humans, behaviors considered appropriate to each sex vary somewhat across history and from culture to culture. (At present, researchers disagree on the extent to which this third category of difference is biologically influenced.)

Although the theoretical implications of current debates on human sexuality are not the direct concern of this book or of the SCID-D, clinicians should be aware that these debates have an indirect affect on patients insofar as they contribute to the making of a social climate in which sexual identity confusion creates high levels of anxiety in those who suffer from it. To begin with, the sheer volume and frequency of discussions of sex in the mass media means that people for whom sexuality is problematic cannot readily put the subject to one side. Second, our culture has made sexuality central to a definition of personal identity to an extent that is historically unprecedented (Turner 1993). What this means is that persons who feel confused about their sexuality are likely to generalize their feelings of confusion and extend them to other dimensions of personal identity. In other words, many patients will interpret sexual identity confusion as an indication that their entire identity is "up for grabs."

Lastly, clinicians should note that sexual identity confusion is often an aftereffect of childhood trauma. When the abuse is sexual in nature, the survivor is particularly likely to experience confusion about sexual identity in adult life because of the belief that he or she may have adopted in childhood that the abuse would not have taken place if his or her sex had been different. For example, a male survivor of incest notes that his mother's anger convinced him that he was "a horrible, little, unwanted monster. . . . Why did I have to be born a disgusting boy!?" (Thomas 1989, p. 3). One researcher in the field of DID reports a case study involving a female patient who developed two male alternate personalities as a reaction to being raped by her father. One alter was potentially homicidal and told the therapists that he was planning to kill the abusive father; the other male alter functioned to keep the would-be killer in check (Wilbur 1985). In this instance, the young woman had interpreted her childhood vulnerability as a direct consequence of her femaleness and developed the male alters to protect herself from further victimization. Although the SCID-D does not include direct questions about childhood sexual abuse, it is not uncommon for patients to volunteer information about a history of trauma. In one instance, a subject in the SCID-D field study mentioned that she had been treated by a previous therapist "for child abuse" in response to one of the early questions about amnestic experiences.

CHAPTER 11

Assessment of Identity Alteration

The last and most overt dissociative symptom assessed by the SCID-D (Steinberg 1994b) is identity alteration. This final section of the instrument includes questions such as question 113: "Have you ever felt as if, or found yourself acting as if you were still a child?" question 114: "Have you ever acted as if you were a completely different person?" and question 116: "Have you ever been told by others that you seem like a different person?" These and similar questions ask about the behavioral and environmental manifestations of identity alteration. The symptom's behavioral manifestations include referring to oneself by different names and acting like a different person. Environmental manifestations of identity alteration, which result from the patient's identity alterations, include feedback from people or objects in the environment. For example, one of the patients in the SCID-D field study cited in Chapter 10 reported being criticized by a new employer who could not understand why it seemed that the patient had apparently lost all her secretarial skills. Feedback from objects in the environment covers phenomena such as finding items in one's possession that one does not remember having purchased, or discovering documents in one's handwriting that are written in a language one does not recall having studied.

Environmental feedback from identity alteration is frequently reported by patients with dissociative disorders. Often, there is a sense of discomfort or anxiety that people experience when confronted with evidence of identity alteration. As with other dissociative symptoms, the patient may fear that the symptom is an indication that he or she is going insane or that others will make harsh misjudgments of his or her mental competence. In addition, manifestations of identity alteration may include for some people a sense of the supernatural or uncanny. Given the dominance of the scientific mindset in our society as a whole, these people may fear misunderstanding or ridicule from medical professionals if they describe their symptoms in religious or spiritual terms. The fact that the SCID-D's format allows for the spontaneous emergence of material related to identity alteration can be helpful to clinicians who are sensitive to this particular feature of dissociative disturbance.

∎ Assessing the Spectrum of Identity Alteration

Levels of identity alteration can run from absent to severe (see Figure 11–1 and Table 11–1). What differentiates the various degrees of severity are the distinctness and complexity of the personality states involved and the ability of these states to control a person's outward behavior. *Mild* identity alteration is widespread in the general population. Many, perhaps most, people are aware of occasions in their lives in which they have assumed different roles or demeanors but remained conscious of their role-switching or alteration, and perceived themselves having been in control of the transition. An example of mild alteration would be a medical professional on emergency room duty who is called on to treat someone he or she recognizes, such as a next-door neighbor or social acquaintance. It would be well within the normal range of behavior for the nurse or physician to be explicitly aware that he or she is dealing with a friend in a professional rather than a personal capacity and to consider the role switch as an intentional decision. This form of identity alteration is generally not associated with dysfunction or dysphoria and is not considered pathological or problematic. By contrast, moderate identity alteration differs from its milder counterpart in that the alterations are not always under the person's control. In addition, moderate identity alteration does not always manifest the presence of distinct alter personalities. Someone who experiences moderate identity alteration may present with mood changes and behaviors that they perceive as uncontrollable. Patients with nondissociative psychiatric disorders (e.g., manic depressive illness) may report moderate alterations in behavior/demeanor that they cannot control; for example, one patient diagnosed as manic depressive mentioned being bothered by his inability to "keep his mind from racing" (SCID-D interview, unpublished transcript). However, these alterations do not coalesce around distinct personalities. Similarly, individuals who have borderline personality disorder tend to fluctuate rapidly between radically different behaviors and moods; however, these changes do not involve different names, memories, preferences, distinct ages, or amnesia for past events. As Kluft (1987a) points out, borderline patients display constant anger and/or frequent temper outbursts, whereas the patient with dissociative identity disorder (DID) has relegated anger to one or

Table 11–1. The spectrum of identity alteration in the SCID-D

	No psychiatric disorder	Nondissociative and personality disorders	DID and DDNOS
Nature of episode	Role changes occur within their control	No use of different names; no alternate identities	Different names linkedto alternate identities with different behaviors and relationships
Amnesia for different behaviors	No	No	Yes
Severity of episodes	None–mild	None–mild	Recurrent–persistent

Note. SCID-D = Structured Clinical Interview for DSM-IV Dissociative Disorders; DID = dissociative identity disorder; DDNOS = dissociative disorder not otherwise specified.

more alters, and the anger is rarely as prevalent.

Severe identity alteration involves the patient's shifting between distinct personality states that take control of his or her behavior and thought. Indicators of severe identity alteration include the patient's use of different names as well as significant variations in memory recall. Individuals in this category may have experienced spontaneous age regressions, considered the possibility of a sexchange operation, or have been told by others that they sometimes act like a completely different person. Severe identity alteration is also accompanied by marked distress or dysfunctionality. Many such patients are chronically unemployed, have a history of unstable personal relationships, or have been involved with the criminal justice system. Involvement with the criminal justice system may be predominant among men with dissociative disorders; in fact, one common explanation of the present sex-ratio imbalance in diagnosis of the dissociative disorders (9 females:1 male) is that many men who have dissociative disorders are sent to prison for some form of antisocial behavior before they ever come to the attention of a therapist (Tyson 1992). However, the extent to which

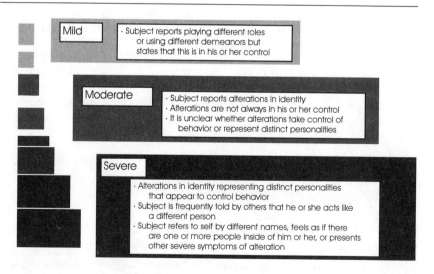

Figure 11–1. Severity range of identity alteration.

men who have DID are more likely than women to "act out" against society as a result of sex expectations and socialization awaits further research (Schetky 1990). Kluft (1987a) has stated that many patients' alters are capable of antisocial behavior. In addition, North et al. (1993) have noted that a significant number of female subjects in the 21 popular accounts of DID that they surveyed had committed antisocial acts, ranging from shoplifting, destruction of property, and killing animals, to child abuse and physical assaults on others.

With respect to the impact of severe identity alteration on an individual's employment, one patient described having an internal conference in which her primary personality explained to her alters why it was important that they not come out while she was on the job:

> I sensed that all the personalities were there. So I had a talk with the personalities, each one of them that I could think of. We have a chart because there are so many. For each one of them I explained to them how I could lose my job if you come to work. You've got to promise to stay home tomorrow and if you stay home and you're good, I will tell you what happened at work. Kind of like how you talk to a child. And it worked, 'cause since then they have never come to work. (SCID-D interview, unpublished transcript)

Another patient reported that the emergence of an angry alter at work affects his relationships with coworkers, who treat him as if he is either immature or unstable:

> Something tells me to "End it, man," and I say, "No, I'm not going to end it, I'm going to fight, I'm going to keep going, I'm going to keep going." Like a lot of times, if I have a hammer or something, like at work, or a broom stick, I'll pick it up and go like this with it, "Hit it, man, hit it, break the hand, break the hand [gestures]," and I throw it down, you know. And guys look at me and they say, "Something is wrong with this kid," and they call me "kid." I'm older than about 25% of the guys in that shop. (SCID-D interview, unpublished transcript)

▌ Identity Alteration in Schizophrenia: Issues of Differential Diagnosis

In psychiatric patients with nondissociative disorders, identity alteration tends to fall within the mild-to-moderate range and does not exhibit the clarity or complexity that characterizes personality changes in the dissociative disorders. It is important for clinicians to pay particular attention to these characteristics of the nondissociative disorders because patients with DID are often misdiagnosed as having schizophrenia (Chu 1991). Table 11–2 provides a compact summary of symptoms for schizophrenia and DID. The primary distinction between the two disorders is the nonpsychotic, nondelusional nature of identity alterations in the dissociative disorders (i.e., the patient's reality testing remains intact). Whereas schizophrenic subjects manifest evident mental decompensation and disintegration, subjects with DID retain a greater degree of mental compartmentalization and organization.

Identity alteration in schizophrenia can be either mild or moderate and usually accompanies psychotic episodes. Moreover, the type of identity alteration that characterizes schizophrenic subjects is less distinct than identity alterations in those with dissociative disorders (Steinberg et al. 1994). Although many schizophrenic patients hear voices emanating from other individuals (e.g., commands from supernatural or extraterrestrial beings) or machines (e.g., radios, tape decks), these auditory hallucinations are perceived as originating *outside* the body rather than from internal personalities. One patient with schizophrenia who was interviewed for the SCID-D field study reported the following:

> I thought that I was talking to Mr. and Mrs. God, and somebody else, and they gave me a new name, and I had to live up to that name. . . . It was "Chastity," and they were telling me what it meant, and I had to do that. . . . One time I thought I was Mrs. Santa Claus, things like that, it was not me. I thought I was Mrs. Santa Claus. I met this guy Lennie who was a ghost. I know it was not me. (SCID-D interview, unpublished transcript)

Table 11–2.   Review of symptoms in the context of schizophrenia and
dissociative identity disorder (DID)

Symptoms characteristic of schizophrenia	Overlapping symptoms potentially present in both schizophrenia and DID	Symptoms characteristic of DID
Usually isolated symptoms (none to mild–moderate ratings on the SCID-D). Symptoms occur in the context of bizarre delusions or other psychotic symptoms.	**Dissociative symptoms**	Recurrent to persistent dissociative symptoms (moderate to severe severity ratings on the SCID-D).
Lack of sense of identity and one's role in society.	**Identity confusion/ disturbance**	Recurrent and consistent alterations in one's identity.
Hallucinations other than the voices of alter personalities. These are perceived as occurring primarily outside the patient's head.	**Auditory hallucinations and internal dialogues**	Auditory hallucinations reflect dialogues between alter personalities. These voices are perceived as occurring inside the patient's head. Often described as similar to thoughts.
Bizarre delusions, paranoid delusions, and any other delusions that do not involve the other personalities, e.g., "The CIA is out to get me."	**Schneiderian symptoms and delusions**	Only delusions are "delusions of several personalities" or of other bodily changes representative of the different personalities
Thinking characterized by incoherence or marked loosening of associations.	**Other psychotic symptoms**	Absent in DID.
Catatonic behavior.		Absent in DID.
Chronic flat affect.		Absent in DID.
Impaired reality testing.	**Reality testing**	Intact reality testing; "as if" descriptions of dissociative symptoms are typical.
"If mood episodes have occurred during active-phase symptoms, their total duration has been brief relative to the duration of the active and residual periods" (DSM-IV, pp. 285–286).	**Comorbid diagnoses**	The full depressive or manic syndrome may coexist with the dissociative syndrome.
"One or more areas of functioning such as work, interpersonal relations, or self-care are markedly below the level achieved prior to the onset" (DSM-IV, p. 285).	**Impairment in functioning**	Any impairment in functioning is usually temporary,, with eventual full return to premorbid level of functioning.

(continued)

Table 11–2. Review of symptoms in the context of schizophrenia and dissociative identity disorder (DID) *(continued)*

Symptoms characteristic of schizophrenia	Overlapping symptoms potentially present in both schizophrenia and DID	Symptoms characteristic of DID
"Continuous signs of the disturbance for at least 6 months" (DSM-IV, p. 285).	**Course of symptoms and syndrome**	Signs of the disturbance may be intermittent. Rapid fluctuations in symptoms, mood, and degree of impairment may occur.

Note. Reprinted with permission from Steinberg M: *Interviewer's Guide to the Structured Clinical Interview for DSM-IV Dissociative Disorders (SCID-D), Revised.* Washington, DC, American Psychiatric Press, 1994, p. 51. Copyright 1994, Marlene Steinberg, M.D.

Another schizophrenic patient described that she was hearing voices from "the Lord" and "the Devil," respectively; she experienced the Devil's conversation as consisting of curses heaped upon her. The external quality of her voices is obvious in her comment that the Devil "put thoughts in" her head (SCID-D interview, unpublished transcript).

As was previously mentioned, there is usually a delusional context to identity alteration in the schizophrenic population, such as *folie de grandeur* (e.g., being in possession of blueprints for saving the world) or paranoid ideation of some kind (e.g., being spied on by the FBI). Identity alterations in schizophrenic subjects are typically relatively primitive, lacking the distinctness and complexity of the personalities manifested in people with DID. And although schizophrenic patients may experience auditory hallucinations, these hallucinations usually do not take the form of the ongoing internal dialogues that characterize identity alteration in people with DID. In addition, psychotic identity alteration may involve the assumption of mythical or celebrity identities; this is connected to the comparatively undeveloped quality of identity alteration in these patients. It is as if, by assuming the identity of a famous person, the schizophrenic subject has taken over a ready-made identity without the need to develop the full and coherent personality that the real celebrity possesses. In other words, a schizophrenic might claim to be Joe DiMaggio or Michael Jordan without having any of the personality traits of a professional athlete in general or of these men as individuals. By contrast, patients with DID manifest relatively well-developed alter personalities and usually coin distinctive names for them, such as "The Wise One," "The Nurse," or "The Commander." In this respect, the names that DID patients attach to their alters are similar to the names that people give to parts of themselves in some therapeutic exercises for getting in touch with their disowned capacities. Clinicians who are familiar with the work of Virginia Satir and the self-help literature influenced by her may recall instances in which patients were encouraged to give names to parts of their personalities to reintegrate these parts into their mature identity (Bradshaw 1988; Fishel 1987). This is, of course, not to suggest that inner parts therapy causes DID or other forms of dissociation; it is only to point out that DID has more in common with the splitting (or partial disowning) of personality that occurs in the general population than it does with schizophrenia. In cases of DID in which one of the alters does borrow the name or title of another, identifiably real, person, the relationship between the two is symbolic rather than one of identification.

A hypothetical example of this distinction as it pertains to differential diagnosis is included in Chapter 10 of this book. In some instances, the alter may assume the name of a mythical, biblical, or fictional character to underscore the symbolic nature of the reference. For example, Christine Sizemore's first therapists thought that two of her alters assumed the names "Eve White" and "Eve Black," respectively, to dramatize her conflicted sexual feelings. The split between the quiet and conventionally virtuous Eve White and the flirtatious and sexually provocative Eve Black could hardly be better demonstrated than by the choice of the first name. Eve is, after all, the archetypal biblical example of primordial femaleness, created innocent but vulnerable to temptation. In any case, the kind of symbol formation that may influence the naming of alters in DID has a demonstrably different clinical "feel" from the delusional borrowing of identity that characterizes schizophrenia.

▮ Identity Alteration in DID

Identity alteration, in its severe form, is the *sine qua non* of DID. In DID, identity alteration is characterized by its complexity, distinctness, the ability of the alters to take control of the patient's behavior, and interconnection with other dissociative symptoms. Patients with DID switch among their various identities, changing such markers of personality as speech patterns, clothing styles, handwriting, and sometimes even physical ailments such as headaches and allergies. There is no substitute for careful observation of these markers on the clinician's part. Although certain aspects of identity switching, such as dress styles or speech patterns, will not be evident as a *pattern* of identity alteration until the therapist has had a number of interviews with the patient, one should be aware from the outset of the importance of noting these external details and their potential significance. In particular, it is well to be aware of a commonplace tendency to overlook clothing as a marker of identity switching in female patients. Because of a widespread cultural assumption that experimenting with different clothing styles is an acceptably "feminine" form of self-expression, one may fail to register changes in a female patient's dress, accessories, and use or nonuse of cosmetics. In addition to clinical observation of the patient's external behaviors in assessing the presence and severity of identity alteration, the therapist will also need to gather information from other direct and indirect sources. A categorical summary of these sources follows.

Direct Sources of Information

The simplest way to obtain information concerning identity alteration is to ask the patient direct questions. The SCID-D contains a number of questions intended to elicit information that is *accessible to the patient's own memory* regarding name changes, perceptions of acting like a different person, visual images of alter personalities, and the presence of internal dialogues. If the patient endorses any of these symptoms, the interviewer can use the optional follow-up sections at the end of the SCID-D to obtain additional direct information. *Indirect* sources of information, which will be discussed later in this chapter, do not depend on the patient's memory for evidence of identity alteration. As a general rule in evaluating cases of DID, a patient's ability to remember an episode of identity alteration implies that there are fewer amnestic barriers between the different personalities.

Acting Like a Different Person

In most cases, a person experiencing severe identity alteration knows of this symptom primarily through reports from other people, but occasionally he or she will have a distinct memory of the transition. One male patient in the SCID-D field trials appeared to recall this type of experience:

> **Interviewer:** Have you ever acted as if you were a completely different person?
>
> **Patient:** Yeah, sure. In the trance I'm completely different.
>
> **Interviewer:** How do you act differently?
>
> **Patient:** Well, I do a lot of things I wouldn't normally do. I'll walk back and forth, I'll mutter, say stuff, I'll knock things over, bang into things, smash things. You know, I'm not the same person. I haven't harmed anyone, but I'm certainly different. (SCID-D interview, unpublished transcript)

Another patient remembered one occasion on which her identity switching involved a change in vocal pitch and dynamics:

> I can make a decision to do something and one or more people [her alters] won't like my decision; they will voice that very loudly so that somebody sitting there reacts and I feel like I am a jerk trying to cover up what they said loud, very loudly. . . . One time I made a decision not to go see the doctor 'cause it was snowing, the roads were horrendous, trucks couldn't move; I made the decision to call home. I went to the phone and called up and said, "I can't come because of the weather," and the doctor said, "Fine," and I went into the car and [the alter] started screaming that we had to go. And I said, "No, we don't

have to go," and then she started screaming and there was a man in a truck or car who looked. And his eyes caught my eyes and I realized that he could hear them. (SCID-D interview, unpublished transcript)

Clinicians should note that patients who are not amnestic for this particular symptom often react to it with anxiety. One patient reported that she had something like a "town meeting" from time to time with her alter personalities as a way of coping with the anxiety caused by personality switches:

Well, for example, if one of the kids mouthed off, say, and did something, you know, um, we'd all sit there and figure what we're going to do about it, and who was the best person to try to undo the damage that was done. Then we'd choose which personality was best to cope with the situation, and they'd go out and try to take care of it. (SCID-D interview, unpublished transcript)

Use of Different Names

The use of different names in direct self-reference suggests severe identity alteration because a name is a core element of personal identity. In many cultures, knowing a person's name represents having power over that person. Even in our own society, the importance of the personal name is indicated by major religious groups having rituals for the naming of a child, for example, or by the desire of many immigrants to take a new name as symbolic of their becoming citizens of the United States. Thus when a person in this society gives evidence of referring to him- or herself by a number of different names, the clinician should consider the presence of severe identity alteration. A typical instance of this symptom follows:

Interviewer: Have you ever referred to yourself by different names?

Patient: Yeah.

Interviewer: Would you feel comfortable sharing some of those names?

Patient: Um, yeah, I have the part that's called Eve and a part that's called Susan. I've integrated a part that was called Becky, I have a part called Alison, um, I have a part that's called Jane. (SCID-D interview, unpublished transcript)

In some cases, patients will associate the different names with particular behaviors or affects, as in the following excerpt of a woman with DID:

Interviewer: Do Andrea or Cindy or Jill ever take control of your behavior or your speech?

Patient: Oh yeah.

Interviewer: What's that like? How does that occur?

Patient: Um, I don't know how it occurs, but I go inside. Sally will have sex. Sally eats. Sally grocery shops. Sally has friends at the law school. Sally has had a relationship, a friendship, relationship with some junior professor from the law school. Um, things like that.

Interviewer: So when Sally is in control, you're more . . .

Patient: Andrea went to school, you know, went to college.

Interviewer: Cindy?

Patient: Cindy burned me.

Interviewer: What did she burn you with?

Patient: Kerosene and a cigarette lighter.

Interviewer: So each one has different things that they may like to do and be involved in and have different activities.

Patient: Yeah. (SCID-D interview, unpublished transcript)

People who do *not* have significant symptoms of identity alteration may respond to these particular SCID-D questions with descriptions of nicknames, aliases, or derogatory names, such as in this example:

Interviewer: Have you ever referred to yourself by different names?

Patient: No, but I hate my name.

Interviewer: Have other people referred to you by different names?

Patient: Well, of course my husband refers to me by derogatory names, like stupid and asshole, and words like that.

Interviewer: Other than that?

Interviewer: Other than that, no. (SCID-D interview, unpublished transcript)

However, as the previous excerpt shows, the interviewer should not overlook the possibility that the subject's description of derogatory names may indicate a history of verbal and/or psychological abuse by a spouse, relatives, or peer group members. As has been mentioned at other points in this book, the majority of persons with dissociative symptoms have experienced some form of trauma in childhood. Even when the subject's description of family names or nicknames does not indicate the presence of identity alteration per se, it may nonetheless suggest a history of abuse. For example, one of the patients in the SCID-D study had obviously been hurt by a nickname that originated from teasing by schoolmates:

Interviewer: Have other people ever called you by different names, or are these names more or less names that you have called yourself?

Patient: Yes. I had the nickname "Fishy" when I hung around with a street gang. I was called Fishy because I have a weak chin, so I was made fun of all the time. I was always called, "Hey, Fishy, Fishy, Fishy, Fishy." Even the girls started calling me Fishy all the time—"Hey, Fishy, how're you doing, Fishy?" And it hurt inside, I wanted to cry. But afterward I'd act macho and a tough guy and [say] "Good, how're you doing, man?," you know, and those things. I just wanted to cry, that's all. (SCID-D interview, unpublished transcript)

Another patient commented that her frequent amnestic episodes resulted in her parents and siblings tagging her with names like

"Space Case" and "Ditzy" (SCID-D interview, unpublished transcript).

It is also true that a patient's failure to endorse the use of different names on direct questioning may result from denial of the symptom. The possibility of denial must be ruled out via thorough interviewing, including the use of indirect evidence, as will be indicated later in the Indirect Sources of Information section.

Visual Images of Alter Personalities

In addition to the use of other names, one of the strongest indicators of severe identity alteration is the patient's reference to detailed visual images in describing internal alters. In the excerpt that follows, the patient presents some striking visual descriptions of her alter personalities, together with some of their other attributes (e.g., age, personality traits). Questions regarding visual images will often elicit descriptions of these other attributes:

Interviewer: Do you have a mental picture of Linda?

Patient: Fun. She looks like a teenager, fun person, fun on the bus. Fun in class, fun in school.

Interviewer: What about Lady Shadie?

Patient: Um, looks like somebody who is about ready to get their head creamed.

Interviewer: Frightened.

Patient: More defiant than frightened.

Interviewer: How old is she?

Patient: Fourteen, or 15, that is what she looks.

Interviewer: What does she look like?

Patient: She has her hair up in a French roll.

Interviewer: Does she look like you?

Patient: I think so.

Interviewer: At a younger age.

Patient: I think so.

Interviewer: Is it an image of you at a younger age?

Patient: I think so.

Patient: . . . I now have pictures of [Lucy] and she really looks like, she really looks closer to a saint than a devil.

Interviewer: What does she look like?

Patient: She sort of looks like a ghost. Like you can see through her. She, is not like a "person" person. She is tall, she looks like she could be 9 or 10 feet tall and capable of maybe getting larger and smaller, but she's huge, she's big. And she looks like the outline of the statue of the Virgin Mary with the flowing outfit. (SCID-D interview, unpublished transcript)

Another patient with DID described the visual images she had of the personalities inside her in the following way:

Interviewer: What does she [the personality] look like?

Patient: She wears jeans, she never wears a dress . . .

Interviewer: Does she look like Josie?

Patient: Yes, they look identical except that their manners and their clothing and their hair. . . . Josie's hair is curly with ribbons and Julie has braids and could care less what she looks like. She's tomboy looking.

Interviewer: Do they look like you?

Patient: I think they look like me. Without the glasses. They don't wear glasses . . .

Interviewer: Do you have an image of Diane?

Patient: Blonde hair, she looks older. (SCID-D interview, unpublished transcript)

In some instances the patient will have a visual image of a contrasexual alter. For example, one female patient endorsed the presence of two male alters with the same name, one a boy of about age 10 wearing a baseball cap and the other a slightly older but still aggressive adolescent. Because a patient's use of visual images provides rich evidence for the degree of identity alteration, each of the SCID-D's follow-up sections incorporates questions about visual images to allow the patient to elaborate on this symptom.

Particular Ages of Alter Personalities

Patients who ascribe specific ages to their alters are likely to be experiencing severe identity alteration. People in the general population, particularly those with strong moral convictions, may describe themselves as conversing with their conscience but would not ordinarily think of this internal monitor as being personified to the point of having a particular age. It is not at all unusual for patients with DID to describe their alters as covering a wide age range; some can be as young as infants, and others may be elderly. Often, the alter personalities represent the patient at different ages, including ages that the patient has not yet attained. The following is an excerpt from a patient with alters of many different ages:

Patient: Kitten is a teenager, I mean that's a child to me.

Interviewer: And Baby?

Patient: Baby's younger.

Interviewer: How old?

Patient: Somewhere between 6 and 11.

Interviewer: ... And Fred and Sal, how old are they?

Patient: Uh, Fred somewhere around 50, and Sal's in his late 20s ...

Interviewer: How old is Martha?

Patient: In her 30s. (SCID-D interview, unpublished transcript)

In addition, some persons with DID report the presence of dead alters. For example, the Portuguese poet Fernando Pessoa once described one of his parts as having been born in 1889 and dying in 1915. Later, he maintained that this supposedly dead person published a book of poetry in 1919. Although the phenomenon of dead alters is often startling to clinicians, and has not yet received much systematic attention from researchers, it has a variety of possible meanings and must be interpreted on an individual basis. Some possible meanings could be that the alter represents that the patient was abused in the past and had to "play dead" to avoid attracting the attention of the abusive parent, or that the dead alter represents an extremely depersonalized aspect of the patient.

Lastly, some DID patients do report the presence of alters who represent internal helpers, guides, or counselors, and are described as ageless or timeless rather than having a specific age. Putnam (1989a) regards this type of "guru" alter as analogous to the *observing ego function* in non-DID patients. Some patients may describe an alter of this type in religious terms or categories. For example, Mayer (1988) cites the case history of a Jewish patient who had a trinity of Christian angels as her internal ageless alter. These figures emerged when the therapist asked his patient about the presence of an inner helper:

> "Who are you?" I asked, amazed that I was maintaining my calm.
> "We are the Dark Ones."
> We? I started to question them carefully. They were not a part of Toby, they claimed. Rather, they said they were sent by the Archangel Michael to help her. They claimed that there were three of them, interchangeable but different, and that they spoke as one. They often paused, as if they were consulting one another. They kept themselves "cloaked" from the other personalities, they said, for fear they would scare them. They were, to use their own description, "awesome." (Mayer 1988, p. 87)

Other patients may describe an ageless alter with references to science fiction or parapsychology. Glass (1993) discusses a patient who had a timeless alter named for a star; this contrasexual alter compared himself to a character in a popular science fiction TV series.

Indirect Sources of Information

The preceding sections have discussed aspects of severe identity alteration in which the patient's own memory can assist the interviewer. However, many patients who manifest severe identity disturbances are unaware of the external manifestations of these disturbances; consequently, the relevant information must be retrieved by indirect questioning. Lack of awareness of identity alteration is usually due to amnestic barriers between the different personalities. Although the format of the SCID-D was designed to elicit reports of identity alteration, it does not encourage descriptions of identity alteration from people who do not have that specific symptom. The open-ended nature of the SCID-D's questions, as well as its assessment of a cluster of dissociative symptoms that typically occur together, is intended to minimize the chances of a patient's confabulation. Indirect sources of information for identity alteration involve feedback from the environment that the patient may have received. He or she may be aware of the manifestations themselves but unaware of their connection with identity alteration. Indirect evidence includes reports from friends and relatives regarding behavior that has confused or upset them as well as the presence of objects or materials in the patient's possession that were acquired under the influence of an alter personality.

Difficulties in Personal Attribution

The use of indirect environmental evidence in clinical assessment is crucial to the establishment of accurate diagnosis of DID because of patients' difficulties with personal attribution. It is not uncommon for a patient to respond negatively to question 118: "Have you ever referred to yourself by different names?" and then refer later in the interview to alter personalities by name. This type of intra-interview inconsistency may occur if the person switches personalities during the interview. The patient may disavow or be amnestic for the activities or existence of particular alters. In the example that follows, the patient initially replies in the negative to a question about identity alteration and then changes her response when the question is re-addressed to her alter personalities and not just to her:

Interviewer: Have you ever experienced rapid changes in your capabilities, or ability to function?

Patient: I don't think so. No. Not in the way that I think you're asking.

Interviewer: Let me put it another way. For instance, does Melanie, do you have different capabilities than Carol, for instance?

Patient: Oh yeah. Yeah. (SCID-D interview, unpublished transcript)

Clinicians should also be aware that many patients are quite defensive about a possible diagnosis of DID because they feel stigmatized by it, and so may react with irritation or anxiety when the interviewer inquires about sudden mood changes or other possible indications of DID. One patient in the SCID-D study made comments in the context of the interviewer's questioning about unexplained purchases that indicated considerable defensiveness:

Interviewer: How do you understand how you happen to have these certain things that you don't remember purchasing?

Patient: I can sit and I can listen to somebody like you, OK, and you can sit there and tell me something about being, like having a split personality . . . to me that's being, um, totally imperfect, and if I had to sit there and listen to you and believe you, then I couldn't survive. You know what I'm saying? It's not something that I can accept or deal with. . . . Speaking of that, I had to go to a, um, an appointment at Harrisburg Hospital . . . the doctor's name was Dr. Weisskopf . . . and he sat there, I thought he was getting extremely frustrated trying to explain the situation to me about, um, multiple personalities, and he's sitting there insisting that that was what my problem was and that unless you, um, believe it or accept it, you know, you can't be cured. It's like having a doctor tell you you're dying, but you feel perfectly well. You know what I mean?

Interviewer: It must be very confusing.

Patient: Just because this guy is supposed to have a degree and he has no obvious reason for telling me something that wouldn't be true, but there's a point of whether you accept it or not, and I choose not to. (SCID-D interview, unpublished transcript)

Unexplained Purchases/Possessions

The discovery of items in one's possession that one cannot recall having bought, received as gifts, or otherwise acquired is a characteristic experience for patients with DID. It is also indirect evidence of severe identity alteration. Question 122 asks, "Have you ever found things in your possession (e.g., shoes) which seemed to belong to you, but you could not remember how you got them?" Objects that have been acquired by one personality will often seem strange to another alter if there is an amnestic barrier between the two personalities. The most common items that patients mention in this category are clothes and similar personal belongings (e.g., jewelry, toiletries, combs, handbags). It is possible that alter personalities are more likely to notice unexplained objects that are associated with dress or personal grooming (as opposed to general household supplies, office supplies, and the like) because people often regard these items as extensions or expressions of their personality. For example, one patient clearly noticed the presence of "strange" accessories in her closet because they represented a certain kind of taste in clothing that was alien to her dominant personality:

Interviewer: Have you ever found things in your possession which seemed to belong to you, but you could not remember how you got them?

Patient: Yes [in the past] . . .

Interviewer: Would that have been a daily or weekly experience?

Patient: Weekly. Like I'd go shopping. I'd buy things. I'd remember that I'd purchased it. I had the receipt. So I know I didn't steal it or something. But why I bought it, where I bought it . . . I buy things that I don't even wear . . . wouldn't be caught dead wearing. Totally strange items . . . a thousand scarves, ponchos, and shawls. And I've never worn one of them. But I have a whole mess of them. It's like none to my knowledge. My mom says I wear them a lot, but I don't know of ever wearing one of them. It's odd. (SCID-D interview, unpublished transcript)

Another patient with DID in the SCID-D study commented not only about the presence of jewelry and minor purchases in her house that did not suit her but also about the mysterious acquisition of a car:

Interviewer: Have you ever found things that obviously belong to you, but that you didn't remember buying or bringing home?

Patient: I bought a Toyota.

Interviewer: What?

Patient: I have a Toyota, a 1990 Toyota that I don't know how I purchased it or where it came from.

Interviewer: Do you own it? I mean, is your name . . .

Patient: On the registration, yes [laughs]. That's a nice present. I mean I love it. It's great.

Interviewer: Are there other things that you find that belong to you that you don't remember?

Patient: Well, yeah . . . jewelry. I mean I have clothes like in my closet that I wouldn't be caught dead in. I have like a ton of silver jewelry and I hate silver. I like gold and I have like a lot of silver, a lot of American Indian pieces and stuff like that. I'm not too into jewelry. I have a lot of things, like a china teacup collection, and I mean I don't believe in collecting things; they collect dust. They're all over. But I keep them. You know, it's not like I go get rid of them. I don't know what to do with them. (SCID-D interview, unpublished transcript)

In another case study of multiple personality, a patient whose primary personality was "neat, timid, and prudish," reported to her therapist that "she would find a number of skimpy, sexy bathing suits in her closet which her husband stated she insisted he buy for her, along with clothes that were too tight and short" (Confer and Ables 1983, p. 51). It should be added that, although an interest in different styles or fashions is usually considered a feminine characteristic, male patients also sometimes endorse having made unexplained clothing purchases, as in the following example of a man who was diagnosed as having dissociative disorder not otherwise specified (DDNOS):

Interviewer: Do you ever find things, let's say, in your closet that you can't recall buying, but they are obviously yours?

Patient: Hmm [pauses]. Yeah [laughs]. I bought two shirts at Sears, put them in my closet and a week later said, "How the hell did you get here, man? I don't remember buying these things." Then the bill came and it was quite obvious my name was on it; I did buy it.

Interviewer: I see. And you can't remember buying them?

Patient: And I didn't remember buying them. (SCID-D interview, unpublished transcript)

Clinicians should be aware that the type of unexplained possession that is characteristic of dissociative identity alteration is qualitatively different from that which characterizes most cases of compulsive spending or compulsive shopping. These so-called shopaholics are essentially people who use shopping as a form of mood alteration; many of them will describe themselves as surprised by the contents of their closets when they are forced by some circumstance (usually because of financial problems or confrontations with family members) to recognize that they have a compulsive disorder. However, the shock or surprise has to do with the quantity and duplication of objects purchased or the total amount of money that has been spent, not with the style or nature of the items. Although there is some overlap between the dissociative population and people with compulsive disorders—as was explained at the beginning of this chapter—in that some people with DID can have alter personalities who are shopaholics, the disorders as such are not identical. One patient interviewed in the SCID-D study mentioned the presence of a shopaholic alter— "Somebody in there likes to go shopping"—but added, "We try to keep that one under control" (SCID-D interview, unpublished transcript).

Unexplained Changes in Literary/Linguistic Abilities or Training

Another manifestation of severe identity alteration that frequently startles or upsets patients is written evidence of some kind (e.g., letters, notebooks, diaries) for the presence of alter personalities. This category of indirect information for identity alteration includes a variety of items, ranging from documents written in different scripts to poetry or prose written in a language that the patient cannot recall having studied. One patient in the SCID-D field study, diagnosed as having DID, found troubling evidence of identity alteration in her diary:

> **Patient:** In my diary, you can see. I had things that happened during the day, and it was like a conversation or something with two different handwritings and people arguing. And it's like *I* wrote this. I don't remember writing it. But it was like an argument. You know, it's plain view, you read it, and it's like, what's going on, you know? . . . I was going out with a couple of guys at the same time, and it's like this one doesn't like this one, this one doesn't like that one. They go back and forth arguing about which guy. It's like, this one hates this class and that one, it's like totally weird. But I know I wrote it. I must have. It was my diary. No one else knew about my diary.
>
> **Interviewer:** Do you still keep a diary?
>
> **Patient:** No. It got too confusing, I didn't like reading it. (SCID-D interview, unpublished transcript)

One manifestation of DID in childhood is inexplicable variations in school performance. Kluft (1984b) notes that a history of irregular school performance, including sudden failure or amnesia for material in a good student (or the reverse), or the child's sense that the rest of the class has been taught something that he or she has not, raises the index of suspicion for DID. One DID subject recalled a fluctuating level of academic ability during her school years:

> **Interviewer:** Have you ever experienced rapid changes in your ability to function? . . . Can you give me an example of some?

Patient: When I was younger, tests, I would take tests and . . . I didn't know where the answers were coming from, but they would come; and then at other times I wouldn't be able to do it at all.

Interviewer: It would be the same course all the time?

Patient: Oh no.

Interviewer: Different courses.

Patient: Yeah. I would get an A in math, and then I would get the exam and I wouldn't be able to tell you how I got that A. (SCID-D interview, unpublished transcript)

Though a patient may be amnestic for an episode of identity alteration, and thus be consciously unaware of her illness, finding written artifacts provides a clue to the true situation. In a similar episode, another patient with DID received a publication in the mail that she had written yet initially failed to recognize as hers:

Interviewer: Have you ever found things in your possession that seemed to belong to you but you could not remember how you got them?

Patient: Um, did I tell you about the books? About a month ago, or a month and a half ago, I got in the mail an envelope, and it was author's copies of this pamphlet with my name as the author, and I didn't remember *anything* about having written this pamphlet. And I was really upset and I took it home and read it and sure enough it was my style . . . but I had a chapter in there about miscarriage, and I know that when I wrote it I said, "Hmm, I wonder if they're gonna think this is too intimate" and toss it out. And when I saw the word *miscarriage* in there I realized, yes, I did write this book. (SCID-D interview, unpublished transcript)

When DID patients are multilingual, some of their alters may manifest as personalities who can speak only one language or who are fluent in a language that the primary personality claims not to know. Fernando Pessoa, for example, developed two subpersonalities in childhood, the "Chevalier de Pas," who spoke only French, and "Alexander Search," who wrote poetry only in English. Pessoa kept a journal in which he noted experiences such as the following:

> Once again, I have found something of mine, written in French, over which fifteen years must have flown now. I've never been to France, never dealt face-to-face with the French, never, therefore, exercised that language in which I had ceased to be fluent. Today I read as much French as ever . . . [but] the French in that passage from my distant past possesses a confidence which today I do not possess. The style is fluid, but in a way I could never be today in that language, with entire passages, complete sentences, forms and modes of expression that demonstrate a control over that language that I lost without ever remembering I had it. How is it possible to explain that? Whom did I substitute inside myself? . . . At other times I have found things I've written that I don't remember having written—which is shocking—things I don't even remember being capable of writing—and that does frighten me. (Pessoa 1991, p. 16)

What comes through very clearly in this journal entry is the silent suffering that severe identity alteration inflicts on people with dissociative disorders. In some cases, one of a patient's alters may concoct a private language, and the patient's anxiety is focused on the problems that arise when the alter allows the private language to slip out. A well-known autobiographical account of a dissociative illness includes an episode of this sort:

> . . . her name became Januce, because she felt like two-faced Janus—with a face on each world. It had been her letting slip this name which had caused the first trouble in school. She had been living by the Secret Calendar . . . and had returned to the Heavy Calendar in the middle of the day, and having then that wonderful and omniscient feeling of changing, she had headed a class paper: NOW JANUCE. The teacher had said, "Deborah, what is this mark on your paper? What is this word, Januce?" And, as the teacher stood by her desk, some nightmare terror coming to life had risen in the day-sane schoolroom. . . . The mark on the paper was the emblem of coming from Yr's time to Earth's, but, being caught while still in transition, she had to

answer for both of them. Such an answer would have been the unveiling of a horror—a horror from which she would not have awakened rationally; and so she had lied and dissembled, with her heart choking her. (Green 1964, p. 20)

It is true that the discovery of a document written by an alter does occasionally allow a patient to retrieve memories rather than remaining completely amnestic. However, in the majority of cases, the person with DID simply concludes that they must be insane:

Patient: There used to be notes of stuff that I would find, and once in a while I would see a name. But I used to find notes, and tracings, and scrawlings. I used to doodle a lot and I always attributed it to that. And anyway, crazy people do those kinds of things. So when I thought I was crazy, it seemed perfectly OK.

Interviewer: So initially you thought that was just something that made no sense whatsoever, what you were doing.

Patient: Oh yeah. (SCID-D interview, unpublished transcript)

As a result of the tendency of patients and observers to judge symptoms of severe identity alteration very negatively, clinicians should be careful not to confuse these indicators with the symptoms of psychosis. The follow-up sections in the SCID-D for "Different Names" and "Different Person" are designed to aid in assessment and evaluation of documentary evidence of identity alteration.

Observations by Other People

Information that the patient has obtained from other people is a very important indirect source for the assessment of identity alteration. The following patient in the SCID-D field study only became aware of her alter personalities because of feedback from friends:

Sarah is vicious and Terry is mean. This sounds really stupid. Frank, my friend, told me, "Just let me know when Sarah arrives. She has a black belt in karate and I don't want to deal with it." I mean, how can your friend tell you that you have a black belt, and I don't even know karate? I'm not very athletic either. (SCID-D interview, unpublished transcript)

Another patient reported that a friend had remarked on her alters' speaking in different American regional accents:

Patient: One of my friends who is really into linguistics could tell exactly . . . where in my past I was thinking about by the accent I used.

Interviewer: How would your speech vary?

Patient: Well, varying from a Bostonian accent, which was the children, and the accent of me when I was a child. I sometimes spoke like California where I went to college and stuff like that. (SCID-D interview, unpublished transcript)

Questions regarding evidence of identity alteration supplied by others in the patient's life can help the therapist with the issue of personal attribution, insofar as changes in behavior or demeanor are usually noticed by people in the patient's social circle or family. Their feedback often provides clues to the magnitude of the symptom, as the following excerpt indicates:

Interviewer: Have you ever been told by other people that you seem like a different person?

Patient: Yes. Guys that I've dated, my family, people that I work with.

Interviewer: Do you know what they've meant by that?

Patient: Well some of them even said that, it's like, different ways, different opinions . . . my opinion might change right in the middle of a conversation. One way definitely over here, and then the next time, just within seconds, over here. . . . They'll make reference to the way in which I behaved. Something I did which didn't seem like what they knew of me.

Interviewer: What would they say?

Patient: Drinking, if I had a drink. Because I don't drink. I rarely ever drink. Or eating certain foods, the way in which I talk.

> Being extremely friendly as opposed to being somewhat quiet
> and withdrawn. (SCID-D interview, unpublished transcript)

In some instances, particularly when the person suffering from
identity alteration is a child or adolescent, family feedback may be
harsh and punitive. Many young people who have dissociative
disorders find themselves repeatedly punished for behavior they
cannot recall, let alone understand. Kluft (1985b) lists "being called
a liar" and "disavowed witnessed behavior" as indicators of childhood DID. The following excerpt from Hannah Green's (1964) account of her adolescent illness contains some vivid examples of
these mystifying accusations:

> But every time mere dislike turned to active anger or hate, I
> never knew why. People would come to me and say, ". . . after
> what you did, . . ." or ". . . after what you said, . . . even I won't
> defend you any more. . . ." I never knew what it was that I had
> done or said. The maids in our house left one after another, until
> it was like a continuous procession, and I kept having to "apolo-
> gize," but I never knew for what or why. Once I greeted my best
> friend and she turned from me. When I asked why, she said,
> "After what you did?" She never spoke to me again, and I never
> found out what had happened. (p. 69)

One of the patients in the SCID-D study reported similar episodes
from her childhood:

> **Interviewer:** Can you give any examples of what you might have
> been told you did that you didn't have memory of or that you
> realized you did?
>
> **Patient:** Constantly. I mean, throughout my . . . you know, from the
> time I was a kid I was always being yelled at and getting in
> trouble for stuff I hadn't done and I didn't know who had
> done it. (SCID-D interview, unpublished transcript)

Consequently, clinicians should note that feedback from others in
the patient's life may be more than a source of diagnostically relevant information; it may also represent an element of emotional

trauma in the patient's history. Some patients may react with anger or annoyance to feedback from others, believing that their friends or relatives are playing a very unfunny game with them, or "gaslighting" them (i.e., invalidating their perceptions in order to cause them to doubt their sanity; named for an Ingrid Bergman film of the 1940s), as in the following example:

Interviewer: So what have other people told you?

Patient: I don't know what you want me to say. You know, I don't keep a list of them. If I kept a list of them. . . . I have a friend who sat there and said, he keeps a list, and like his list has . . . he started reading names off. It's like 22 names, and I'm like, and he's saying, "No, really, this is the truth," you know, and I'm like [sighs], you begin to wonder who your friends are.

Interviewer: Are you saying that other people have told you that you're using different names and what do the other people say?

Patient: Well, they don't really say that I'm using different names, but they said, "Yesterday your name was Renee," or you know, whatever, and "Your hair was done in a punk style," and you know, it's like a big joke, a joke that I don't find amusing.

Interviewer: So do you think they are teasing you?

Patient: Well, I have two choices. OK. I mean they are my friends, but I have two choices. I can either choose to believe they're pulling my leg or I can choose to believe I'm nuts. (SCID-D interview, unpublished transcript)

With regard to the particular problem of name changes, patients' friends and colleagues may be the only source of information that they are answering to a variety of different names. In patients whose alter personalities are amnestic with regard to one another, the primary personality may be completely oblivious to name changes. The following excerpt indicates how confusing the situation can become:

Other people tell me that, you know, "You're using this name," and I'd say, "No I wasn't!" and they'd say, "Yes you were." And it was funny cause I used to do that . . . in grammar school; they would tell me, kids would tell me, "Oh, you're name is Shelly," or this, and they'd tease me about it because I used that name or whatever. And I'd say "No it's not, my name's Denise!" and I'd argue back and forth with them. And when I went to high school, I was with totally new kids. And then, you know, I didn't even have any of the people that I used to hang around with, that would know me as whatever the names were, and they'd turn around and say "Why are you calling yourself this name?" And it would be freaky to me, cause it's like, "What do you mean?" Because I didn't do it, you know, I didn't remember doing it. I had no idea that I was using different names, or acting differently or anything else. That's when I realized there was something to it, more than they were just teasing me, because, you know, how would they know those names? (SCID-D interview, unpublished transcript)

It is not unusual for patients with DID to meet people and form relationships while they are under the influence of alter personalities; these relationships are often kept separate from those of the primary personality. The following patient occasionally meets people that she knows only through a specific alter. She finds herself in awkward situations when one of her alter's acquaintances addresses her by the wrong name.

Interviewer: Have you ever referred to yourself by different names?

Patient: Yeah.

Interviewer: What names did you refer to yourself by?

Patient: Um, Susan, Becky, Eve, Jeanne, Alison, and Betsy.

Interviewer: Have other people referred to you by some of these different names?

Patient: Yeah.

Interviewer: Are some of those nicknames? How did you get those names?

Patient: I haven't the slightest idea.

Interviewer: Who would call you by those other names?

Patient: Um, I've been in places where people have called me by those names, but I cannot tell you who they are. Um, I've gotten phone calls from people and I'll always say, "No, you have the wrong number." It wasn't until therapy that I realized that these people do *not* have the wrong number. I have gone over to the medical center and have had people call me and I don't know who they are. . . . They'll come up and say "Hi, Eve," and I just pretend that I know exactly what they're talking about. In fact I was on a skiing trip in Vermont, and somebody came up to me and said, "Hi, Alison," and I had pretended I knew exactly who they were, and I haven't the slightest idea who they were. (SCID-D interview, unpublished transcript)

Again, it is important for therapists to be sensitive to the distress that symptoms of severe identity alteration inflict on those experiencing them. Whereas some of the potential consequences of separate friendship or acquaintanceship circles are only a matter of temporary social embarrassment, others are much more serious. Some patients may be concerned about the possibility of having violated their moral standards or ideals during the period of an alter's emergence and control. For example, one patient in the SCID-D study mentioned her concern that she might have shoplifted some drugstore items that she found in her possession with no apparent explanation:

Interviewer: What sorts of things have you found in your closet?

Patient: Well, shirts, blouses, pretty blouses, um, jeans, dresses and shoes, sandals. And then there's personal items, things like, um, shampoo and stuff like that. Like one day I went home and I found a whole bag of stuff from Rite-Aid, all kinds of things that I could use and I didn't know where they were from. This happened about a year ago.

Interviewer: So they were things that you were able to use and so you used them.

> **Patient:** Um hmm. I felt kind of guilty using them, though, like what happens if I stole them or something? (SCID-D interview, unpublished transcript)

Lastly, female patients may express some anxiety about the possibility of having met or formed a relationship with a dangerous or predatory individual while under the influence of an alter personality. Although the probability of any one particular individual's being victimized by a psychopath is relatively low, the rising rate of crimes against women in our society is not a subject for complacency. It may well surface as a factor contributing to a patient's overall anxiety level. It is not uncommon for hostile alters to "set up" the host personality for a compromising and potentially dangerous situation with a stranger. As Putnam (1989a) has remarked, persecutor alters may place a patient in debt, alienate the patient's friends by obnoxious or irresponsible behavior, or place the patient in a situation in which rape or physical violence at the hands of a stranger is likely.

PART III

Clinical Applications

CHAPTER 12

Differential Diagnosis of the Dissociative Disorders

I wander with my thoughts and I'm sure that what I'm writing now I already wrote. I remember . . . My God, my God, whose performance am I watching? How many people am I? Who am I? What is this space between myself and myself?

—Fernando Pessoa, *The Book of Disquiet*

■ The Five Dissociative Disorders

The dissociative disorders are a circumscribed set of syndromes that are grouped together by DSM-IV (American Psychiatric Association 1994). These disorders include dissociative amnesia, dissociative fugue, depersonalization disorder, dissociative identity disorder (DID), and dissociative disorder not otherwise specified (DDNOS). Because recent research indicates that the dissociative disorders occur more frequently in the patient population than was previously recognized, it is more important than ever that clinicians be familiar with these disorders and their diagnostic criteria. The primary distinguishing feature of the dissociative disorders, eloquently expressed in Pessoa's words above, is a fragmentation of consciousness manifested in a variety of ways, including memory loss and feelings of detachment from self and surroundings. (The reader may consult the figures in each of the following subsections for summaries of DSM-IV's criteria for these disorders.) DSM-IV (American Psychiatric Association 1994) defines the dissociative disorders in the following way:

The essential feature of the Dissociative Disorders is a disruption in the usually integrated functions of consciousness, memory, identity, or perception of the environment. The disturbance may be sudden or gradual, and transient or chronic. (p. 477)

Because the dissociative disorders were once thought to be comparatively unusual in both the general and the psychiatric population, most practitioners thought of these syndromes as a diagnosis of last resort for florid or spectacular cases. This stereotype has unfortunately been reinforced by dramatizations of a few well-known cases by the mass media, such as the movie versions of *Sybil* (Schreiber 1973) and *The Three Faces of Eve* (Thigpen and Cleckley 1957). As a result, clinicians frequently overlook or misdiagnose less colorful presentations of the dissociative disorders (Kluft 1985a, 1985c). The majority of cases do in fact fall into this category. Consequently, there has been little clinical awareness of the need to screen the general psychiatric population for the presence of dissociative pathology.

Differential diagnosis is a painstaking process in the dissociative disorders because of some complicating factors: 1) an overlap of symptoms, 2) the variable presentations of the disorders, 3) the fact that none of these disorders is commonly the patient's presenting complaint (Kluft 1984a; Putnam et al. 1986), 4) frequent comorbidity with substance addictions and other compulsive disorders, and 5) difficulties in precise description of dissociative symptoms. Some of the symptoms of dissociative pathology are difficult to put into words, even for highly educated and articulate patients. In spite of the importance of careful diagnosis, at present few medical professionals routinely take a history of dissociative symptoms as part of an intake interview. However, amnesia, fugue, derealization, and depersonalization may occur as secondary, isolated dissociative symptoms within a wide variety of major psychiatric disorders. Complications in diagnostic evaluation due to the additional presence of addictions or compulsive disorders have already been mentioned. In addition, the close connection between the dissociative disorders and severe trauma, child abuse, or incest may also complicate assessment because patients may deny or be amnestic for these stressors (Kluft 1987c; Putnam 1985; Stern 1984; Wilbur 1984a). Fluctuations in the data available on incest, physical abuse, neglect, and emotional abuse of children (Ellerstein and Canavan 1980; Emslie and Rosenfelt 1983; Gelinas 1983; Husain and Chapel 1983; Krener 1985; Sansonnet-Hayden et al. 1987) directly affect the accuracy of histories taken in connection with the diagnosis of the dissociative disorders. Histories of abuse have been noted in 82%–98% of all reported cases of the dissociative disorders (Coons et al. 1988; Kluft 1988a; 1991; Putnam et al. 1986; Schultz et al. 1989) and are currently noted in 50%–75% of psychiatric patients (Ellerstein and Canavan 1980; Emslie and Rosenfelt 1983; Husain and Chapel 1983; Myers 1991; Sansonnet-Hayden et al. 1987). It is not known whether this high percentage is due to clinicians' increased awareness or to a rising rate of occurrence. One researcher observes that "in incest victims who consciously use dissociative phenomena in the service of defense, the tendency toward dissociation under stress continues" (Gelinas 1983). Lastly, of course, the observant professional will note that histories of trauma also predispose survivors to various forms of substance abuse and compulsive behaviors that may well overlap with dissociative symptomatology. It cannot be stressed too often that patients who endorse a history of abuse and/or a history of substance addictions or compulsive disorders during an intake interview should be screened for the presence of dissociative symptoms as well.

Clinical assessment of the five dissociative disorders involves consideration of the patient's manifest symptoms as well as determination of their underlying patterns. Each disorder manifests a variety of dissociative symptoms to some degree. Each is also characterized by a predominant symptom or specific symptom constellation, such as amnesia in dissociative amnesia and fugue and depersonalization in depersonalization disorder.

The particular constellations of symptoms in each dissociative disorder constitute symptom profiles that can be plotted visually. Figures 12–1 through 12–4 in the sections that follow indicate the symptom profiles for each of the five dissociative disorders. Each dissociative symptom is evaluated according to severity from a low severity of 1 (none) to a high severity of 4 (severe).

Dissociative Amnesia

Dissociative amnesia is the most common of the dissociative disorders and is regularly encountered by emergency room personnel (Nemiah 1985). It is typified by an inability to recall important personal information, usually of a traumatic or stressful nature (American Psychiatric Association 1994). To meet DSM-IV criteria, 1) the amnesia must be too extensive to be accounted for by ordinary forgetfulness; 2) it must not occur exclusively during the course of DID, dissociative fugue, posttraumatic stress disorder (PTSD), acute stress disorder, or somatization disorder, or due to the effects of a substance or a general medical condition; and 3) it must cause significant impairment in functioning (see Table 12–1). Dissociative amnesia is often seen in combat veterans, members of high-stress occupations such as police officers and firefighters, and in the victims of single severe traumas such as transportation accidents, natural disasters, or sexual assault. For example, an air force chaplain ministering to survivors of a civilian plane crash noted that a businessman who had come to the airport to identify his dead wife's effects could not remember his own address or telephone number without the help of the airline agent's registration

---

Table 12–1. DSM-IV criteria for dissociative amnesia

A. The predominant disturbance is one or more episodes of inability to recall important personal information, usually of a traumatic or stressful nature, that is too extensive to be explained by ordinary forgetfulness.
B. The disturbance does not occur exclusively during the course of Dissociative Identity Disorder, Dissociative Fugue, Posttraumatic Stress Disorder, Acute Stress Disorder, or Somatization Disorder and is not due to the direct effects of a substance (e.g., a drug of abuse, a medication) or a neurological or other general medical condition (e.g., Amnestic Disorder due to head trauma).
C. The symptoms cause clinically significant distress or impairment in social, occupational, or other important areas of functioning.

Source. Reprinted with permission from American Psychiatric Association: *Diagnostic and Statistical Manual of Mental Disorders*, 4th Edition. Washington, DC, American Psychiatric Association, 1994. Copyright 1994, American Psychiatric Association.

list (Hicks 1993). This syndrome may also occur in some people as a defense against guilt (i.e., the amnesia may follow an action that the patient considers morally repellent).

Because dissociative amnesia may be subtle or have features in common with amnesia of organic etiology, its presence may be easily overlooked (Coons and Milstein 1992; Loewenstein 1991). In a study (Kiersch 1962) conducted at two general military hospitals, the researchers carefully reviewed all cases of amnesia in the patient population and found that 20% were of dissociative origin. They described most of the cases in this group as "classical psychogenic dissociative or fugue-like state." In another example, an investigation (Kirshner 1973) of 1,795 consecutive psychiatric admissions to Wright-Patterson Air Force Medical Center between 1968 and 1970 indicated that 1.3% of all patients had dissociative episodes accompanied by varying degrees of amnesia and/or fugues leading to their admission.

Dissociative amnesia is usually marked by sudden onset (American Psychiatric Association 1987), and the patient is usually aware of his or her loss of memory. Unlike DID, in which amnestic episodes may be chronic and recurrent, dissociative amnesia typically resolves as suddenly as it manifests. The precipitating trauma for dissociative amnesia is more commonly a single psychosocial stressor, in contrast to DID, whose antecedents usually include ongoing, severe abuse or trauma. To compare dissociative with organic amnesia, patients suffering from dissociative amnesia frequently fail to recall their own name. In organic amnesia, the personal name is usually the last item to be lost, and the patient rarely recovers memory fully. Abrupt and full return of memory suggests dissociative amnesia. Lastly, dissociative amnesia has a low rate of recurrence.

Differential Diagnosis of Dissociative Amnesia

The reader should note that the SCID-D's (Steinberg 1993b) assessment of the five dissociative symptoms allows for accuracy in differential diagnosis. Dissociative amnesia is marked by amnesia in the absence of significant depersonalization, derealization, identity confusion, or identity alteration, and in the absence of organic etiology. If any of the other four dissociative symptoms are present to a significant degree, the diagnosis of dissociative amnesia should be excluded (see Figure 12–1).

The amnesia characteristic of dissociative amnesia has several distinctive features: 1) abrupt onset, 2) presence of severe stress prior to onset, and 3) abrupt termination with full recovery and rare recurrences. If a patient experiences *recurrent* amnestic episodes, one should rule out the presence of another dissociative disorder such as DID and DDNOS.

Dissociative amnesia is usually associated with frustration and dysfunction. A male patient in the SCID-D field study presented with a severe case of dissociative amnesia: One day he had fallen to the ground and was taken to the emergency room by his wife. He was evaluated for organic problems, his medical workup was negative, and yet he could not remember his name or recognize his wife. He had no recall of any events prior to June 1990 and was

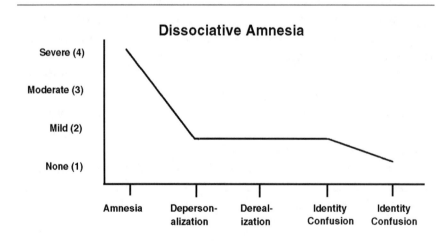

Figure 12–1. SCID-D symptom profile of dissociative amnesia.
Source. Reprinted with permission from Steinberg M: *Interviewer's Guide to the Structured Clinical Interview of DSM-IV Dissociative Disorders (SCID-D), Revised.* Washington, DC, American Psychiatric Press, 1994. Copyright © 1994, Marlene Steinberg, M.D.

thereupon briefly hospitalized. At the time of the SCID-D interview, he was in outpatient therapy. The following excerpts illustrate some of the distinctive features of dissociative amnesia:

Interviewer: What led to your stopping work?

Patient: I had a . . . I don't know if you really want to call it a seizure . . . I fainted, like I fainted. When I woke up, when I got to the hospital I lost all recall, memory, that I had, of the previous 42 years that I had lived. And the only thing I remembered was the dog. And the four kids.

Interviewer: . . . What did they say when they took you to the hospital at that time? What did they find?

Patient: I don't think they found really anything, physically. I was OK. I just kind of dropped out of sight. Mentally. Big time. You know.

Interviewer: So you lost memory for your whole past?

Patient: I lost it all. Most of it. I'd say 98% of it anyway. And I was still shaky, but I went home. What would be called home, if I remembered. . . . Every time you see somebody that you used to know, or someone talks about the past, or, "Do you remember this guy?" "Do you remember that guy?" Even TV people, songs. It's loaded. 'Cause everything's in there. . . . After June I was being told certain things, what I was doing, where I was living, who I was, basically what I was. You know all kinds of things that I didn't know. . . .

Interviewer: Prior to June of '90, did you ever have a similar experience in which you had trouble with your memory that you were aware of?

Patient: I don't remember. (SCID-D interview, unpublished transcript)

One feature of amnesia that emerges quite clearly in this citation is its elusive, "black hole" quality. When asked about episodes of amnesia in the past, the patient answered, "I don't remember." He then proceeded to describe the anxiety and dysfunctionality associated with global amnesia.

If a patient with dissociative amnesia later proves to manifest severe identity confusion and alteration, one would want to rule out a DID diagnosis. Amnesia is typically severe in patients with DID. In all patients, a dissociative amnesia diagnosis should be made after an assessment of the other dissociative symptoms (i.e., depersonalization, derealization, identity confusion, and identity alteration) and the clinician has ruled out possible organic etiology.

Dissociative Fugue

The primary symptom of dissociative fugue is sudden, unexpected, travel or wandering, usually accompanied by confusion about personal identity or even the assumption of a new identity (American Psychiatric Association 1994). According to DSM-IV's classification, "The predominant disturbance is sudden, unexpected travel away from home or one's customary place of work, with inability to recall one's past" (p. 484). Other criteria include "Confusion about personal identity or assumption of new identity (partial or complete)." and "The disturbance does not occur exclusively during the course of DID and is not due to the direct psychological effects of a substance . . . or a general medical condition" (see Table 12–2). In dissociative fugue, the patient ordi-

---

Table 12–2. DSM-IV criteria for dissociative fugue

A. The predominant disturbance is sudden, unexpected travel away from home or one's customary place of work, with inability to recall one's past.

B. Confusion about personal identity or assumption of new identity (partial or complete).

C. The disturbance does not occur exclusively during the course of Dissociative Identity Disorder and is not due to the direct effects of a substance (e.g., a drug of abuse, a medication) or a general medical condition (e.g., temporal lobe epilepsy).

D. The symptoms cause clinically significant distress or impairment in social, occupational, or other important areas of functioning.

Source. Reprinted with permission from American Psychiatric Association: *Diagnostic and Statistical Manual of Mental Disorders*, 4th Edition. Washington, DC, American Psychiatric Association, 1994. Copyright 1994, American Psychiatric Association.

narily remains alert and oriented, although he or she is amnestic for the former identity. Sophisticated social adaptation is one feature that distinguishes dissociative fugue from fugues seen in organic disorders (i.e., in dissociative fugue the patient is able to seek employment, make new friends, and so on). The disorder is distinguished from dissociative amnesia by unexpected travel in connection with the amnesia. Dissociative fugue is distinguished from DID by its sudden onset, the presence of a single severe stressor or trauma, and the lack of struggle between different partial or complete personalities for dominance. Unlike DID, dissociative fugue usually consists of a single, nonrecurrent episode. Recovery is usually complete, spontaneous, and rapid.

Prior to DSM-III, dissociative fugue did not constitute a separate diagnostic category. Its incidence and prevalence are unknown. Akhtar and Brenner (1979) suggest that "in times of great and generalized stress, e.g., during a war, such fugues are common." Two case reports describe a familial pattern in dissociative fugue (McKinney and Lange 1983), but at this time there are no reliable statistical data that confirm any of the theoretical hypotheses advanced in connection with the disorder.

Dissociative fugue is characterized by total retrograde memory loss but usually no anterograde loss. The fugue state itself resolves in a matter of days in most instances, and the patient is subsequently amnestic for events that occurred during the fugue state. Patients usually do not complain of defective memory during the state, and their memory loss is confined to the time lost during the actual travel and its accompanying altered state of consciousness (Croft et al. 1973). People who undergo fugue episodes are capable of highly complex behavior requiring intelligence and good coordination; they can drive cars, operate computers, perform difficult pieces of music, and so on. As Pierre Janet said, "They are mad people in full delirium; nevertheless, they take railway tickets, they dine and sleep in hotels, they speak to a great number of people" (qtd. in Rowan and Rosenbaum 1991, p. 364).

Dissociative fugues are usually precipitated by severe stress and are most commonly reported in wartime (Kopelman 1987). Other occasions that may precipitate fugue are marital discord, financial difficulty, and suicidal ideation (Kopelman 1987). Fugue episodes may represent an attempt to escape depression and anxiety on the one hand or intolerable situations and relationships on the other (Croft et al. 1973). Perhaps the best-known case of dissociative fugue in the American literature is that of Ansel Bourne, a nineteenth-century itinerant lay preacher who fled from his home in Rhode Island in January 1887 and who lived for 6 weeks in Norristown, Pennsylvania, as Mr. Brown, a variety store owner. William James (1890) made Bourne the subject of a landmark case study. James' examination indicated that his patient had two completely separate stores of memory for his different identities. Bourne's case is a clear example of fugue precipitated by personal stress, in this instance adjustment to a recent second marriage.

Differential Diagnosis of Dissociative Fugue

A diagnosis of dissociative fugue is made when an individual presents with significant amnesia in combination with either identity confusion or identity alteration. Dissociative fugue is generally an acute, brief, and self-limited episode. If an individual has recurrent fugue states, the clinician is advised to rule out DID or DDNOS. Questions assessing occurrences of dissociative fugue are included in the amnesia section of the SCID-D because of the predominance of amnesia in this disorder.

Dissociative fugue and fugue episodes thus represent a combination of several dissociative symptoms. Fugue involves a change or loss in identity, amnesia for personal information, and finding oneself at a location far from home or one's customary workplace (see Figure 12–2). One patient recalled an episode of fugue as a stressful experience:

> Probably the most significant thing that ever happened in the last few years was that I was on a bus and ended up all of a sudden looking out the window and not knowing where I was or how I got there in that bus and ended up like in Boston or something. I was in a panic state because I said, "How did I get on this bus?" (SCID-D interview, unpublished transcript)

It is true that mild dissociative episodes resembling fugue are not uncommon in the general population. For instance, many drivers have had the experience of missing a highway exit due to "highway hypnosis," or of arriving at a destination without conscious recall of the decisions and maneuvers involved in the actual driving. In a similar fashion, the poet Pessoa experienced a kind of mild dissociative trance in watching the passing landscape from a train window during a business trip for his employer:

> I couldn't describe the slightest detail of the trip, the smallest bit of what I'd seen. . . . I don't know if that is better or worse than the contrary, which I also do not know how to define. The train stops bouncing . . . I've reached Lisbon, but I haven't reached any conclusion. (Pessoa 1991, p. 77)

However, the fugue or amnestic episodes that afflict patients with dissociative disorders are more severe than these benign forms in that they involve significant amnesia for travel behavior and distress.

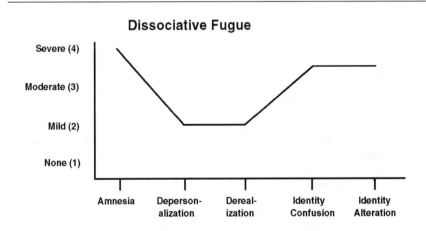

Figure 12–2. SCID-D symptom profile of dissociative fugue.
Source. Reprinted with permission from Steinberg M: *Interviewer's Guide to the Structured Clinical Interview of DSM-IV Dissociative Disorders (SCID-D), Revised.* Washington, DC, American Psychiatric Press, 1994. Copyright © 1994, Marlene Steinberg, M.D.

Some of the more dramatic instances of fugue involve an individual's sudden "waking up" after a considerable period of absence from home to find that he or she is living and working in a completely unfamiliar environment. The case of Ansel Bourne has already been mentioned. This type of episode, when not recurrent, suggests a diagnosis of dissociative fugue.

On the other hand, a patient endorsing numerous fugue episodes warrants the consideration of DID and DDNOS. Multiple episodes may involve identity alteration with associated amnesia in an individual with multiple personalities. One patient in the SCID-D field study with DID reported a number of fugue episodes:

> **Interviewer:** Have you ever found yourself in a place and been unable to remember how or why you went there?
>
> **Patient:** Yes.
>
> **Interviewer:** Where did you find yourself?
>
> **Patient:** I found myself in the therapist's office, not knowing how or why I got there. I found myself in the grocery store. I found myself at the movies. (SCID-D interview, unpublished transcript)

Another patient with DID mentioned recurrent fugue episodes that took her on lengthy trips across state lines:

> **Interviewer:** Have you ever had days that seem to be missing that you couldn't account for?
>
> **Patient:** [Pauses] Yeah.
>
> **Interviewer:** OK. How much time was missing and how did you become aware of that fact?
>
> **Patient:** It's not easy to simplify the answers to these questions. When you end up in another state 5 days from the time that you last saw, or the date that you last saw, and you don't know how you got there or what you're doing there, and you have absolutely no recollection of it.

Interviewer: How often has that occurred?

Patient: Well, it happens quite frequently. It makes it very difficult to keep a job. (SCID-D interview, unpublished transcript)

Fugue states of this type are frequent occurrences in patients with DID, and their apparent "wandering" *is* intentional and purposeful activity from the viewpoint of the personality engaged in making the travel arrangements. It seems inexplicable or strange only to the other personality(ies).

Interviewer: Have you ever found yourself away from your home and been unable to remember how or why you went there?

Patient: Yeah.

Interviewer: Can you tell me where you found yourself and what happened?

Patient: I'd be at a store. I'd have no idea what I was supposed to get, and I don't even remember getting there. I also remember, this is something Dr. Simpson asked me, I'm very embarrassed about it. I do remember waking up when I was younger, with a hangover, but I don't remember drinking. I've also woke up with strangers.

Interviewer: By strangers you mean people who you are unable to identify?

Patient: I guess I picked them up. (SCID-D interview, unpublished transcript)

If a person experiences recurrent episodes of fugue, a diagnosis of DID should be ruled out. Furthermore, a patient who comes to a hospital or to therapy after a fugue episode may have DID and may have similar episodes of identity changes in his or her history. Many people with DID are unaware of their fugue episodes or identity alterations. Others, however, experience considerable distress connected with identity confusion resulting from fugue episodes. One patient with DID in the SCID-D study made a direct connection between her inexplicable geographical relocations and experiences of identity confusion:

Interviewer: Have you ever felt as if there was a struggle going on inside of you as to who you really are?

Patient: [Pauses] Who I really am. I'm not sure that I can even answer that. I don't even know who I am. My life is like too up and down, up and down, up and down. I don't . . . there is . . . there is like nothing solid to grasp. I don't even know how I got in Camden, where I'm living now. I mean I was living in Trenton, now I'm living in Camden. It's OK; I'm not . . . but, um, if I knew who I was, I suppose I could stay where I wanted. (SCID-D interview, unpublished transcript)

Depersonalization Disorder

Depersonalization disorder involves persistent and recurrent episodes of severe depersonalization, associated with significant distress and/or dysfunction (see Table 12–3). The symptom of depersonalization can be defined as a feeling that one's body or self is unreal. Patients may perceive their minds or bodies as detached, observed from the outside, existing in a dream, or robot-

---

Table 12–3. DSM-IV criteria for depersonalization disorder

A. Persistent or recurrent experiences of feeling detached from, and as if one is an outside observer of, one's mental processes or body (e.g., feeling like one is in a dream).
B. During the depersonalization experience, reality testing remains intact.
C. The depersonalization causes clinically significant distress or impairment in social, occupational, or other important areas of functioning.
D. The depersonalization experience does not occur exclusively during the course of another disorder, such as Schizophrenia, Panic Disorder, Acute Stress Disorder, or another Dissociative Disorder, and is not due to the direct physiological effects of a substance (e.g., a drug of abuse, a medication) or a general medical condition (e.g., temporal lobe epilepsy).

Source. Reprinted with permission from American Psychiatric Association: *Diagnostic and Statistical Manual of Mental Disorders,* 4th Edition. Washington, DC, American Psychiatric Association, 1994. Copyright 1994, American Psychiatric Association.

like. Chronic depersonalization is commonly accompanied by derealization, which is a feeling of unreality regarding the immediate environment. A patient suffering from depersonalization disorder will, however, retain intact reality testing, in that they will be able to distinguish their subjective feelings of unreality from genuine delusions, and will typically describe their experiences with the use of "like," "as if," and similar expressions. For example, one patient in the SCID-D field study who was diagnosed as having depersonalization disorder spoke of her symptoms repeatedly in this "like" or "as if" fashion:

> **Interviewer:** Have you ever felt as if you were a stranger to yourself?
>
> **Patient:** Umhmm.
>
> **Interviewer:** Can you describe what that experience feels like to you?
>
> **Patient:** Well, you just feel like you're never being yourself, uh . . . you're not thinking as you normally do. You just feel strange [pauses]. I don't know. It's really difficult to explain.
>
> **Interviewer:** How often do you have that feeling?
>
> **Patient:** All the time . . .
>
> **Interviewer:** Have you ever felt as if part of your body was unreal?
>
> **Patient:** Yeah, all of it [chuckles].
>
> **Interviewer:** All of it? OK. What does that experience feel like to you?
>
> **Patient:** Um [pauses] . . . it's like [if you were to] touch me or something, like I would have, um, I mean I would have that sensation, but it wouldn't be as strong. It would be dull. It's . . . I don't know. It's a very distinct feeling, but it's just very hard to explain. (SCID-D interview, unpublished transcript)

Differential Diagnosis of Depersonalization Disorder

The criteria for depersonalization disorder have been refined in the course of successive editions of the DSM. Clinicians accustomed to the four criteria of this disorder as outlined in DSM-III-R should be aware that they have been somewhat modified in DSM-IV. In DSM-III-R, criterion A included experiences of detachment or feeling like an automaton/in a dream. The new criterion A omits references to a dreamlike state and adds "feel like an automaton" (American Psychiatric Association 1994, p. 488) as merely an example of feeling detached from one's mental process or body. The revised criterion C adds that depersonalization can result in either stress *or* impaired social functioning for depersonalization disorder to be diagnosed. This revision accounts for the possibility that patients with *chronic* depersonalization may experience little or no *distress* but may indeed experience dysfunction. Criterion D adds DID to the list of disorders that supersede depersonalization disorder (i.e., if depersonalization occurs as part of such a disorder, that disorder replaces a diagnosis of depersonalization disorder). Agoraphobia and personality disorders were omitted from this qualification list because they may coexist with depersonalization disorder. Finally, two new disorders were added that rule out a diagnosis of depersonalization disorder, namely substance-induced disorder and a general medical condition (e.g., temporal lobe epilepsy).

Depersonalization disorder has a chronic, yet variable course. Onset can be gradual or rapid, but disappearance is usually gradual. Depersonalization subsequent to life-threatening situations usually develops suddenly upon exposure to the trauma. Level of functioning is thought to range from slight to severe impairment and may be related to the coexistence of other symptoms and syndromes. Depersonalization disorder is typically thought to begin in adolescence (Kluft 1988a), although it may have an undetected onset in childhood (Shimizu and Sakamoto 1986). (See Figure 12–3 for a symptom profile of depersonalization disorder.)

∎ Dissociative Identity Disorder

DID represents the most chronic and severe manifestation of the dissociative processes (Kluft et al. 1988). DID is believed to result

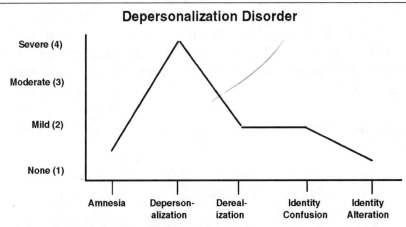

Figure 12–3. SCID-D symptom profile of depersonalization disorder.
Source. Reprinted with permission from Steinberg M: *Interviewer's
Guide to the Structured Clinical Interview of DSM-IV Dissociative Disorders
(SCID-D), Revised.* Washington, DC, American Psychiatric Press, 1994.
Copyright © 1994, Marlene Steinberg, M.D.

from severe and persistent sexual, physical, or psychological abuse
in the patient's childhood (American Psychiatric Association 1987;
Putnam 1985; Stern 1984; Wilbur 1984a). This disorder is characterized by separate identities existing within one individual, which
may control his or her behavior or attitudes, leading to internal
struggle and confusion over the nature of personal identity. The
patient will often remain amnestic for periods when alternate personalities predominate. In other cases, however, patients may be
able to have internal conversations or other interactions with one
or more alters, in much the same way that they would interact
with another person (see Table 12–4).

DID may mimic a spectrum of psychiatric conditions, including
the psychotic, affective, and character disorders (Coons et al. 1988;
Fine 1990; Greaves 1980; Horevitz and Braun 1984; Kluft 1984a,
1987c; Putnam et al. 1986). Patients may experience hallucinations
and endorse first-rank symptoms (e.g., audible thoughts, voices
arguing or commenting, thought insertion or withdrawal, thought
broadcasting, "made" feelings or impulses), which contribute to

confusion with schizophrenia (Bliss 1986; Kluft 1984a, 1987c; Putnam et al. 1986; Rosenbaum 1980). For example, one patient in the SCID-D study with a diagnosis of DID described auditory and visual hallucinations that could be interpreted as symptoms of schizophrenia:

> **Interviewer:** Did you ever hear things that other people couldn't hear, noises or voices of people?
>
> **Patient:** Every now and then, really. It feels like a glimpse of somebody saying something, and a glimpse of the person saying it, who's like a flash.
>
> **Interviewer:** Have you ever heard voices commenting about your behavior or your thoughts?
>
> **Patient:** I don't think about my behavior. I'll have somebody say, "Well, that's crazy." Or they will say that they will call me a liar, or they'll say, "You're stupid if you think that." And it causes a great deal of trouble because it is usually somebody who is trying to . . . I think something and they are giving me reasons why I shouldn't think it, and it is usually negative. Sometimes they say things like, "You shouldn't trust Dr.

Table 12–4. DSM-IV criteria for dissociative identity disorder

---

A. The presence of two or more distinct identities or personality states (each with its own relatively enduring pattern of perceiving, relating to, and thinking about the environment and self).
B. At least two of these identities or personality states recurrently take control of the person's behavior.
C. Inability to recall important personal information that is too extensive to be explained by ordinary forgetfulness.
D. The disturbance is not due to the direct physiological effects of a substance (e.g., blackouts or chaotic behavior during Alcohol Intoxication) or a general medical condition (e.g., complex partial seizures). **Note:** In children, the symptoms are not attributable to imaginary playmates or other fantasy play.

Source. Reprinted with permission from American Psychiatric Association: *Diagnostic and Statistical Manual of Mental Disorders*, 4th Edition. Washington, DC, American Psychiatric Association, 1994. Copyright 1994, American Psychiatric Association.

Smith" or "You shouldn't trust this person or that person." And they will give me reasons . . .

Interviewer: Did you ever feel that certain thoughts that were not your own were put in your head or taken out of your head?

Patient: I don't know. I feel like I am being fed information. I don't know if it is inside of my head. So I guess I usually feel safe by saying I will tell you everything I think and everything I hear; mostly everything I hear seems like it is contradictory. (SCID-D interview, unpublished transcript)

DID patients may also endorse depressive symptoms, which contribute to confusion with affective disorders (Bliss 1986; Coons 1984; Kluft 1987c; Marcum et al. 1985; Putnam et al. 1984, 1986), and a chaotic lifestyle, which contributes to confusion with borderline personality disorder (Clary et al. 1984; Horevitz and Braun 1984; Kluft 1987c). Patients with DID also frequently experience coexisting personality disorders, substance abuse, and somatic complaints, which often mask the underlying dissociative disorder (Coons and Milstein 1986; Kluft 1984a, 1987c; Putnam et al. 1984). An investigation of 100 patients by Putnam reveals that, on average, patients diagnosed with DID receive 3.6 (range = 0–23) diagnoses from the time of first psychiatric presentation until accurate diagnosis. Their previous diagnoses included depression, 70%; neurotic disorder, 55%; personality disorder, 46%; schizophrenia, 44%; substance abuse, 20%; and manic depressive illness, 18% (Putnam et al. 1986). The time between entry into the mental health system and eventual correct assessment and initiation of appropriate treatment of such patients may consume a decade and more.

Differential Diagnosis of DID

In terms of differential diagnosis from other dissociative disorders, both dissociative fugue and dissociative amnesia lack the characteristic recurrence of alternate identities that is a criterion of DID. Although a classic instance of dissociative fugue involves the assumption of a new identity after unexpected but purposeful travel, the alternate identity appears only for the single acute episode and does not reappear or remain consistent over time. Another factor that complicates assessment in cases of DID is that the separate alters may have coexisting psychiatric disorders that are not necessarily shared by all of them. Those cases that do not cross the threshold of severity for DID, yet present with personality fragments or recurrent amnesia associated with changes in identity, would currently be categorized under DDNOS (see Figure 12–4).

Patients with DID present with behavioral manifestations of both severe amnesia and severe identity confusion. Where amnestic barriers exist between the alter personalities, the patient may well be unaware of the relationship between the identity disturbance and the symptomatic behaviors. The improvement of communication between the personalities, and the decrease of amnesia, is one of the most important aspects of therapy for these patients. Amnestic barriers between the personalities are almost universal (Putnam et al. 1986), and amnesia within individual per-

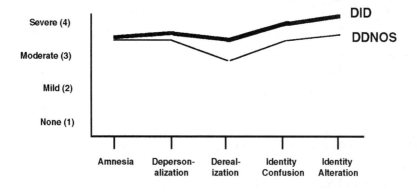

Figure 12–4. SCID-D symptom profile of dissociative identity disorder (DID) and dissociative disorder not otherwise specified (DDNOS). *Source.* Reprinted with permission from Steinberg M: *Interviewer's Guide to the Structured Clinical Interview of DSM-IV Dissociative Disorders (SCID-D), Revised.* Washington, DC, American Psychiatric Press, 1994. Copyright © 1994, Marlene Steinberg, M.D.

sonalities has also been reported. (Schacter et al. 1989). Because the experiences of one personality may not be shared by other personalities, a given alter may have numerous time gaps that represent periods of time during which he or she was not the "host."

Questions in the amnesia section of the SCID-D related to loss of memory for personal information provide diagnostically discriminating clues for DID because patients with dissociative disorders often endorse these experiences with characteristic replies. Patients with DID who are not aware of their other personalities often present to clinicians with subtle cues of amnesia and identity confusion. Asking diagnostically discriminating questions can elicit symptoms of identity alteration behind the amnesia. The following transcript excerpt is an example of the presence of identity disturbance underlying the patient's loss of memory:

Interviewer: Have you ever been unable to remember your name age, address, or other personal information?

Patient: Oh Yeah. Yeah. A lot.

Interviewer: How often would that occur?

Patient: A lot.

Interviewer: What information did you forget?

Patient: Oh, how old I am, my phone number, my address. You know, I pretty much know my name.

Interviewer: Can you give me an example of what might occur when you might forget your age?

Patient: Applications for jobs. I can't fill them out. I have to sit and just think. And sometimes I have to look at my driver's license. Or someone will ask me for my phone number, and I just go blank. (SCID-D interview, unpublished transcript)

In addition to the presence of severe amnesia in cases of DID, this particular dissociative disorder is an example of the interconnection between amnesia and identity confusion and alteration. Moreover, it may cause the patient significant distress, as the following example indicates:

Patient: It's not the losing time, it's not being able to think I have any history that is mine, it's like I don't really exist.

Interviewer: That's very distressing.

Patient: Well, first of all it makes it seem like I'm living somebody else's life. (SCID-D interview, unpublished transcript)

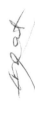

Amnesia is a difficult symptom to detect, and clinicians should make it a routine subject of inquiry when the presence of a dissociative disorder is suspected. In some cases, the interviewer may need to gather information from the patient about amnestic episodes and automatic activity, as well as other data from friends or relatives (Coons and Milstein 1990). Moreover, when amnesia is present, interviewers should note that it may complicate obtaining an accurate history of childhood trauma and abuse (Coons and Milstein 1990).

Dissociative Disorder Not Otherwise Specified

DDNOS covers a variety of dissociative disorders that are increasingly recognized as posttraumatic phenomena (Kluft et al. 1988). For the most part, DDNOS includes syndromes that are very similar to the four dissociative disorders previously described but not severe enough to warrant their diagnoses. DDNOS includes the following: 1) clinical presentations that are similar to DID but that do not meet the full criteria, such as absence of two or more distinct personalities or a lack of amnesia for important personal information; 2) derealization without depersonalization; 3) dissociated states in people who have undergone intense coercive persuasion (e.g., brainwashing); 4) dissociative trance disorder; 5) loss of consciousness, stupor, or coma not attributable to a general medical condition; and 6) Ganser syndrome (American Psychiatric Association 1994) (see Table 12–5).

To assist the reader in acquiring a feel for the sometimes subtle differences between DDNOS and DID, as well as for the range of dissociative disturbances included under the rubric of DDNOS, a few examples from SCID-D subjects are included. SCID-D research indicates that the most common forms of DDNOS appear to be

---

Table 12–5. DSM-IV classifications of dissociative disorder NOS

This category is for disorders in which the predominant feature is a dissociative symptom (i.e., a disturbance in the usually integrated functions of consciousness, memory, identity, or perception of the environment) that does not meet the criteria for any specific Dissociative Disorder. Examples include

1. Clinical presentations similar to Dissociative Identity Disorder that fail to meet full criteria for this disorder. Examples include presentations in which a) there are not two or more distinct personality states, or b) amnesia for important personal information does not occur.

2. Derealization unaccompanied by depersonalization in adults.

3. States of dissociation that occur in individuals who have been subjected to periods of prolonged and intense coercive persuasion (e.g., brainwashing, thought reform, or indoctrination while captive).

4. Dissociative trance disorder: single or episodic alterations in the state of consciousness, identity, or memory that are indigenous to particular locations and cultures. Dissociative trance involves narrowing of awareness of immediate surroundings or stereotyped behaviors or movements that are experienced as being beyond one's control. Possession trance involves replacement of the customary sense of personal identity by a new identity, attributed to the influence of a spirit, power, deity, or other person, and associated with stereotyped "involuntary" movements or amnesia. Examples include *amok* (Indonesia), *bebainan* (Indonesia), *latah* (Malaysia), *pibloktoq* (Arctic), *ataque de nervios* (Latin America), and possession (India). The dissociative or trance disorder is not a normal part of a broadly accepted collective cultural or religious practice. (See p. 727 for suggested criteria.)

5. Loss of consciousness, stupor, or coma not attributable to a general medical condition.

6. Ganser's syndrome: the giving of "inappropriate answers" to questions (e.g., "2 plus 2 equals 5") when not associated with Dissociative Amnesia or Dissociative Fugue.

Source. Reprinted with permission from American Psychiatric Association: *Diagnostic and Statistical Manual of Mental Disorders,* 4th Edition. Washington, DC, American Psychiatric Association, 1994. Copyright 1994, American Psychiatric Association.

variants of DID in which personality states may take over consciousness and behavior but are not sufficiently distinct to qualify as full personalities. One patient diagnosed as having DDNOS described the personality states or fragments inside her as being in an inner competition:

> **Interviewer:** Have you ever felt as if there was a struggle going on inside of you?
>
> **Patient:** Yeah, a fight. I feel that a lot of times, like somebody's punching somebody else out inside of me.
>
> **Interviewer:** What does that feel like?
>
> **Patient:** Kind of like pushing and shoving. It's a lot of turmoil, kind of traumatic, actually. It's very traumatic because that's when I get really scared, because I know I can't control that. I see these two little men with gloves on and they're punching each other [chuckles].
>
> **Interviewer:** Have you ever felt as if this is a struggle as to who you really are?
>
> **Patient:** No, because I really didn't think that anybody knows who I really am. I think I'm starting to find that out now. I think it's just in terms of what's going to get the best of me. (SCID-D interview, unpublished transcript)

The reader may have noted that endorsements of personality states or fragments in patients with DDNOS lack the fullness and complexity that typify DID patients' descriptions of their alter personalities; the "two little men" do not have sharply defined visual images or differentiated personalities.

Lastly, the SCID-D field study included one male patient who endorsed trance states that caused him considerable distress. He had given up driving because of his selectively focused responses to the environment:

> **Patient:** About the trances that I have . . . I become fearful and distrustful of many things. I have had to learn and listen and start really new relationships with everyone. I trust I was not very

... there are times when I can't go out of the house, I can't get behind the wheel. Really scared of a lot of things.

Interviewer: So you are unable to drive?

Patient: Unable to drive ... not able to do much of anything.

Interviewer: What is the difficulty for you to drive at this time?

Patient: I might just go off, I might just go off, go into a trance. I don't know if I could handle that while I was driving. I have a fear of going anywhere alone. Forget it. I also have this fear of running, once you let me out, that I will decide to run and that scares me.

Interviewer: So you are frightened you might run away?

Patient: Frightened that I might. I get that feeling a lot, going someplace and not coming back. (SCID-D interview, unpublished transcript)

DSM-III-R expanded the discussion of DDNOS "to better accommodate recognized dissociative syndromes that do not fall within the four formally defined dissociative disorders," and "perceived this classification as extremely important for contemporary psychiatry" (American Psychiatric Association 1987). Hostages, members of cults, victims of torture or terrorism, prisoners, or survivors of extreme trauma may all present with many dissociative symptoms that do not meet the criteria for other disorders.

▐ Summary

The dissociative disorders are psychological disorders that manifest in distinctive forms of severe dissociation, arising from overwhelming abuse or trauma. Each dissociative disorder represents a particular method, so to speak, by which the person detaches him- or herself from a traumatic past and its capacity to invade the present via memory. Dissociative symptoms range in complexity from amnesia for certain memories to dissociation from one's entire identity and past.

■ New DSM-IV Diagnostic Categories for Dissociative Disorders

Two changes in nomenclature that appear for the first time in DSM-IV are *dissociative trance disorder,* listed as a subheading under DDNOS, and *acute stress disorder,* listed with the anxiety disorders. Dissociative trance disorder has been proposed as a cross-cultural classification for a subtype of dissociative disorder that occurs in some non-Western societies as well as in certain subcultures in the West. Dissociative trance disorder is defined by DSM-IV as "single or episodic alterations in the state of consciousness that are indigenous to particular locations and cultures" (American Psychiatric Association 1994, p. 490). The manual specifies that "the dissociative or trance disorder is *not* a normal part of a broadly accepted collective cultural or religious practice" (p. 490, italics added). In other words, the type of mild self-induced trance that some individuals experience in the course of meditation as it is practiced by mainstream religious groups in the United States does not come under the heading of dissociative trance disorder.

Acute stress disorder has been proposed as a subcategory of anxiety disorder to account for cases that resemble PTSD but have shorter duration. *Acute stress disorder* is described as a reaction to extreme trauma, which includes a brief period (less than 4 weeks) of anxiety and dissociative experiences accompanied by distress and dysfunction. The dissociative symptoms characteristic of acute stress disorder include amnesia, depersonalization, derealization, and flashbacks. Children are equally or more likely to manifest these responses than adults. Acute stress disorder is marked by sudden onset and relatively brief duration, a period of days or several weeks.

The format of the SCID-D allows the clinician to evaluate the presence of these newly classified disorders, insofar as their criteria are addressed by questions included in the normal course of the SCID-D interview. For instance, the interviewer can screen for the presence of acute stress disorder by assessing the severity of any dissociative symptoms endorsed by the patient. Moreover, the clinician should take into account all questions regarding duration and onset of symptoms that are included in the SCID-D. With respect to dissociative trance disorder, the clinician will find questions dealing specifically with possession and culture-specific rituals in one of the follow-up sections of the SCID-D.

The SCID-D assesses dissociative symptoms independently of syndromes. Furthermore, the SCID-D examines different *forms* of the same symptom as well as their associated features and chronicity. In this way, the interviewer can elicit a broad picture of the subject's dissociative experiences and assess the existence of dissociative symptoms or disorders, past or present.

❙ Differential Diagnosis in the Dissociative Disorders

Figure 12–5 lists the primary considerations in differential diagnosis of the dissociative disorders in summary form. In general, the clinician will find that an isolated dissociative symptom may occur in several of the five dissociative disorders. However, rather than focusing attention on a single symptom, the careful interviewer will evaluate the symptom for distinctive features, if any, and the presence of the *entire constellation of symptoms* typical of each specific dissociative disorder. To recapitulate, the five disorders can be distinguished from one another according to the nature of the precipitating stressor, its chronicity, the severity of the symptoms, and, most importantly, according to the characteristic constellations of dissociative symptoms that support their DSM-IV criteria. The reader may also wish to refer to Figures 12–1 through 12–4, which illustrate the characteristic symptom profiles of the five dissociative disorders with line graphs.

❙ Coexistence of Dissociative and Nondissociative Disorders

As the introductory chapter of this book indicates, the five dissociative disorders share overlapping symptoms (e.g., auditory hallucinations, Schneiderian symptoms, mood changes) with some

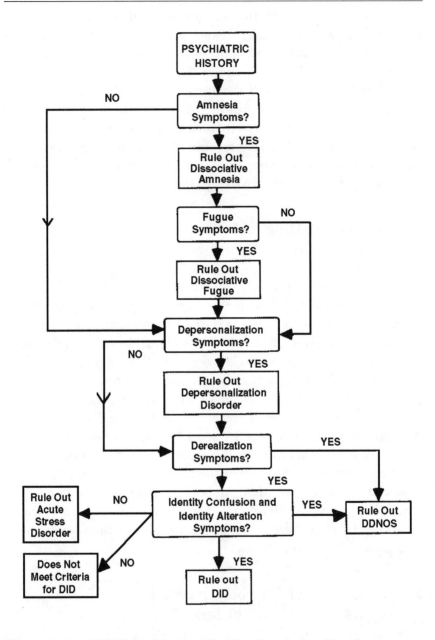

Figure 12–5.   SCID-D decision tree for the dissociative disorders.
Note.   The diagnosis of DID subsumes the diagnosis of any of the four
dissociative disorders.

of the nondissociative disorders and may coexist with them in a given patient. In terms of summary assessment of the possibility of coexisting disorders, clinicians should consider the following major points in evaluating patients:

I Dissociative disorders may coexist with substance abuse and organic disorders (e.g., temporal lobe epilepsy) but only if the dissociative symptoms are not induced by these factors alone.

I In DID, one or more personalities may have a particular symptom or disorder that the other personalities do not share. For example, one of the alters may have major depression, an eating or substance abuse disorder, and so on.

I Because the dissociative disorders are all Axis I disorders, they may coexist with the personality disorders (Axis II). For example, depersonalization disorder or DID may coexist with borderline personality disorder.

I A dissociative disorder *cannot* coexist with a psychotic disorder such as schizophrenia. However, a person with a dissociative disorder may *appear* to have a transient psychotic episode, which is often due to age regression and/or flashbacks of traumatic events. DID is particularly likely to be misdiagnosed as a psychotic disorder because of its characteristic auditory (and sometimes visual) hallucinations.

I Depersonalization disorder is diagnosed if the depersonalization is the primary symptom and if the predominant disturbance is of a dissociative nature. However, depersonalization is often masked by symptoms of anxiety, panic, and/or depression; a thorough investigation of dissociative symptomatology is necessary for correct differential diagnosis.

I Conclusion

Dissociative disorders are posttraumatic disorders that involve the fragmentation of the patient's consciousness. They are difficult to detect because the function of dissociative symptoms is to protect the patient from memories of the abuse and the effects of the disorder itself so that he or she can function without overwhelming anxiety.

The dissociative disorders and symptoms are now receiving greater attention from both clinicians and researchers. In general, the dissociative disorders result from severe trauma, most commonly childhood physical and sexual abuse. Therapy with patients who have dissociative disorders is a process of reintegration: helping people to accept their traumatic past while maintaining control over the emotional responses they have to their memories.

CHAPTER 13

Intra-Interview
Dissociative Cues

How does it FEEL to be MPD? It feels ugly, dirty and repulsive. It feels like being the Elephant Man. Who would ever want to hold a thing like you or love such a deformed creature? Dying would feel better.

You scream and guess what? No one notices anything. You make jokes when your guts are hemorrhaging and guess what? No one notices anything. Your stomach lurches and your bowels loosen because you can't find the answer to that easy question your therapist just asked and guess what? He doesn't even notice the beads of sweat on your lip.

—"Wendy W.," *Multiple Personality Disorder from the Inside Out*[1]

The SCID-D (Steinberg 1993b) has been designed to allow the interviewer to look for and incorporate a number of intra-interview cues in the final assessment. These cues may be collectively defined as a set of behaviors observed during the interview that occur in the course of the subject's responses to the questions but are not assessed through the administered questions. Incorporating these behaviors and symptoms in conjunction with the verbal responses best approximates a clinical *unstructured* interview and is therefore essential to the comprehensive assessment of the dissociative disorders. Some intra-interview cues are themselves verbal; for example, the presence of item 266, intra-interview depersonalization, would be manifested by the subject's explicitly remarking during the interview that he or she "feels unreal," or words to that effect. Other cues are nonverbal; the interviewer is

---

[1] From Cohen et al. 1991, p. 25.

asked to note the subject's changes in body posture, general mood or affect, vocal tone, eye movement, and so on.

The use of intra-interview cues as a supplement to the denotative content of the patient's responses to questions is a standard component of psychiatric examinations. Most introductions or handbooks for clinical interviewers will include an outline or schema of some kind in order to assist the interviewer in organizing his or her impressions of the patient. For example, a British handbook for psychiatrists (Institute of Psychiatry and Maudsley Hospital 1987) groups intra-interview cues under the following headings:

1. Appearance and general behaviour
2. Talk
3. Mood
4. Thought content

With specific regard to dissociative identity disorder (DID), Putnam (1989a) groups intra-interview cues as follows:

Physical Changes

1. Facial changes
2. Postural and motor behavioral changes
3. Voice and speech changes
4. Dress and grooming
5. Behavior during switching

Psychological Changes

1. Affect
2. Behavioral age
3. Thought processes

Kluft (1987c) has drawn up the following condensed list of signs suggestive of DID that consist of a mixture of items from the patient's history as well as intra-interview cues in the strict sense.

Items corresponding to the intra-interview cues as listed by the SCID-D are italicized.

- A history of prior treatment failures
- Three or more prior diagnoses
- Concurrent psychiatric and somatic symptoms
- *Fluctuating symptoms and an inconsistent level of functioning*
- Severe headaches, often refractory to narcotics
- A history of time distortions or time lapses
- The patient's having been told of forgotten behaviors by others
- The patient's having been told by others of observable changes in facies, voice, and behavioral style
- Discovery of unaccountable productions, handwriting, or objects in one's possession
- Auditory hallucinations
- *The use of* we *in a collective sense*
- The elicitability of other alters by means of hypnosis or amobarbital
- Patient has a history of child abuse

In addition to these signs, Kluft notes the possible presence during the interview of *"brief evidences of forgetfulness"* and *"fluctuations of voice, speech, and movement characteristics within the interview."* He then adds, "A surprising number of these patients avert or partially cover their face and lower their voice to minimize the emission of such evidences" (p. 216).

The SCID-D regards intra-interview dissociative cues as supplementary and corroborative information for the clinician-interviewer in that it considers them to be indications of the external manifestations of the five core symptoms of dissociation, rather than independent phenomena. Because these cues are regarded as external behavioral manifestations of the five core dissociative symptoms, the SCID-D booklet enumerates 14 of them, which can be correlated with the five core symptoms. Table 13–1 lists the 14 cues in tabular form, together with the symptoms that they represent or externalize. Because differential diagnosis of the dissociative disorders depends in part on recognizing the symptom

Table 13–1. Intra-interview dissociative cues and the five SCID-D dissociative symptoms

Intra-interview dissociative cue	SCID-D dissociative symptom indicated
Alteration in subject's demeanor	Identity alteration
Alteration in subject's identity	Identity alteration
Spontaneous age regression or childlike behavior in an adult	Identity alteration (often associated with derealization)
Inconsistencies/fluctuations in level of functioning or mood	Identity confusion Identity alteration
Subject refers to him- or herself in the first-person plural *(we)* or third person *(he/she/they)*	Identity confusion Identity alteration
Subject is noted to talk to him- or herself, or reports intra-interview internal dialogues (silently or out loud), though he or she is not psychotic	Depersonalization Identity confusion Identity alteration
Intra-interview amnesia	Amnesia
Intra-interview depersonalization	Depersonalization
Intra-interview derealization	Derealization
Responses such as "I do not know" or "I do not remember" to questions that appear basic, in a subject who is cooperative and genuinely puzzled	Amnesia (possible identity confusion)
Ambivalent responses regarding dissociative symptoms	Identity confusion
Significant emotional response to SCID-D questions regarding dissociative symptoms	Symptom(s) asked about during significant emotional response Identity confusion
Eye movements suggestive of hypnotic state (e.g., lid fluttering, closing eyes for long duration)	Rule out amnestic episode Rule out identity alteration
Trancelike appearance	Rule out amnestic episode Depersonalization Derealization Identity alteration

constellation that characterizes each disorder, a sensitive awareness on the interviewer's part to the presence of intra-interview
cues can assist in accurate identification of the constellation.

■ Intra-Interview Cues as Sources of Supplementary Information

Assessment of intra-interview cues is a partial compensation for
the limitations of the patient's verbal descriptions. As this book has
emphasized, those who are diagnosed as having a dissociative disorder typically suffer their symptoms in silence, often for years.
Their descriptions of their dissociative experiences are often frag-
mentary and hesitant, or metaphorical rather than strictly conceptual. In some cases, such as experiences of depersonalization or
derealization, the episode itself may be intrinsically difficult to verbalize. The pauses in the excerpt that follows indicate the presence
of a significant emotional response (item 270) to the interviewer's
questions:

Interviewer: Have you ever felt as if part of your body . . . was
fading away?

Patient: Hmm [pauses]. Mentally, I felt like my body drifting away.

Interviewer: What is that like?

Patient: It's like . . . it's hard to describe like . . . [pauses] just sitting
there, but yet I'm drifting. That's the best way I can explain it
to you.

Interviewer: OK. Have you ever felt as if part of your body was
unreal?

Patient: Unreal? Hmmm [pauses]. My whole body. My whole
body sometimes seems like it's unreal.

Interviewer: What do you mean by that?

Patient: What do I mean by that? I mean I look at myself [pauses],
just the whole body. I don't know if that's because of being
called fat and ugly when I was a kid all the time and it's just
something mentally . . . [pauses] fat and ugly, fat and ugly,

constantly. And I'm almost in tears, crying and crying and crying and I couldn't take it no more [pauses]. I'm about to cry now. I really don't want to cry right now because a man is not supposed to cry, my father told me. He said it's a sign of weakness. (SCID-D interview, unpublished transcript)

This patient's response is particularly telling as an illustrative example of embarrassment regarding not only the presence of dissociative symptoms but also hesitation to discuss them because of the pressure of sex role expectations—in this case that men should not cry or display "weakness." In other instances a patient may manifest ambivalence (item 269) because some alter personalities may be instructing the person not to disclose their presence or other items of significant information. As Kluft (1987c) has pointed out, "It is not uncommon for the patient to hear an inner voice warning against giving complete answers. The clinician routinely expects deception and dissimulation in a forensic context, but may not be alert to it under more routine conditions" (p. 368). Putnam (1989a) has noted that many DID patients have alter personalities who function as administrators or "gatekeepers," in that they control access to the patient's inner system. Some of the participants in the SCID-D study indicated that their ambivalent responses to certain questions reflected internal dialogues among their alters, as in the following example:

Interviewer: Is there a dialogue that's occurring now, or is there any other side of you that would like to share anything?

Patient: Um, I feel the panic that I feel before I split into Blanche. Um, I have a feeling like I should have kept quiet, I've talked too much, like I'm to punish myself for trying to get out. That's the type of dialogue I hear. (SCID-D interview, unpublished transcript)

Another patient specifically mentioned the presence within her system of a gatekeeper alter who commanded the patient's internal "army" as well as controlling her freedom to speak to the interviewer:

Interviewer: Have you ever felt that there was a struggle going on inside of you as to who you really are?

Patient: As to who is in charge. And I say things like, "Well, you think you're in charge and we can show you differently in about 2 seconds." I am told and I guess maybe it's true, I don't know, I am told that the person who really is in charge is Loretta, who will allow me to come here, allow me to work, allow me to go to therapy. She allows me to do all of those things, unless or until there is reason to call up the army. If there is reason to call up the army, then she will take over and she will command the army because it's a matter of life or death and she will not allow anyone to be killed without putting up one hell of a fight. (SCID-D interview, unpublished transcript)

It should be noted by the reader that patients with internal personality systems of this sort might easily manifest cues such as referring to themselves in the first person plural (i.e., *we)* or third person (i.e., *he, she, they)* (item 263) or talking to themselves in the interviewer's presence (item 264), as well as appearing ambivalent or highly emotional. One patient in the SCID-D study, for example, laughed repeatedly while describing the ways in which her system of alters cost her jobs and otherwise involved her in problematic situations:

Interviewer: Have you ever felt as if words would flow from your mouth as if they were not in your control?

Patient: Yeah. [Laughs] Yeah.

Interviewer: Can you describe what that experience is like?

Patient: Well, usually it means after I've said something, I get in a lot of trouble for saying something stupid, but I don't know what it was. I just know I get in a lot of trouble. I've lost jobs and everything because of that.

Interviewer: And you can't remember what it was that you said?

Patient: I just know I've pissed a lot of people off [laughs]. Or else it was stupid. Like it would be incoherent. People would not understand. . . . I mean, I would apparently be talking and making perfect sense to me, but talking incoherently to other people.

Interviewer: Have you ever felt your behavior was not in your control?

Patient: Oh yes [laughs]. (SCID-D interview, unpublished transcript)

In some instances, intra-interview cues may contradict the verbal content of a patient's response. For example, the subject may answer question 158: "When you experience simultaneous dialogues, does this cause you discomfort or distress?" with a verbal denial. At the same time, his or her face may assume an anxious or worried expression that belies the verbal answer, or the vocal tone may be agitated or jittery. In another example from a SCID-D interview, the patient's smiles and laughs are at odds with his verbal uncommunicativeness:

Interviewer: Have you ever felt as if your surroundings and other people were fading away or disappearing?

Patient: Nnnno.

Interviewer: Have you ever been unable to recognize close friends, relatives, or your own home?

Patient: [Muffled] No.

Interviewer: Have you ever felt as if close friends, relatives, or your own home seemed strange or foreign?

Patient: Mmm, no.

Interviewer: Have you ever felt puzzled as to what is real and what is unreal in your surroundings?

Patient: [Mumbles, shakes head.]

Interviewer: Have you ever felt as if there were a struggle going on inside of you?

Patient: [Long pause] Mmm, No. I don't know. I don't know [smiles].

Interviewer: Well, what makes you . . . what do you think about it?

Patient: [Pause] I don't know. I'm kind of stumped right now [raises arms in an "I don't know" gesture, smiles].

Interviewer: OK. Have you ever felt as if you are still a child?

Patient: [Shakes head and mumbles.]

Interviewer: Have you ever been told you were still a child?

Patient: [Shakes head and silently mouths] No.

Interviewer: Have you ever acted as if you were a completely different person?

Patient: [Pause] I don't know.

Interviewer: You don't know?

Patient: I don't know [smiles].

Interviewer: Well what is it that you don't know? How might that be?

Patient: Well, I mean there are times, I mean you know, I mean [rubs forehead], I guess there are times when I could be two totally different people [loud, nervous laugh]. (SCID-D interview, unpublished transcript)

The SCID-D's scoring system allows the interviewer to note discrepancies of this kind, rather than forcing him or her to decide on the best answer. As the *Interviewer's Guide to the SCID-D* (Steinberg 1993a) explains, a rating of "I" for a particular item indicates that the interviewer has obtained inconsistent or discrepant information from the subject regarding symptoms or experiences described by the question. Rather than choosing the response that seems more valid, the interviewer notes both of the responses that were inconsistent with each other. Figure 13–1 illustrates the proper scoring of the subject's response in the previous transcript excerpt.

In this instance the interviewer has noted that the subject stated that the symptom was absent (a rating of "N") but that an intra-interview cue, in this case the smiling and laugh, implied that the

symptom was present (a rating of "Y"). The interviewer's assessment of "present" would override the subject's negative verbal
response.

▌ Other Considerations

Intra-interview cues are one indication among others of the
SCID-D's cross-class and cross-cultural applicability. Whereas the
verbal content of patients' answers may vary according to general
level of intelligence and education, nonverbal cues are less affected
by these factors. Therapists who are sensitive to visual phenomena
(e.g., facial expressions, body movement, hand gestures) and audible changes in vocal pitch, speed, rhythm, and tone will be able to
derive a great deal of relevant information from a SCID-D interview, even if the patient has difficulties with verbal self-expression,
fluency in English, or intra-interview amnesia. In the following
example, the patient's relative lack of conceptual sophistication
did not inhibit the interviewer's determination of a severe degree
of identity confusion. She displayed facial contortions that indi-

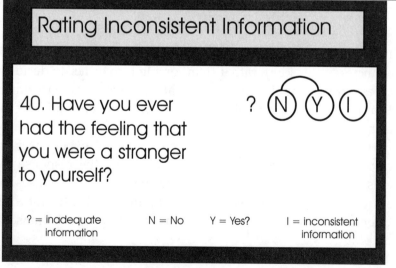

Figure 13–1. Rating inconsistent information in the SCID-D.

cated an internal struggle for control of her body. While the left side of her face was unaffected during this portion of the interview, the right side contracted upward, exposing her teeth, and forming a crease in her right cheek. Her eyebrows also moved asymmetrically.

> **Interviewer:** Have you ever acted as if you were a completely different person?
>
> **Patient:** Yeah [right part of face is contracted upwards].
>
> **Interviewer:** In what way?
>
> **Patient:** [Right side of face contracts again] I don't know. My father used to call me Dr. Jekyll and Mr. Hyde. He said that for years. Ever since I was little he told me . . . from one way to another way. I don't know [sigh].
>
> **Interviewer:** How do you act differently at different times?
>
> **Patient:** I don't know. Different stuff has happened and stuff. It's not me. I think I know who I am. I have an idea, but. . . . Somehow it doesn't come across that way I guess. I don't know.
>
> **Interviewer:** So it feels as if you're doing things that aren't you.
>
> **Patient:** No.
>
> **Interviewer:** And who does it feel as if it is?
>
> **Patient:** They say it's a multiple personality, but I don't think it is. I think it's a possessed feeling, you know, like your body and your eyes, and your mouth, they're *controlling* them. You can't control them. You have episodes and you can't control it. It's somebody taking over you. It's someone, it's like a devil taking over your body or something. And it's scary. You know? (SCID-D interview, unpublished transcript)

In addition, the rating of intra-interview cues can assist therapists in evaluating possible countertransference issues as part of planning the course of therapy. Awareness of intra-interview cues together with the therapist's understanding of his or her own typical reactions can minimize potential problems in treatment planning. It should be noted that therapists who have written case studies of patients with DID for the general public usually mention intra-interview cues as the immediate sources of strong emotional responses, ranging from a sense of the otherworldly to surprise and confusion. One therapist who eventually had to terminate with a patient because he could not deal adequately with his countertransference (Schoenewolf 1991) describes his first experience of the patient's personality switching:

> She stared at the empty chair and the confused expression began to fade and a transformation occurred . . . a small gleam appeared in her face, and her very features underwent a modification—her cheekbones protruded more, her jaw came out, and her eyes grew larger and stronger. Her posture also changed, and she sat upright with her head held straight and her eyes staring confidently and a bit disdainfully at the empty chair. When she spoke her voice was full and angry . . . nothing can compare with the first encounter with a multiple. I understood immediately why centuries ago people like Jennifer were thought to be possessed. It was truly uncanny. The atmosphere in the room seemed to jump with her personality change. . . . (pp. 49–50, 53)

Another therapist/writer (Mayer 1988) had a similar reaction to his patient's vocal and postural changes during her first episode of switching:

> I tried to get a conversation going with this [second] voice. "Where are you located?" I asked it.
>
> I was not prepared for the response.
>
> Toby shut her eyes for a second or two, and when she opened them her posture—no, her whole person—had changed. Her body wiggled and fidgeted like that of a child who just couldn't get comfortable.
>
> "Hi. I'm Beth. I thought you would never get around to talking to me."
>
> A chill started at my toes and rose up my spine. I felt like I had as a kid, hanging around the haunted houses down on the Jersey shore (p. 19).

Examples of personality switching in SCID-D interviews are discussed in the next section.

■ Intra-Interview Switching

As Table 13–1 indicates, many of the intra-interview cues assessed by the SCID-D are related to the symptom of identity alteration although many of them are indicative of other dissociative symptoms as well. In some cases, the cues may be subtle and suggestive of identity alteration. In others, intra-interview cues may be sufficiently striking to indicate that the patient is switching to an alter personality during the conversation with the interviewer. Putnam (1989a), in fact, discusses intra-interview cues within the context of switching. In some cases, the switching may take several minutes before the new alter emerges. The following excerpt from a SCID-D interview is an example of a switch that took 2–3 minutes to complete; the patient went into a trancelike condition (item 272), from which she emerged by "grounding" herself. As Putnam (1989a) indicates, grounding behaviors can include the patient's touching face or temples, clutching the chair in which he or she is sitting, looking around the room, and shifting posture in a restless fashion. In this instance, the patient's grounding included visual scanning and holding the arms of her chair somewhat tensely.

> **Interviewer:** Have you ever had a time when you have had difficulty remembering your daily activities?
>
> **Patient:** [Head is oscillating, eyelids partially closed, mischievous smile, childlike, playful demeanor] Yeah.
>
> **Interviewer:** OK. Can you describe what that was like and how often that occurs?
>
> **Patient:** [Sits back abruptly, smiles, and in a high pitched, childlike voice, asks] What it was like? Let's see. Nothing unusual. I don't understand, "What it was like."
>
> **Interviewer:** OK. Can you describe, let's say, what do you mean by having large gaps in your memory or feeling that time was discontinuous? What do you mean by that?

Patient: What do *I* mean.

Interviewer: Right. Exactly.

Patient: I mean, you know, losing whole weeks, months, uh, from up to months up to 5 minutes.

Interviewer: OK. By losing whole weeks, what do you mean?

Patient: What do I mean?

Interviewer: Right.

Patient: I mean I'm being unable to account for the time.

Interviewer: OK. And how often would you say that occurs?

Patient: A lot.

Interviewer: A lot? OK. Has it just happened to you a few times in your life? Does it happen sort of most of the time—is it an ongoing event? Or does it happen occasionally?

Patient: [Blank stare, long pause, says quietly] Um, kind of ongoing.

Interviewer: OK. Have you ever found yourself in a place and you are unable to remember how or why you went there?

Patient: [Eyes flutter and then partially close. Eyes are moving rapidly under eyelids, *which are partially closed.* Head rocks back and forth. This continues for about a minute.]

Interviewer: What are you feeling now?

Patient: [Eyes jar open, breathing heavily, wide open eyes scanning room and interviewer anxiously.]

Interviewer: Do you understand what's going on here? You look a little surprised.

Patient: [Continues to scan room silently.]

Interviewer: Do you have any questions for me?

Patient: [Looks at interviewer suspiciously.]

Interviewer: Do you know why you are here now?

Patient: [Quietly] What's your name?

> **Interviewer:** My name is Dr. Steinberg. Do you remember coming in here just a few minutes ago and talking with me?
>
> **Patient:** *I* talked to you, on the phone.
>
> **Interviewer:** You did talk to me on the phone. Do you remember just being here for the last 5 minutes?
>
> **Patient:** [Looks around the room *with rapid eye movements*] What time is it? (SCID-D interview, unpublished transcript)

The intra-interview cues involved in the foregoing example include identity alteration, intra-interview amnesia, trancelike appearance, inconsistencies in mood, and alteration in demeanor.

❚ Summary

Although intra-interview cues are epiphenomena of the five core dissociative symptoms, their presence during a diagnostic interview provides the clinician with corroborative or supplementary data that allow an approximation of a clinical unstructured interview. Careful observation and interpretation of these cues will add to the accuracy as well as the completeness of the final assessment. Clinicians should note all relevant intra-interview cues, not only those suggestive of the identity switching that characterizes DID.

CHAPTER 14

The SCID-D in Nondissociative Psychiatric Disorders

The bulk of the material in this book is intended to familiarize the reader with the dissociative symptoms and disorders and with the various applications of the SCID-D (Steinberg 1993b). At this point, however, it is also useful for the reader to have an overview of the relevance of SCID-D assessment to diagnosis and treatment of the nondissociative disorders. Clinicians should note that dissociative symptomatology may manifest in any of the disorders classified under Axis I and Axis II in DSM-IV (American Psychiatric Association 1994). These include affective disorders, personality disorders, substance abuse and eating disorders, and psychotic disorders. The relationship between dissociative symptoms and the nondissociative disorders will fall into one of two basic patterns: 1) the primary disorder is nondissociative but co-exists with some dissociative symptoms, or 2) the nondissociative disorder has been masking the presence of an underlying, previously undetected dissociative disorder. Because accurate diagnosis is essential to the planning and implementation of appropriate treatment, selective administration of the SCID-D is crucial to prevent misinterpretation of a patient's dissociative symptoms. As a general rule, patients who exhibit suspected dissociative symptoms should be screened even when their primary diagnosis is one of the nondissociative disorders. The clinician can ask one or two questions from each of the 5 SCID-D symptom areas as an informal office screener. Those who endorse dissociative symptoms should then be evaluated by administration of the full SCID-D to ascertain whether they meet criteria for a dissociative disorder. The following sections discuss the relationship between dissociative symptomatology and some selected non-dissociative disorders in further detail.

∎ The SCID-D and Dissociative Symptoms in Eating Disorders

As described in the foreword of this book, a connection exists between the SCID-D and the eating disorders because there is an overlap between compulsive behaviors of various sorts and dissociative symptomatology. With respect to eating disorders in particular, many persons with bulimia nervosa or anorexia nervosa report alterations in mood, brought about by their bingeing/purging or self-induced starvation, that verge on dissociative symptomatology. Roth (1992) has described the dissociative dimension of a typical eating binge from her own experience:

> Today would be a good day to go shopping, you tell yourself . . . so you get in the car and begin driving to your favorite store, but as you come to a stoplight, you realize that something is wrong. Something is gnawing at you. You can't put it into words, but as you sit there, it grows more and more oppressive until you feel you'll suffocate under the weight of it. You're having a hard time breathing, the anxiety is rising and you want it to stop. All you care about is having it stop, and you begin thinking about the eclairs in the bakery next to the clothes store. Suddenly you are relieved. Something will take this feeling away. . . . With the determination of a samurai, you steer the car to the parking lot, click click click go your shoes on the pavement. You look at the man with the tortoiseshell glasses who is passing on your left but you don't really see him, you don't see anything, your mind is a laser beam of intent. You want the food. Then you are standing in front of the glass case, hearing yourself order not one but four eclairs, five cookies, and a marzipan cake. . . . Click click click on the pavement, the sound of car door opening, the thud of its slamming shut and finally, finally

you are alone with your blessed relief. Quickly, frantically, and
without tasting them, you inhale two eclairs. (pp. 102–103)

Roth's account incorporates the numbing of painful sensation and
the loss of overall sensory awareness—the writer doesn't "really
see" the other pedestrians around her, "hears" another part of herself order the baked goods, doesn't "taste" the food she wolfs
down—that border on experiences of depersonalization and derealization. A patient with an eating disorder and underlying dissociative identity disorder (DID) who was cited by Torem (1986)
described her experiences of binge eating as follows: "I don't know
why I do it. I am so confused. It is not like me" (p. 141). Another
patient reported a sense of emotional struggle in connection with
binge eating: "It feels like a part of me wants to binge and part of
me hates it" (p. 141). Male patients with eating disorders have also
endorsed a connection between dissociative symptoms and binge
eating. One man cited by Hunter (1990) remarked on this connection: "I could 'run' to this faraway corner in my mind where I
could huddle up with myself and no one could hurt me. . . . The
first clue that I'm not dealing with something going on in my life is
a desire to binge. I swear that I could binge on rocks and it
wouldn't matter" (p. 199).

The SCID-D field study uncovered previously undetected dissociative disorders in two patients with past diagnoses of eating
disorders, even though the relationship between compulsive behavior and dissociation was not the main subject of the study.
These two subjects fit the criteria for dissociative disorder not otherwise specified (DDNOS) and endorsed a history of eating disorders. One subject had been in outpatient therapy for bulimia; the
other had experienced episodes of binge eating. The first patient
associated her eating disorder with symptoms of identity confusion—that is, with an internal struggle between a part of herself
that she defined as "successful" and another part that she considered "unsuccessful" (SCID-D interview, unpublished transcript).
This self-description would be consistent with a widespread tendency in popular culture to associate slenderness in women with
success and to associate obesity in women with failure. There are

also men who have eating disorders. However, Goodwin reports that all-male samples of patients with eating disorders indicate that men are "less pressured toward abnormal eating by societal preoccupations"; rather, anorexia and bulimia in men reflect childhood trauma (Goodwin and Attias 1993). It is also not surprising that other researchers have discovered cases of DID in women in which the patient's weight was affected by the alter that was dominant at the time. Torem (1990), in fact, specifically includes the following item in his checklist of clues for early detection of DID: "The patient wearing significantly different styles of clothing from session to session to the point that therapists may feel as if they were dealing with a new person" (p. 360). In some instances, these changes in clothing styles may represent adaptations to weight fluctuations and corresponding alterations in self-image. Coons and Bowman (1993) recommended the use of the SCID-D in patient assessment in their discussion of three separate patients (1 male, 2 female) who failed to lose weight in spite of adherence to exercise regimes and calorie-restricted diets. It was found that all three patients had alter personalities who binged surreptitiously. In the SCID-D field study, one patient with DID responded to question 138, concerning identity disturbance, with a description of an internal dialogue among her alters regarding an eating binge:

Interviewer: Do you ever talk to yourself or have ongoing dialogues with yourself?

Patient: Oh, constantly.

Interviewer: What's that like? How might a dialogue go?

Patient: . . . I'm trying to remember. Well, an example might be in the grocery store [between] The Anorexic and The Fat Person. The Fat One is having an argument in front of the freezer counter. The Fat One is wanting to buy chocolate Jello pudding bars; The Anorexic is saying, "You got to be kidding, you're going to take these home and eat all 12 at once." The Fat One says, "No, I promise I will be good, I will only eat 2 a day." The Skinny One says, "You gotta . . . you're, you're, you're crazy, you're going to go home and eat every one of

> them." They get into an argument . . . they finally compromise. She said, "Yes, I promise," and I said "OK." She bought the chocolate pudding bars. She went home that night, she put them in the freezer, and The Fat One came out after dinner and ate all 12. (SCID-D interview, unpublished transcript)

Another patient in the SCID-D study, diagnosed with DID, was upset by indirect evidence from a friend that she had an alter who was a compulsive eater:

> All I know is I have a very good friend and he's like . . . like he buys Hershey bars . . . I don't eat candy, OK. He buys Hershey bars because Marsha [the alter] loves them and he keeps them in his refrigerator. And every time I go over there he hands me a whole supply and says, "Those are for you; oh excuse me, those are for Marsha." Now come on, after awhile you . . . I try to, like, stay away from him because I think he's cracking up and sick. (SCID-D interview, unpublished transcript)

In a Dutch study concerning the coexistence of eating disorders and dissociative symptoms, Havenaar et al. (1992) interviewed 25 women with eating disorders. Fourteen of these women presented with diagnoses of anorexia nervosa and 14 had diagnoses of bulimia nervosa; 3 patients were diagnosed as having both disorders. Each was given the SCID-D and the Dissociative Experiences Scale. All 25 patients had fairly high total scores on the SCID-D and endorsed a number of dissociative symptoms. No dissociative disorders were diagnosed, however. The two most common symptoms reported were depersonalization and derealization, which parallels Roth's anecdotal self-description. Identity confusion was also present but in lesser severity. Amnesia and identity alteration were uncommon. The authors found a history of physical or sexual abuse in 4 of the 25 patients (16%).

A number of researchers have found an etiologic connection between sexual abuse in childhood and eating disorders in later life. Putnam (1990) relates the high incidence of DID, "with its alternation of radically different identities," in incest survivors, to the presence of eating disorders "with their distortions of body image" in the same population. In many cases, the incest survivor begins to binge on food both to numb the immediate painful feelings and to protect herself against further molestation by making herself unattractive to the perpetrator (Roth 1992; Stone 1989). Although most recent studies on the connection between eating disorders and dissociative disturbances have been conducted in populations of female patients, insofar as eating disorders are widely regarded as a women's health issue, other accounts suggest that eating disorders are not uncommon in male incest survivors (Thomas 1989). Hunter's (1990) study uncovered several male survivors who were bulimic, including one man who began to remember his history of sexual abuse only after joining a 12-step group for overeaters. This particular survivor suggests that abused males may, like females, gain weight as a form of protection in that the fat helps to hide or cover their genitals. In this particular subpopulation, sexual dysfunction is quite common. In one study (Goodwin and Attias 1993) involving 27 male survivors with eating disorders, 26% were homosexual and "almost all had problems with sexuality and sexual behavior." Questions concerning the overlap between dissociative symptoms and other mood-altering compulsions that are not related to substance abuse, such as compulsive spending, gambling, compulsive religiosity (Booth 1991), and relationship addiction await further research.

▮ Dissociative Symptoms in Substance Use Disorders

Present standards of diagnosis and treatment of substance abuse disorders provide a useful clinical example of the complicated relationships between dissociative symptoms and Axis I substance-related disorders. Until recently most investigators assumed that drug or alcohol abuse generated dissociative symptomatology. However, recent research indicates that many persons with a primary dissociative disorder turn to mood-altering substances to self-medicate the distress caused by the dissociative symptoms (Steinberg et al. 1989–1992). Two patients in the SCID-D field study, both with DDNOS, endorsed having been in treatment for alcohol and cocaine abuse, respectively. In both cases, the substance abuse began as a response to dissociative symptoms, amnesia in the second patient and episodes of depersonalization (i.e., feeling "like a robot") in the first patient (SCID-D interviews, unpublished transcripts). Whereas the development of standardized tools for the diagnosis of a range of Axis I and Axis II disorders has aided in the evaluation of comorbid diagnoses in substance abusers (Endicott and Spitzer 1978; Spitzer et al. 1990), these tools are unable to detect the presence of dissociative symptoms and disorders in substance abuse populations. SCID-D field trials have found that the SCID-D is an effective instrument in detecting previously undiagnosed dissociative disorders in substance-abusing patients. Of 27 patients referred for evaluation with referring clinician diagnosis of alcohol abuse (including 4 referred with suspicion of dissociative disorder), 2 patients were newly detected as having dissociative amnesia, and 9 subjects were diagnosed as having DDNOS. No cases of dissociative fugue, depersonalization disorder, or DID were uncovered in this group (Steinberg et al. 1989–1992).

It is characteristic of substance-abusing patients with a coexisting dissociative disorder not only to endorse, but to elaborate on the symptom of identity alteration. As was mentioned in Chapter 12, patients with DID may well have alter personalities with substance abuse problems, even though the dominant personality may have no difficulty maintaining sobriety or abstinence.

One patient diagnosed with DID indicated the presence of an alcoholic alter even though she herself was abstinent:

Interviewer: Can you give an example of what you can't account for that you don't normally do?

Patient: I don't drink. OK, I've been in numerous bars and people have told me that I'm like, you know, "You can't have another drink because you're totally wiped out." Well, that is their opinion and I don't drink, so me, it's like, "What are you talking about?" I don't even drink and yet I'm supposed to be totally drunk. I didn't feel drunk. As a matter of fact, I never even felt like I had anything to drink, but people are telling me, around me, that I was acting totally blitzed just a few minutes before that. You know, it leaves you totally unsettled. (SCID-D interview, unpublished transcript)

One diagnostically discriminant feature that clinicians should note in the assessment of patients with coexisting dissociative and substance abuse disorders is the richness of description that characterizes patients with dissociative disorders. Descriptions of dissociative symptoms from patients without dissociative disorders tend to be unelaborate and one-dimensional. It will be evident that the open-ended format of the SCID-D facilitates the emergence of this discriminant characteristic. For example, one SCID-D subject whose primary diagnosis was substance abuse interpreted one of the interview's questions on derealization in terms of her family's behavior surprising her:

Interviewer: OK. Have you ever felt puzzled as to what is real and what is unreal in your surroundings?

Patient: I think I really know the difference, but . . .

Interviewer: But what?

Patient: But I'm not sure [laughs].

Interviewer: You're not sure?

Patient: Yeah.

Interviewer: Can you describe an instance to me where that's happened? Where you haven't been sure?

Patient: Like what [gestures]? I mean . . . ?

Interviewer: Between what is real and what is unreal in your surroundings?

Patient: Like . . . I don't understand.

Interviewer: Well, we can use the example that we had just used, like when I asked you, "Have your close friends ever seemed unreal?" And you had said, "Yeah."

Patient: Well, sometimes you think you know people. And then they totally surprise you. Like, I get surprised all the time [chuckles].

Interviewer: What happens?

Patient: Um . . . well [pauses]. Like I never know what's going to go off from day to day. You think you do, but you don't. I mean, I could go home now and . . . [pauses] I don't know, it's just . . . I kind of like don't trust the people I live with.

Interviewer: OK. (SCID-D interview, unpublished transcript)

The reader will note that this response lacks the metaphorical content and intensity of affect that typify dissociative patients' descriptions of this symptom.

In addition, professionals should note that dissociative symptoms caused solely by substance use tend to be transient, "ceasing with the elimination of the causative agent" (Good 1989). If dissociative symptoms are caused solely by the use of alcohol or drugs, a diagnosis of dissociative disorder is excluded (American Psychiatric Association 1987); on the other hand, if the dissociative symptoms are experienced at least occasionally apart from substance use, a dissociative disorder can be included in the differential diagnosis. To summarize, patients with underlying dissociative disorders may resort to drugs or alcohol to alleviate the distress, typically anxiety or depression, resulting from experiences of dissociative symptoms such as depersonalization or derealization. Accurate differential diagnosis requires assessment of the temporal relationship between the drugs or alcohol and the dissociative symptoms (see Table 14–1).

■ Dissociative Symptoms in Obsessive-Compulsive Disorder

Obsessive-compulsive disorder (OCD) is classified as an anxiety disorder in which the patient experiences repetitive, intrusive thoughts that are accompanied by compulsions to repeat them or to perform some ritual to relieve the anxiety associated with these thoughts. An example would be that of an outpatient who reported persistent and unreasonable fears of developing AIDS. The person was not engaging in any high-risk practices; nevertheless

Table 14–1. Dissociative symptoms in patients with substance abuse and in patients with dissociative disorders—dissociative identity disorder (DID) and dissociative disorder not otherwise specified (DDNOS)

Substance abuse only	Dissociative disorders (DID and DDNOS)
Context	
Five dissociative symptoms occur only in context of drug or alcohol use (e.g., alcohol induced blackouts).	Five dissociative symptoms occur in the absence of drug or alcohol use.
Content	
∎ Descriptions of dissociative symptoms are unelaborate and unidimensional.	∎ Descriptions of dissociative symptoms are elaborate and multidimensional.
∎ Depersonalization occurs in the absence of ongoing internal dialogues.	∎ Ongoing, internal dialogues. between observing and partici- pating selves can occur during episodes of depersonalization.
∎ Depersonalization and derealization episodes consist mainly of perceptual alterations involving distortions in color and shape of objects.	∎ Depersonalization and derealiza- tion episodes are described in terms of perceptual, affective, and cognitive alterations.
∎ Amnesia usually occurs for events occurring during the episode of intoxication.	∎ Amnesia may occur for complex behaviors and talents such as having acquired the skill of playing the piano.
∎ Derealization may involve the loss of the sense of familiarity for a variety of people, including strangers.	∎ Derealization experiences typically involve one's friends, family, or home.
∎ Identity alteration involves unidimensional shifts in character limited to the period of intoxication.	∎ Identity alteration consists of complex shifts in demeanor, behavior, memories, and sense of identity; it often includes the use of different names.
Course	
Dissociative symptoms are transient and temporally related to the alcohol or drugs. They may occur during intoxication and/or withdrawal states.	Dissociative symptoms are recurrent or persistent, and usually associated with dysphoria.

he washed his hands repeatedly and showered 3 times a day to "stay clean and avoid contamination" (McGlynn and Metcalf 1989). Patients with OCD, unlike patients with dissociative disorders, score low on hypnotizability scales. However, dissociative symptoms have been found in this disorder, as has been found among patients with anxiety disorders in general (Goff et al. 1992; Roth 1960). One common link between obsessive-compulsive symptoms and dissociative symptoms is patients' fears of a negative response from the interviewer. McGlynn and Metcalf (1989) report that OCD patients are aware that their rituals and/or obsessions are excessive and are often reluctant to reveal them to clinicians for fear of being judged "goofy, stupid, silly, irrational, insane, dumb, crazy, or bizarre." As a response to the anxiety, the obsessive-compulsive individual may dissociate while performing his or her rituals or compulsive behavior. Booth (1991) has noted that this connection between OCD and dissociation is particularly strong when the patient's ritualized behavior centers on religious practices, such as reciting prayers, fasting, handwashing, private confession, the wearing of phylacteries, or other ceremonials or rituals. One patient with OCD in the SCID-D field study was diagnosed as having previously undetected DID. He mentioned having been compulsive about his bedtime prayers in childhood. Some researchers have found instances of derealization in patients who experience anxiety disorder (Cassano et al. 1989; Trueman 1984a). As the reader may recall from the discussion of anxiety in the chapter on derealization, it is not unusual for patients with an anxiety disorder such as OCD to manifest a cyclical pattern of anxiety attacks and dissociative symptoms that has been labeled *phobic anxiety–depersonalization syndrome*. As was mentioned in that context, researchers are not yet certain whether underlying anxiety precipitates the episodes of derealization or whether the derealization generates the anxiety. This depersonalization-anxiety syndrome has been investigated by Ambrosino (1973) and Roth (1959). At present, a number of researchers consider anxiety as central to the microgenesis of dissociation (Cassano et al. 1989; Nemiah 1989a; Oberndorf 1950; Shorvon et al. 1946)

One group of researchers drew upon the SCID-D to assess dissociative symptoms and disorders in a sample of 100 OCD patients. Goff et al. (1992) found that these patients had dissociation scores higher than those of normal control subjects and comparable to those of patients with other anxiety disorders. Patients with high dissociation scores were also more likely to have severe OCD symptoms. The most common dissociative disorder diagnosed was depersonalization disorder ($n = 7$), followed by dissociative amnesia ($n = 3$) and DDNOS ($n = 3$). No cases of DID were diagnosed. One interesting finding of Goff et al.'s research is that OCD symptoms can mask dissociation.

In addition, Goff et al.'s study indicated that OCD patients had a surprisingly high rate of amnestic episodes, as assessed by the SCID-D, which the patients "considered . . . to be unrelated to their OCD symptoms."

In contrast to the absence of cases of DID in Goff's subject population, the SCID-D field study found one case of previously undiagnosed DID in a patient who presented with OCD. This patient, who was mentioned earlier in this section, had obsessions that included sadistic thoughts and feelings connected with experiences of identity confusion and identity alteration. The patient reported states of coconsciousness with one alter identified as "The Persecutor," and another as "The Witness," who was visualized by the patient as "starting off as a body and ending as a fluid substance or brown cloud" (SCID-D interview, unpublished transcript). The patient also experienced the presence of childlike alters of preschool age. He endorsed occasional experiences of hearing his mother's voice scolding him in the same tones as The Persecutor. As is commonplace for patients with DID, this subject reported a number of difficulties in his personal relationships and his educational and employment history (SCID-D interview, unpublished transcript).

▮ Dissociative Symptoms and Compulsive Sexual Behavior

The growing consensus in the literature regarding the connection between a history of sexual abuse in childhood and dissociative symptomatology in adult life indicates the importance of further research in the area of sexual compulsions and addictions in adults. As has been mentioned at several points in this book, patients will often spontaneously volunteer histories of childhood trauma in the course of responding to the SCID-D's questions regarding dissociative symptoms. One patient specifically mentioned that she had entered therapy in the first place to deal with her memories of molestation. The SCID-D study suggests that, just as with dissociation and anxiety, there may be a similar cyclical pattern between dissociation and sexual compulsivity. More specifically, whereas some adult survivors of abuse dissociate from their bodies during sexual activity, others sometimes engage in sexual activity as a reaction to episodes of dissociation. Whereas the first pattern is commonplace in survivors' self-help materials as well as guidebooks for therapists, the second has received less attention.

Dissociation as a survivor's learned response to sexual overtures from another person is frequently reported in the literature. Both men and women describe their dissociative reactions to their adult partners in terms of "freezing," "numbing out," "blanking out," "going out of my body," or having flashbacks during intercourse (Briere 1992; Gil 1988; Hunter 1990). However, although many survivors seek couples therapy to resolve their sexual dysfunction, most do not present with an initial history of childhood sexual abuse. Follette's (1991) study indicates that many survivors use dissociation as a coping mechanism when confronted with the partner's anger as well as with his or her desire for sex.

Clinicians who specialize in the treatment of DID have noted that some patients with DID combine a host personality who is "rigid, frigid, and compulsively good" (Putnam 1989a, p. 107) with one or more promiscuous personalities who act out sexually and often involve the host in compromising or potentially dangerous situations. Several patients in the SCID-D study endorsed the presence of alters who handled their sexuality for the entire personality system. One referred to her sexualized alter as "The Fox," and felt anxious in the presence of men because this alter might emerge and behave inappropriately. When asked if she ever suffered from panic attacks, she replied, "When I do have panic, it's as though I'm suffocating, and that's usually associated with being with a person of the opposite sex" (SCID-D interview, unpublished transcript). A male patient with DID acknowledged the existence of a promiscuous alter named "Don Juan" (SCID-D interview, unpublished transcript). A woman with DID in Cohen's (1991) anthology of first-person accounts of DID spoke of the impact of sexual compulsivity on her friendship network as well as on her personal life:

> I couldn't keep a boyfriend because on the first date, I would switch and one of the other personalities would come out and seduce my date. Of course, my date would think I was easy . . . and there would be no more dates. I had to stay away from the sports car club, the band, and my friends because the other personalities would seduce the girls' husbands or boyfriends. Soon, people began to avoid me. And I was ashamed of the situations I would end up in . . . . I fear I will live the rest of my life alone and unwanted because of a disorder that is very strange and hard for others to understand. (qtd. in Cohen et al. 1991, p. 53)

Some researchers interpret seductive behavior as a reenactment of childhood abuse. When sexual acting-out is directed against the therapist, Putnam considers it a form of aggression, "equivalent to violence or the threat of violence toward the therapist" (p. 192). Kluft (1989), on the other hand, believes that sexual acting-out may proceed from a variety of other reasons, including the wish to actualize a fantasy, a reaction formation against anger, an expression of dependency needs, an evasion of more threatening material, a narcissistic desire to be special to the therapist, and a way of rejecting the therapy. However, Kluft also mentions the motivation of *anxiety release*, which is consistent with the second pattern of connection between dissociation and sexual behavior, namely that sexual acting-out may be a response to anxiety generated by dissociative episodes or experiences.

This pattern is somewhat analogous to self-mutilation in that the patient engages in it to regroup following a dissociative experience. Hunter (1990) has discussed self-mutilation as "a method of dissociation termination" in which victims "bring themselves back to reality through the use of pain" (p. 83). In addition, *sexual masochism* and *sexual sadism* are classified under sexual and gender identity disorders by DSM-IV, combining the infliction or endurance of physical pain with the sexual act. DSM-IV also incorporates a category called *sexual disorder not otherwise specified*, which includes "distress about a pattern of repeated sexual relationships involving a succession of lovers who are experienced by the individual only as things to be used" (American Psychiatric Association 1994, p. 538).

Though the SCID-D was not designed to be a sexual history questionnaire, it may elicit accounts of sexual behavior that are distressing to patients in the course of exploring dissociative symptoms. Further research into the connections between dissociative symptoms and disorders, and sexual disturbances is needed.

■ Dissociative Symptoms in Posttraumatic Stress Disorder and Acute Stress Disorder

Posttraumatic stress disorder (PTSD) and acute stress disorder are categorized in DSM-IV as anxiety disorders, although those with these disorders experience numerous dissociative symptoms. More specifically, the first three dissociative symptoms assessed by the SCID-D (i.e., amnesia, depersonalization, and derealization) are embedded in the DSM-IV criteria for acute stress disorder. Specifically, acute stress disorder criterion B specifies the presence of three of more dissociative symptoms during or following the person's experience of severe trauma (see Tables 14–2 and 14–3).

Because criterion B specifies that the person manifest three or more symptoms of depersonalization, derealization, or amnesia, the SCID-D allows for the diagnosis of acute stress disorder as well as the five DSM-IV dissociative disorders. Acute stress disorder can generate several characteristic SCID-D profiles. As a result, persons suffering from acute stress disorder may present with several different combinations of these three core symptoms at a high level of severity, combined with a low or moderate severity level for identity confusion and identity alteration (see Figure 14–1).

Table 14–2. DSM-IV diagnostic criteria for posttraumatic stress disorder

A. The person has been exposed to a traumatic event in which both of the following were present:

    (1) the person experienced, witnessed, or was confronted with an event or events that involved actual or threatened death or serious injury, or a threat to the physical integrity of self or others

    (2) the person's response involved intense fear, helplessness, or horror. **Note:** In children, this may be expressed instead by disorganized or agitated behavior

B. The traumatic event is persistently reexperienced in one (or more) of the following ways:

    (1) recurrent and intrusive distressing recollections of the event, including images, thoughts, or perceptions. **Note:** In young children, repetitive play may occur in which themes or aspects of the trauma are expressed.

    (2) recurrent distressing dreams of the event. **Note:** In children, there may be frightening dreams without recognizable content.

    (3) acting or feeling as if the traumatic event were recurring (includes a sense of reliving the experience, illusions, hallucinations, and dissociative flashback episodes, including those that occur on awakening or when intoxicated). **Note:** In young children, trauma-specific reenactment may occur.

    (4) intense psychological distress at exposure to internal or external cues that symbolize or resemble an aspect of the traumatic event

    (5) physiological reactivity on exposure to internal or external cues that symbolize or resemble an aspect of the traumatic event

C. Persistent avoidance of stimuli associated with the trauma and numbing of general responsiveness (not present before the trauma), as indicated by three (or more) of the following:

    (1) efforts to avoid thoughts, feelings, or conversations associated with the trauma

    (2) efforts to avoid activities, places, or people that arouse recollections of the trauma

    (3) inability to recall an important aspect of the trauma

    (4) markedly diminished interest or participation in significant activities

    (5) feeling of detachment or estrangement from others

    (6) restricted range of affect (e.g., unable to have loving feelings)

    (7) sense of a foreshortened future (e.g., does not expect to have a career, marriage, children, or a normal life span)

D. Persistent symptoms of increased arousal (not present before the trauma), as indicated by two (or more) of the following:

    (1) difficulty falling or staying asleep

Table 14–2. DSM-IV diagnostic criteria for posttraumatic stress disorder *(continued)*

    (2) irritability or outbursts of anger

    (3) difficulty concentrating

    (4) hypervigilance

    (5) exaggerated startle response

E. Duration of the disturbance (symptoms in Criteria B, C, and D) is more than 1 month.

F. The disturbance causes clinically significant distress or impairment in social, occupational, or other important areas of functioning.

    Specify if:

    Acute: if duration of symptoms is less than 3 months

    Chronic: if duration of symptoms is 3 months or more

    Specify if:

    With Delayed Onset: if onset of symptoms is at least 6 months after the stressor

---

Table 14–3. DSM-IV diagnostic criteria for acute stress disorder

A. The person has been exposed to a traumatic event in which both of the following were present:

    (1) the person experienced, witnessed, or was confronted with an event or events that involved actual or threatened death or serious injury, or a threat to the physical integrity of self or others

    (2) the person's response involved intense fear, helplessness, or horror

B. Either while experiencing or after experiencing the distressing event, the individual has three (or more) of the following dissociative symptoms:

    (1) a subjective sense of numbing, detachment, or absence of emotional responsiveness

    (2) a reduction in awareness of his or her surroundings (e.g., "being in a daze")

    (3) derealization

    (4) depersonalization

    (5) dissociative amnesia (i.e., inability to recall an important aspect of the trauma)

C. The traumatic event is persistently reexperienced in at least one of the following ways: recurrent images, thoughts, dreams, illusions, flashback episodes, or a sense of reliving the experience; or distress on exposure to reminders of the traumatic event.

D. Marked avoidance of stimuli that arouse recollections of the trauma (e.g., thoughts, feelings, conversations, activities, places, people).

Table 14–3. DSM-IV diagnostic criteria for acute stress disorder
              (continued)

E. Marked symptoms of anxiety or increased arousal (e.g., difficulty
    sleeping, irritability, poor concentration, hypervigilance, exaggerated
    startle response, motor restlessness).

F. The disturbance causes clinically significant distress or impairment in
    social, occupational, or other important areas of functioning or
    impairs the individual's ability to pursue some necessary task, such
    as obtaining necessary assistance or mobilizing personal resources by
    telling family members about the traumatic experience.

G. The disturbance lasts for a minimum of 2 days and a maximum of
    4 weeks and occurs within 4 weeks of the traumatic event.

H. The disturbance is not due to the direct physiological effects of a
    substance (e.g., a drug of abuse, a medication) or a general medical
    condition, is not better accounted for by Brief Psychotic Disorder, and
    is not merely an exacerbation of a preexisting Axis I or Axis II disorder.

Individuals with PTSD may also manifest dissociative symptoms
in the form of dissociative amnesia regarding the trauma as well as
depersonalization in the form of numbing. SCID-D field trials indicate that individuals experiencing flashbacks are often experiencing
age regression (identity disturbance) and derealization (Steinberg et
al. 1989–1992). Moreover, SCID-D field trials indicate that some patients diagnosed with PTSD have underlying dissociative disorders,
particularly DID. One subject with a referring clinical diagnosis of
PTSD endorsed high levels of identity confusion and identity alteration that appeared to intensify her symptoms of amnesia, depersonalization, and derealization. The subject met DSM-IV criteria for DID.
Virtually identical dissociative symptom profiles were noted in subjects with a referring clinician diagnosis of PTSD who were identified
as having DID as compared with subjects with a referring clinician
diagnosis of DID (Steinberg, in press [a]).

The predominance of dissociative symptoms in individuals
with PTSD and acute stress disorder raise the possibility that PTSD
and acute stress disorder may be best classified as a dissociative
disorder. Further research using the SCID-D in subjects diagnosed
with PTSD and acute stress disorder will clarify the frequency of
dissociative symptoms and disorders in this patient population, as

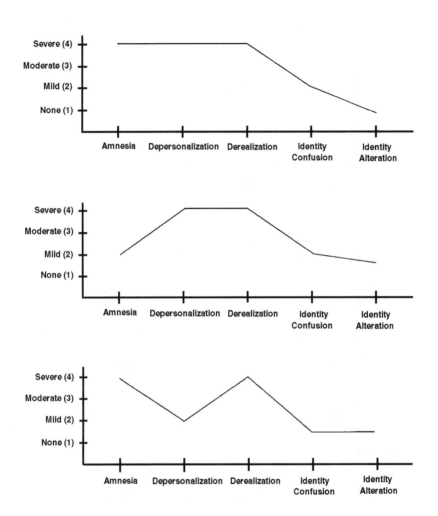

Figure 14–1. Profiles for acute stress disorder.
Source. Reprinted with permission from from Steinberg M: Interviewer's Guide to the Structured Clinical Interview of DSM-IV Dissociative Disorders (SCID-D), Revised. Washington, DC, American Psychiatric Press, 1994. Copyright © 1994, Marlene Steinberg, M.D.

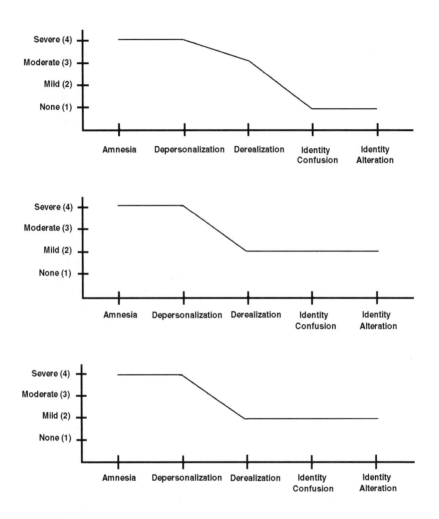

Figure 14–1. Profiles for acute stress disorder. *(continued)*

well as shed light on their classification for future revisions of DSM-IV.

Because PTSD is by definition a posttraumatic syndrome, all persons diagnosed with PTSD should be evaluated for underlying dissociation. In addition, because many persons with PTSD may be seeking government or workmen's compensation insurance, the clinician may be asked to provide symptom documentation. The SCID-D summary score sheet, along with the patient's responses to the entire interview, can be used to document the patient's baseline level of dissociative symptom severity. Such comprehensive documentation serves as the clinician's first line of defense against potential allegations of iatrogenic symptom production.

■ The Relation of Schizophrenia to Dissociative Identity Disorder

The reader may wish to consult Chapter 11 for a tabular presentation and more detailed account of the differential diagnosis of DID and schizophrenia. As was mentioned in that context, patients with DID have been frequently misdiagnosed as having schizophrenia because the occurrence of hallucinations and other first-rank symptoms in the dissociative disorders may be misinterpreted as psychosis (Kluft 1987c).

To summarize, the basic difference between the overlapping symptoms of DID and schizophrenia is the psychotic and delusional context of the latter compared with the intact reality testing that characterizes the former (Steinberg et al. 1994). For instance, identity alteration in DID occurs in the context of other dissociative symptoms (e.g., amnesia and depersonalization), whereas identity alteration in schizophrenia occurs in the context of psychotic disturbances such as a delusional identification with another person. In addition, the severity of all dissociative symptoms is higher in DID (Steinberg et al. 1994).

CHAPTER 15

The SCID-D in Clinical Practice

A Sample Interview

Interviewer: Do you have any questions about anything I've asked?

Patient: Well, what do you think about what I've told you? What do you think so far about some of the stuff I've told you?

Interviewer: I think that the symptoms you're describing are symptoms I commonly hear from people who have lived through high stress or trauma as a child.

Patient: [Skeptical] Yeah?

Interviewer: And that they're very adaptive, and they occur in very bright individuals, to help them cope.

Patient: [Nodding] Are you going to be able to help me?

Interviewer: Well, I think I can help give you a clearer understanding of your diagnosis, and help discuss it with your therapist.

Patient: Yeah? You think I'll get better?

Interviewer: I think you can.

Patient: [thoughtfully] Do you think the days will come when I won't be as scared?

Interviewer: Mmhmm, I do. (SCID-D interview, unpublished transcript)

The sample interview in this chapter is a representative case study of the use of the SCID-D (Steinberg 1993b) in diagnosing and assessing a patient with a dissociative disorder. The patient whose interview was selected for this chapter was chosen because her case is instructive on a number of different levels:

1) as an example of the length of time that can elapse between the onset of symptoms and the correct diagnosis; 2) as an instance of typical human reactions to dissociative symptomatology, both on the patient's part and on her family's; 3) as an indication of the relationship between the dissociative disorders and a history of trauma; and 4) as a case study in the use of the SCID-D in patient education as well as in diagnosis and assessment. The interviewer conducted a feedback interview with the patient 1 week after the administration of the SCID-D, during which the patient indicated that she had done a considerable amount of reflection following the assessment interview and had a more accurate perspective on both her symptoms and their significance.

In addition to a verbal summary and analysis of the interview, this chapter refers to two figures, the Differential Diagnosis Decision Tree of Amnesia (Figure 15–1) and the SCID-D Decision Tree for the Dissociative Disorders (Figure 12–5), that provide a visual representation of the diagnostic process described in this chapter. A formal evaluation protocol has also been included at the close of the case history as an example of an appropriate summary record, based on the use of the SCID-D, for inclusion in a patient's file.

Lastly, another decision tree outlining considerations relevant to forensic evaluations has been included (see Figure 15–2). The patient in the sample interview was in no way involved with the criminal justice system. However, to demonstrate the clinical and evidentiary applications of the SCID-D in evaluation and assessment of patients who are suspects in criminal cases, a brief explanation of this third decision tree has been provided. Although clinicians who frequently serve as expert witnesses in the courtroom will find this section of particular interest, it is hoped that all readers will find it instructive. The reader is referred to Appendix 2 for a sample SCID-D diagnostic report, which can be filed with patient's records and admitted in court as evidence.

❚ Case Study

Carol was referred to the author for diagnostic consultation by the patient's therapist, who suspected the presence of dissociative

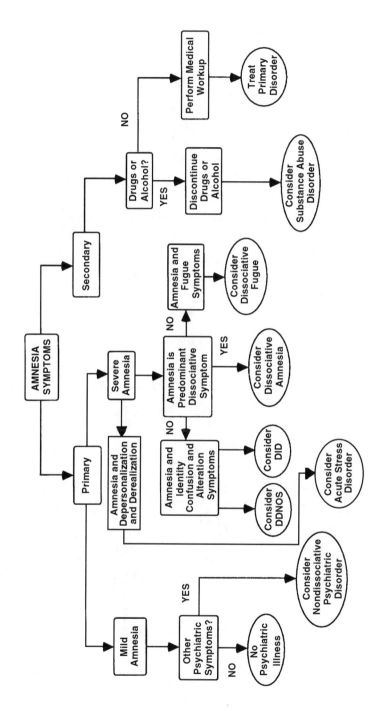

Figure 15–1. Differential diagnosis decision tree of amnesia.

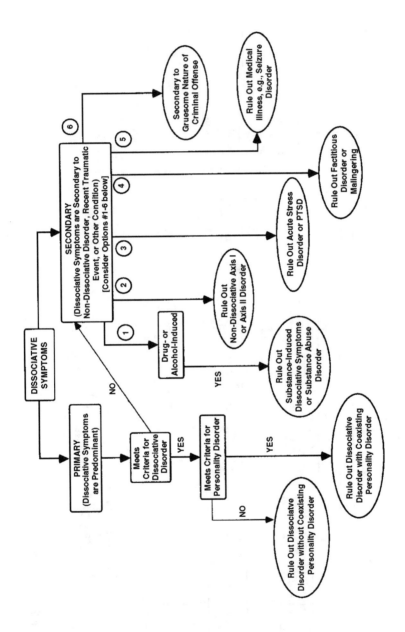

Figure 15–2. Differential diagnosis of dissociative symptoms.

symptoms. Carol's responses to SCID-D questions will be used to illustrate and review the use of the instrument in differential diagnosis and assessment, from the assessment of the severity of her dissociative symptoms to the final diagnosis.

▌ Sample SCID-D Diagnostic Interview

Demographic History, History of Present Illness, Psychiatric History

Carol is a 25-year-old, white, single woman who lives with her parents in a remote area of California. She had been diagnosed in infancy as having petit mal seizures but was referred to the author for diagnostic evaluation by her therapist and neurologist because of symptoms that were atypical of epilepsy. (See Table 5–1 in Chapter 5 for a tabular summary of the symptomatic differences between epilepsy and psychiatric disorders.) According to the patient, her seizure symptoms discontinued at the age of 18 months and returned when she was 12. At the time of the interview, she described her symptoms as "uncontrolled"; she reported experiences of "jolting awake," with "body shaking," about 4 nights per week. The patient expanded on these experiences as including feelings of "being suffocated," "feeling like I'm having a heart attack," "feeling paralyzed," and "screaming 'No!.'" In addition to her seizure symptoms, Carol had also had one experience of head injury, again in childhood, when she fell off a bed in the course of roughhousing with her siblings. She required stitches for the cut in her scalp but denied loss of consciousness.

The patient presented as a pleasant but subdued young woman, fashionably attired with a shawl, jewelry, and dark nail polish complementing her dress. She occasionally twisted the ends of the shawl during the interview. Her voice was soft, high-pitched, and slightly childlike. Although Carol's general speech patterns and vocabulary were those of a well-read and articulate person, her self-descriptions throughout the interview indicated a persistent underestimation of her intelligence and talents. She indicated that she had dropped out of college after her second year.

The patient had been hospitalized once at age 24 for psychiatric reasons. Her first deeply frightening encounter with her dissociative symptoms occurred after her discharge from the hospital, when she walked to a shopping plaza from her parents' house, wrote checks recorded in her checkbook for items that she could not recall purchasing, and wandered the area for some time unable to remember her name, address, or telephone number. She was able to be identified by the personnel department from the hospital where she had been committed. At the time of the SCID-D interview, Carol had been in outpatient therapy with a psychiatric social worker for 10 months.

Medications

The patient was taking the following medications daily at the time of the interview: carbamazepine (an anticonvulsant), 400 mg/day; fluoxetine (an antidepressant), 20 mg/day; lorazepam (an anxiolytic), .5 mg/day. She had been treated with phenobarbital to control her seizures at the time she was first diagnosed as epileptic; the medication was discontinued several years later, after her seizures stopped temporarily, and was restarted when they reappeared.

Family History

The patient endorsed a history of alcohol abuse in both parents, which began when they were separated for a year because of the father's employment, although neither parent was ever hospitalized for substance abuse. The patient remarked that her father has been drunk several times since she was in her 20s. Carol also indicated that her mother had a history of depression, which was never treated, and that her father is "maybe a little paranoid." Both parents have never been treated for their psychiatric symptoms.

During the feedback interview the following week, the patient indicated that she had been reflecting on her symptoms during the interval by asking the interviewer whether more than one member of a family could experience such symptoms. Upon follow-up questioning, Carol mentioned that her mother has mood swings and sometimes "talks in different accents," ranging from a Down East twang to an Australian accent. She also commented that her sister alternates between periods of "partying" and compulsive working. Neither the mother nor the sister is presently in treatment. The patient summarized the situation by stating, "Treatment isn't valued in our family." Clinicians should note the importance of the family history in assessment and diagnosis of the dissociative disorders, particularly since recent research has uncovered the presence of intergenerational patterns of incidence in families (Braun 1985; Kluft 1990b).

Carol spontaneously supplied some details of her family's verbal abuse of her during the SCID-D interview, such as her parents' calling her an "airhead" and their other derogatory comments about her intelligence and maturity. In addition, she endorsed a history of significant trauma during the second part of the assessment interview as well as in the feedback interview the following week. Carol's volunteering of additional information during the second interview suggests that the SCID-D may be beneficial to patients in assisting them to recall and work through traumatic events.

Carol described her parents' temporary separation and the beginning of her mother's heavy drinking as occurring when she was 10. However, she endorsed a history of verbal abuse by her parents as a constant since childhood; she added that they abused her siblings in this way as well. The patient used the metaphor of a "mine field" to define the emotional atmosphere of her household. She also reported having been sexually abused although she was unsure of her age at the time of the assault(s) or of the perpetrator's identity. A number of her symptoms suggest that the abuse may have started when she was 6 because she reported that her feelings of being smothered as well as a number of self-destructive behaviors began at that age. When asked to describe what she meant by "trying to harm herself," Carol specified drinking liquid soap, attempting to jump out of a moving car, and running in front of cars. In addition, a pattern of revictimization is present in her history; she indicated that she was raped by a former landlord and two of his friends when she was 22. She added during the feedback interview that she became pregnant by her boyfriend when she was 23 and had an abortion, which she described as a "very traumatic experience."

The material that follows includes a review of Carol's dissociative symptoms as assessed with the SCID-D, severity ratings of her symptoms, and the considerations relevant to differential diagnosis, including substance use, organic disorders, and psychotic disorders.

▌ Assessment of the Five Dissociative Symptoms

To assess the five dissociative symptoms, the interviewer used the Severity Rating Definitions of Individual Dissociative Symptoms (Steinberg 1993b, pp. 23–27, see Appendix 1 of this book), the Summary Score Sheet for the SCID-D (see Figure 15–3), and the *Interviewer's Guide to the SCID-D* (Steinberg 1993a).

Amnesia

The Symptom of Amnesia

In response to question 1: "Have you ever felt as if there were large gaps in your memory?" the patient reports experiencing significant memory deficits. She found herself "not remembering weekends, weeks, months, years—people ask questions and you don't remember being with them, don't remember childhood occurrences that everybody else seems to remember." When asked about her educational history, she indicated that she had no recollection of large blocks of her schooling, from junior high school through college. She could not remember how many times this occurs: "I really can't determine time." She reported that her time gaps were "really scary," and that she would call a crisis hotline when "coming to" (i.e., regaining consciousness), not being able to remember what she had been doing for the last several hours. On one occasion she came to in a local shopping mall, realized that she

Subjects initials __C. S.__   Date _____
Interviewer _____   Total SCID-D score __20__

SUMMARY SCORE SHEET FOR THE SCID-D

A. OVERALL DIAGNOSTIC IMPRESSION	☐ No evidence of a Dissociative Disorder
	☐ Meets criteria for a Dissociative Disorder
	    ☐ Past episode
	    ☑ Present
	☐ Meets criteria for Acute Stress Disorder

B. TYPE OF DISSOCIATIVE DISORDER	☐ Dissociative Amnesia ☐ Dissociative Fugue ☑ Dissociative Identity Disorder (Multiple Personality Disorder) ☐ Depersonalization Disorder ☐ Dissociative Disorder Not Otherwise Specified

C. DISSOCIATIVE SYMPTOMS	Severity*	
AMNESIA	1 ☐ Absent 2 ☐ Mild 3 ☐ Moderate 4 ☑ Severe	☐ Only with alcohol or drugs ☐ Sometimes with alcohol or drugs ☑ Not associated with alcohol or drugs
DEPERSONALIZATION	1 ☐ Absent 2 ☐ Mild 3 ☐ Moderate 4 ☑ Severe	☐ Only with alcohol or drugs ☐ Sometimes with alcohol or drugs ☑ Not associated with alcohol or drugs
DEREALIZATION	1 ☐ Absent 2 ☐ Mild 3 ☐ Moderate 4 ☑ Severe	☐ Only with alcohol or drugs ☐ Sometimes with alcohol or drugs ☑ Not associated with alcohol or drugs
IDENTITY CONFUSION	1 ☐ Absent 2 ☐ Mild 3 ☐ Moderate 4 ☑ Severe	☐ Only with alcohol or drugs ☐ Sometimes with alcohol or drugs ☑ Not associated with alcohol or drugs
IDENTITY ALTERATION	1 ☐ Absent 2 ☐ Mild 3 ☐ Moderate 4 ☑ Severe	☐ Only with alcohol or drugs ☐ Sometimes with alcohol or drugs ☑ Not associated with alcohol or drugs

*See Severity Rating Definitions in the *Interviewer's Guide to the SCID-D, Revised*, pp. 18–22.

Figure 15–3. Summary Score Sheet for the SCID-D.
Note. Scoring of the Summary Score Sheet for the SCID-D should be performed using the guidelines described in the *Interviewer's Guide to the Structured Clinical Interview of DSM-IV Dissociative Disorders (SCID-D), Revised.* Washington, DC, American Psychiatric Press, 1994. Copyright ø 1994, Marlene Steinberg, M.D.

had missed an appointment with her therapist, and called him in a state of considerable anxiety.

She reported frequent episodes of finding herself in a place and not knowing how or why she went there (question 7). She found herself in "San Diego, coming to in a barbershop getting my hair cut. Why or how, I don't know." She said this type of experience occurred "at least a few times a week." When asked if she had ever found herself away from home, not knowing who she was (question 11), she reported that she has experienced this often. She described being found wandering around town not knowing who she was and remembered often needing to look at her identification to determine her name, age, or address. She could not remember how many times this happens. When asked if she has ever been unable to remember this basic personal information (question 15), she said that it occurred "many times . . . every week." During the feedback interview 1 week later, Carol remarked that her fear of these amnestic episodes is her primary reason for continuing to live at home with her parents rather than attempting to find her own apartment in another town. She felt that the location of their house in an isolated spot, "in the boondocks," offered her some protection from the risks of "coming to in bars" or other unsafe places.

The patient mentioned that she compensates for her memory gaps by pretending that she recognizes people who claim to know her. In the follow-up section, later in the interview, she remarked, "I don't really have memories. I can basically tell you what people have told me, and then I have a memory of that, but it's not the actual memory."

These amnestic episodes have occurred without the use of drugs or alcohol and in the absence of acute medical illness, because the patient reports abstention from drugs or alcohol. The patient was consistent in her answers on both occasions that the interviewer asked her about her substance use. In addition, the patient's symptoms occur independently of her epilepsy and in fact were present even when she was seizure-free.

Amnesia severity rating—severe. Carol's amnesia is rated as severe because of its nature (e.g., not remembering weekends, weeks, months, years; not knowing who she was); frequency (weekly to daily gaps in her memory); and degree of accompanying distress ("really scary"). (See Appendix 1 in this volume for more information.)

The Syndrome of Dissociative Amnesia

The presence of severe amnesia warrants the consideration of two possible diagnoses: dissociative amnesia and dissociative fugue. DSM-IV criterion A for dissociative amnesia states,

> The predominant disturbance is one or more episodes of inability to recall important personal information, usually of a traumatic or stressful nature, that is too extensive to be explained by ordinary forgetfulness. (American Psychiatric Association 1994, p. 481)

Criterion B states,

> The disturbance does not occur exclusively during the course of Dissociative Identity Disorder [DID], Dissociative Fugue, Post-traumatic Stress Disorder, Acute Stress Disorder, or Somatization Disorder and is not due to the direct physiological effects of a substance (e.g., a drug of abuse, a medication) or a neurological or other general medical condition (e.g., Amnestic disorder due to Head Trauma). (p. 481)

This patient has had numerous episodes that appear to meet criterion A for dissociative amnesia, such as losing years of time and not being able to remember her age. However, this patient's amnesia symptoms are not isolated symptoms; they occur in conjunction with other dissociative symptoms. Therefore, dissociative amnesia cannot be viewed as her *predominant* disturbance. As to whether or not Carol would meet criterion B, we can only say that at this point in the interview we have information indicating that her symptoms are *not* due to alcohol/substance use or to medical illness. However, an interviewer would need to wait until the end of the interview to determine whether Carols's symptoms are due to DID.

The Syndrome of Dissociative Fugue

Dissociative fugue involves the interaction of three symptoms assessed by the SCID-D, namely amnesia, identity confusion, and identity alteration. The criteria for dissociative fugue as specified by DSM-IV (American Psychiatric Association 1994, p. 484) are as follows:

A. The predominant disturbance is sudden, unexpected travel away from home or one's customary place of work, with inability to recall one's past.
B. Confusion about personal identity or assumption of new identity (partial or complete).
C. The disturbance does not occur exclusively during the course of Dissociative Identity Disorder and is not due to the direct physiological effects of a substance (e.g., a drug of abuse, a medication) or a general medical condition (e.g., temporal lobe epilepsy).
D. The symptoms cause clinically significant distress or impairment in social, occupational, or other important areas of functioning.

The patient endorsed question 11 (traveling away from home and forgetting who she was), in support of criteria A and B. However, the fugue episodes in this patient are not isolated events; they occur in the context of the other dissociative symptoms assessed by the SCID-D. As a result, fugue cannot be described as this patient's *predominant* disturbance, and therefore she does *not* meet criterion A for dissociative fugue. In addition, the interviewer should explore possible symptoms of identity alteration in order to rule out DID, and subsequently, criterion C for dissociative fugue.

Depersonalization

The Symptom of Depersonalization

Carol endorsed numerous manifestations of depersonalization. She reported feeling as if she were watching herself from a point outside of her body (question 38): "It's like sitting on my shoulder or like standing back, watching the scene." This occurred "daily." When asked how long ago she could remember this happening, she replied, "I don't know . . . ages."

She answered question 40, whether she felt as if she were a stranger to herself, in the affirmative: "It's a little weird, feeling that your body doesn't belong to you . . . someone else's face, someone else's face in the mirror, someone else's voice, someone else's thoughts. It's frustrating. You feel trapped." Carol also endorsed the feeling that part of her body is foreign (question 41): "The hands look strange, or the arms look strange. . . . The touch . . . It didn't feel like *I* was touching me. It was someone else that was touching me. The perceptions were different. It just didn't seem right."

She mentioned feeling that her whole being was unreal (question 44). That it was "scary, depressing, very depressing. . . . It felt like just going through the motions, like the whole world was foreign or I was foreign to the whole world. It was just different." Lastly, Carol answered she felt that she was going through the motions of living but that the real self was far away (question 46). She experienced this as "watching us having a conversation with somebody . . . like watching a movie . . . like you're on the movie screen or something. It's hard to explain." She mentioned that this occurred weekly.

The patient's answers to the depersonalization section of the SCID-D are of interest to clinicians because they exemplify the ways in which the instrument's open-ended format allows patients to provide additional relevant information. For instance, Carol reported a headache during this part of the assessment interview and added that she usually experiences such headaches "right before things become strange . . . you know, tunnel vision, increased hearing, and things like that." Carol appears to be describing perceptual distortions that occur in conjunction with a derealization episode. Second, she begins to describe the impact of dissociative symptomatology on her self-esteem: she has found her symptoms "puzzling, very puzzling," but that it has taken her years to realize that "everybody doesn't feel this way. I thought it was just one of the quirks of life." The reader should note that this attitude of resignation and helplessness is one reason why so many persons with dissociative disorders have been misdiagnosed as depressives. In addition, Carol's comments exemplify the fact that many patients with dissociative disorders become habituated to their symptoms to the extent that they no longer feel disquieted by them. Carol stated that she was "not really uncomfortable [with a feeling of depersonalization] because I've felt it so often. I'm only uncomfortable now that I realize it's not normal." Third, Carol also remarks in more detail about the effects of her disorder on her relationships and consequent negative feedback from significant others. She reports not only that episodes of depersonalization interfere with her relationships because she has "to work hard at concentrating" when they occur but also that she has "heavy mood swings, radical mood swings that people complain about." During the feedback interview the following week, Carol expanded on her family's negative reactions to her illness, commenting that they call her "airhead" and "stupid" to her face and that they tell her repeatedly that she is "a pain to live with."

The patient's episodes of depersonalization have occurred without the use of drugs or alcohol and in the absence of acute medical illness. Again, she reports never using drugs or alcohol, and her symptoms are not related to her epilepsy.

Depersonalization severity rating—severe.   Carol's depersonalization is rated as severe due to its frequent recurrence ("weekly"), its extreme nature (e.g., she experienced "someone else's thoughts"), the degree of distress caused ("scary, depressing"), and the extent of dysfunctionality (difficulty concentrating). (See Appendix 1 in this volume for more information.)

The Syndrome of Depersonalization Disorder

The DSM-IV (p. 490) criteria for depersonalization disorder are as follows:

A. Persistent or recurrent experiences of feeling detached from, and as if one is an outside observer of, one's mental process or body (e.g., feeling like one is in a dream).

B. During the depersonalization experience, reality testing remains intact.

C. The depersonalization causes clinically significant distress or impairment in social, occupational, or other important areas of functioning.

D. The depersonalization experience does not occur exclusively during the course of another mental disorder, such as Schizophrenia, Panic Disorder, Acute Stress Disorder, or another Dissociative Disorder, and is not due to the direct physiological effects of a substance (e.g., a drug of abuse, a medication) or a general medical condition (e.g., temporal lobe epilepsy).

Criterion A is satisfied by Carol's multifaceted episodes of depersonalization, including feelings of unreality, foreignness, and being an external observer. Her reality testing was intact during these episodes, thus meeting Criterion B, as indicated by her lucidity and lack of delusions during her experiences of depersonalization. Marked distress and social impairment was evident in her descriptions, satisfying criterion C. Criterion D is met to the extent that Carol has no history of substance use, panic disorder, or schizophrenia, and that her depersonalization symptoms occur independently of her epilepsy. However, this patient may also meet the criteria for DID, in which case the manifestations of depersonalization disorder would be subsumed under the latter diagnosis.

Derealization

The Symptom of Derealization

On the third section of the assessment interview, Carol endorsed derealization episodes in which familiar surroundings and people felt unreal or unfamiliar (question 79). She stated, "My room seems unreal, unfamiliar, my closet, my family . . . mother, father, brother, sister. . . . They seem unfamiliar." These experiences occurred on a weekly basis. When asked if anyone in particular seemed unreal to her, she replied, "My father." She discussed her family in terms of the phenomenon of *jamias vu*, as if they were "someone you've never met, yet you know everything about them."

Carol also described being unable to recognize close friends, relatives, and her own home (question 82). She recounted "walking down the street towards a group of friends and not recognizing them until they stop and . . . start talking to me and then I realize that oh, maybe I know these people." In other instances, she remembers, "I don't drive . . . my friends drive me places . . . going home, saying they haven't been to my house before, and I can't find it. You stall and drive around for a little while until you remember which one it is, or you say, 'Oh, I have to do a chore,' and do something else, you know, without telling them." Episodes like these occur "monthly." In addition, Carol reported feeling puzzled as to what is real and unreal in her surroundings (question 84): "It's like I'm in a dream sometimes. Knowing that it's real but it doesn't seem unreal." She could not recall how often that particular form of derealization occurred.

Again, it is significant that the patient expressed harsh self-judgments during this section of the interview. When asked by the interviewer, "How do you understand that feeling [of not recognizing family members]?" Carol replied, "I don't [understand it]. I just thought I was an airhead . . . some strange psychotic person or something." Derealization enables individuals to distance themselves from their family, as can be gauged from her remark that "a lot of times it seems like I'm not a part of the family." She indicated that she felt that way at least once a week.

These derealization episodes have occurred without the use of drugs or alcohol and in the absence of acute medical illness, since she reports never using drugs or alcohol, and her symptoms are not related to her epilepsy.

Derealization severity rating—severe. This symptom is rated as severe because her derealization is recurrent and results in significant social dysfunction as is shown, for example, by her reluctance to drive. In addition, the *nature* of her derealization (she has been unable to recognize her father, close friends, and her home) is also rated as severe. (See Appendix 1 for more information.)

The Syndrome of Derealization (Dissociative Disorder Not Otherwise Specified)

When evaluating the symptom of derealization, the interviewer should include the possibility of dissociative disorder not otherwise specified (DDNOS) in the differential diagnosis. DSM-IV lists "derealization unaccompanied by depersonalization in adults" (American Psychiatric Association 1994, p. 490) as example 2 under the heading of DDNOS, which is described more fully as "disorders in which the predominant feature is a dissociative symptom (i.e., a disruption in the usually integrated functions of consciousness, memory, identity, or perception of the environment) that does not meet the criteria for any specific Dissociative Disorder" (p. 490).

Although this patient is experiencing derealization, she also has persistent episodes of severe depersonalization. Therefore, the classification *derealization unaccompanied by depersonalization in adults* is not applicable.

Identity Confusion

The Symptom of Identity Confusion

The fourth section of the SCID-D interview indicates that Carol has persistent confusion regarding her identity. When asked if there was a struggle going on inside of her (question 101), she replied, "Yes . . . A struggle for identity, who I am, what I'm like, attitudes, beliefs, knowledge . . . not knowing who I am . . . identity . . . you know, our name is Carol, but it doesn't seem like our name. Does that make sense? We're trying to figure out what that is." This struggle occurs "almost daily." She experienced these feelings as "threatening, scary, and very frustrating. Sort of like being in a candy store and not being able to decide which candy." To some extent, Carol's identity confusion was connected to her doubts about her basic intellectual capacities. During the feedback interview, there were some repeated exchanges between Carol and the interviewer regarding her intellect; she seemed surprised that the interviewer regarded her as a "bright" person:

Patient: We were never bright, though.

Interviewer: What do you mean by that?

Patient: Not intelligent.

Interviewer: What do you mean?

Patient: I don't feel . . . that I am . . . bright.

Interviewer: Perhaps the people at home couldn't appreciate your brightness.

Patient: Maybe. It's a new concept.

Carol also responded that she felt confused as to who she really was (question 102). Her descriptions included experiences of sexual identity confusion

> Not knowing even what it's like to be a woman. Not even really knowing. I know I have all the body parts, but what is that? Not knowing what I truly feel, not being able to decide on . . . just . . . a lot. . . . Well, I know, on forms, we checked "female," because we have, you know, those parts, but not knowing really what it's like to be a female? Not even really the slightest idea.

The difficulty patients often have in expressing symptoms of identity confusion is exemplified by her comment, "I'm totally puzzled—neutral. I can't even describe it. I just don't know. I just don't know. I don't." The reader should note that sexual identity confusion and a general numbing of sexual feelings are typical sequelae of the childhood sexual abuse that the patient endorsed. In the fifth section of the assessment interview, Carol mentioned her boyfriend's incomprehension mixed with anger when she could not recall their sexual activity during one of their dates. Although her comment is in reply to a question concerning identity alteration, it clearly reflects her sexual identity confusion as well.

Lastly, Carol's episodes of identity confusion occurred in the absence of substance or alcohol use and were unrelated to her epilepsy.

Identity confusion severity rating—severe. Due to the persistent/recurrent nature of her identity confusion, as well as its associated distress, this symptom is rated as severe. The nature of the identity confusion (regarding all aspects of her identity, including sexual) also yields a rating of severe. (See Appendix 1 in this volume for more information.)

Syndromes That Should Be Included in the Differential Diagnosis

When a patient experiences a moderate-to-severe level of identity confusion, the interviewer should include DID and DDNOS in the differential diagnosis. To explore this symptom and these syndromes further, refer to the SCID-D's section on identity alteration, the associated features of identity disturbance, and follow-up sections on identity confusion and alteration.

Identity Alteration

The Symptom of Identity Alteration

Carol endorses several significant subjective and behavioral manifestations of identity alteration. When asked if she ever felt as if or found herself acting as if she were still a child (question 113), she responded, "Yes," and described it as "very puzzling. Very confusing. You know, realizing that you shouldn't go around carrying a teddy bear." She reported that others criticized her childlike views and behaviors: "People saying to 'Grow up! Why are you behaving like this?' things like that." She also remembers "coming to in a toy store playing with toys, things like that." She reported that episodes of this nature occur "weekly."

When the interviewer asked her if she ever acted as if she were a completely different person (question 114), she responded, "Yeah ... Coming to in a bar, talking to a bunch of guys, that I had no idea who they are. Things like that. And then withdrawing, you know, going back, again, where you're watching. And that's the last memory." That occurs "every once in a while, that I'm, you know, aware of." In addition, she reported being told by others that she seemed like a different person (question 116): "Yes ... A friend of mine, Doug, he'll often say, 'Who are you? I don't know this Carol. Who are you?'" particularly when she doesn't remember experiences they had together that were important to him. She experienced his reactions as "distressing" and "scary." She then mentioned that "family, friends remark on mood changes that had happened that day, 'Why are you doing that? I don't understand you. Who are you?' type of thing."

Carol endorsed having referred to herself by different names (question 118) but only through confirmation from others: "Recently we've . . . we [laugh] . . . have been told that [we] refer [to ourselves] in the plural sense once in a while, and Carol is a common one at work that the girls hear. But I don't remember doing it." The patient reported that co-workers and fellow students had occasionally called her by different names (question 120): "They've called me Jamie, Vinnie, Carol, Anne, Gloria, things like that." Additionally, "Carol and Vinnie receive mail." She could remember being called these names since grade school. Her family also called her those names. When the interviewer asked if she knew the people who sent mail to the other names, she replied, "Sometimes I do, sometimes I don't. There are still a few letters that I haven't figured out who's what." When she gets the mail, "I take it upstairs to my room. Sometimes I read it and try to figure out what it is. I believe I wrote back a couple of times trying to figure out who was what, but I keep getting mail, so, I don't know . . . I would say it's an even third of the mail." She added that mail addressed to her other names has been coming to her house over a period of years.

Carol also recalled finding things in her possession that seemed to belong to her but that she could not remember purchasing (question 122). She described, "There are a lot of different toiletries. Several different perfumes. You know, lingerie that I would never imagine getting. Clothes, dresses, that I would never consider buying . . . all different styles. Young, old, tacky, tacky as in cheap." This occurs "a lot" although she believes she's not conscious of many of her shopping expeditions. Again, the stereotypically feminine character of the items in question suggests a need to resolve her sexual identity confusion through purchasing such items.

At one point in this section of the interview, the patient mentioned that she felt "controlled" (question 124). She described

> There's one I refer to as "The Screamer," which is totally scream-
> ing. Can't stop it . . . [I] Get mad at somebody and blow up more
> than you should but watching myself yell at this person and
> realizing that this isn't the way it should be. Scaring friends
> when that happens. They don't know who I am. You know, they
> jump back.

In this context also, the reader can discern the negative effects of
identity disturbance on the patient's relationships.

Carol's symptoms of identity alteration did not occur in the
context of drugs or alcohol. In addition, her medical condition
(epilepsy) was not related to these symptoms.

Identity alteration severity rating—severe. The use of several
different names to refer to oneself is listed in the SCID-D's Severity
Rating Definitions of Individual Dissociative Symptoms as a manifestation of severe identity alteration. Receiving mail addressed to
these names is another indication of severe identity alteration.
Other endorsements indicating severe identity alteration include
acting like a different person and finding unfamiliar items in her
room. (See Appendix 1 in this volume for more information.)

Syndromes That Should Be Included in the Differential Diagnosis

When a patient endorses moderate-to-severe identity alteration,
the clinician should include DID and DDNOS in the differential
diagnosis. To explore this symptom and these syndromes further,
one would refer to the associated features of identity disturbance
and the follow-up sections included in the SCID-D interview. The
diagnosis of DID subsumes the diagnosis of DDNOS as well as the
other three dissociative disorders.

Associated Features of Identity Disturbance

Mood Changes

Carol mentioned having rapid mood changes at several points
during the assessment interview but gave the most detailed an-

swer to question 134 ("Has your mood ever changed rapidly, without any reason?"). She reported that her moods fluctuated "from very calm and peaceful to very violent, angry, to crying, temper tantrums, like a little kid." When asked how often these mood changes occurred, she responded, "I would say daily." In the feedback interview, she mentioned her mood swings as one of the characteristics that her family labeled negatively as "another weird part of me."

Internal Dialogues

The patient also reported the presence of ongoing internal dialogues (question 138). She remarked that these dialogues "help me with information. Just talk. How to do things, what to do, little squabbles with myself. I've never really thought about it." These dialogues occurred "daily." When asked at this point if she was having an internal dialogue during the interview itself, she replied, "Off and on." Responses of this type should be noted for the scoring of a patient's intra-interview dissociative cues after the interview has been concluded. These endorsements, including frequent mood fluctuation and age regression, are further indications of a severe degree of identity confusion and alteration.

Summary of Dissociative Symptoms

This patient suffers from each of the five dissociative symptoms at a severe level. She has large gaps in her memory, reports weekly episodes of depersonalization and derealization, daily episodes of identity confusion, and a marked degree of identity alteration. Her endorsement of identity alteration includes the use of several names, accompanied by daily internal dialogues, a feeling of being controlled, and daily rapid mood changes. The existence of all five dissociative symptoms at a high level of severity are typical of DID or DDNOS, both of which require additional information on identity confusion and identity alteration. The necessary supplemental material can be obtained by administration of the appropriate follow-up sections.

Follow-Up Sections on Identity Confusion and Alteration

The interviewer first administered the follow-up section on *different names* (questions 192–201), because it seemed to be the most appropriate section for further elaboration of the extent of identity confusion and alteration, based on the patient's previous responses. The interviewer said, "Earlier you did mention that others have referred to you by different names, right? Vinnie and Jamie and Carol, and Gloria. Can you say some more about these names?" (elaboration on question 192). She replied, "Going along with a stranger, yes. Trying to figure out what's going on, yes."

When Carol was asked if she felt as if the names she mentioned ever controlled the way she acted or talked (question 193), she answered, "Yeah . . . Being out of control of your voice, and things like that . . . your thoughts. Racing to get a thought out, but someone else gets the voice first." When asked how her voice changed, she replied, "Whiny, up and down, you know, deep low." When the interviewer inquired as to whether she had visual images of the names (question 194), she replied, "Different variations. Sometimes of me, sometimes of I don't know who. This is really touchy. I can't say." The patient then mentioned that she was having internal dialogues at this point, which were interfering with her responses to the interviewer. Carol added that there were different ages associated with the names (question 195):

> I'd say it's 4 to 8 to 13 to 15, different stages. . . . Anne [is age 4] . . . Jamie would be 8 to 13 [pause]. Now it's getting all muddled . . . I can't grasp it. It's really weird. Sometimes thoughts come in and then they go away. It's like I'm not supposed to know or something.

She mentioned earlier in the interview that she pictured one of her child parts as "scared, lonely, and hurt," and that Anne was "scared." The interviewer then asked, "If Anne could speak, what would be said?" (question 197). Carol replied, "Anne would cry." She also mentioned that Vinnie and Jamie could talk to her therapist directly (question 198). She then described Jamie as "athletic . . . and he likes wood."

The patient was then asked if the memories, behaviors, or feelings of the names were different from her own, and she replied, "different." She mentioned that the voices inside made her aware of that as well as the letters she received that were addressed to the different names, and were written in different styles. She noted, "Vinnie is a more spiritual, asexual type, and Carol seems to be more flirtatious." She felt that the names were separate as opposed to part of her personality (question 200). At this point, the interviewer concluded the interview, having decided that a second set of follow-up questions was unnecessary; the patient had already provided responses indicating severe levels of identity confusion and alteration.

It is worth noting that the patient volunteered further information on her different names and their associated characteristics during the feedback interview the following week. (The issue of control reemerged about two-thirds of the way through the session when the interviewer asked at one point, "Who is in control?" and the patient responded, "I don't know, I don't know. . . . Whoever wants to be.") It became evident that Carol's alter personalities were not a harmonious group even though she had referred to them in passing during the initial assessment interview as her "system." Her internal conflicts surfaced in a variety of forms. One was the fear, repeatedly expressed, that integration implied the "death" of one or more alters. At one point she asked the interviewer directly whether "integration means that various parts will die" and added, "It's kind of creepy thinking that your body will be walking around but you'll be dead." At a later point, she interjected, "We just don't want to die" and explained herself more fully by indicating her assumption that integration represents the triumph or domination of one alter over the others, rather than cooperation among them: "Whoever is the strongest will take over." The reader should observe that Carol's ideation here reflects the distorted interpersonal dynamics within dysfunctional families; it is typical of such families that relationships are understood in terms of hierarchical control rather than shared power and appreciative affirmation of all family members

In addition, the competitive, conflictual attitudes of Carol's alters emerged in her description of her inner "house." As was mentioned in Chapter 9, it is not uncommon for patients with DID to use the metaphor of a house with many rooms to describe their internal personality organization. Carol introduced this image about 20 minutes into the feedback interview when she indicated that she went elsewhere while one of her alters was talking to her therapist. When the interviewer asked where she went during the alter's conversation, she replied, "This is going to sound silly. There's a house inside. Sounds weird. I go hang out in the house." She added that she had her own room in the house, which she described as "very comfortable." The interviewer then inquired, "How is it decided when you should go to that room?" and Carol responded symptomatically: "When I have a really bad headache." Following her account of the house, the patient then asked the interviewer about the possibility that her "different sides" could do harmful things to one another. When the interviewer followed up with questions concerning self-injury, Carol endorsed having come to on several occasions with self-inflicted cuts on her stomach, left part of the chest, and extremities. She described these wounds as "leaving a mark, but not enough for stitches . . . I don't know how it happened . . . I'd come to in the shower and the soap would sting in the cuts." When asked what her thoughts were at present about these experiences, the patient mentioned that she was afraid of "losing control . . . it feels like I'm at war with myself . . . [and] I wonder how high the stakes will get."

The final item of additional information concerning Carol's identity disturbance that surfaced during the feedback interview was the emergence of a previously unmentioned alter, "Gray," who seemed to represent the patient's depression and feelings of hopelessness. Toward the close of the interview, Carol became very quiet and withdrawn. She told the interviewer that Gray was speaking. The patient's inability to specify Gray's age may suggest a timeless, age-old sense of sadness and inner pain.

In summary, we learn from both interviews that Carol associates "the names" (or the personalities) with consistent behaviors, memories, and feelings that are different from her own. She reports that some of the identities have spoken with her therapist and that they seem separate from her personality. The follow-up sections of the interview have now ended.

Intra-Interview Dissociative Cues

After the conclusion of the interview, the interviewer rated the patient for intra-interview dissociative cues—that is, behaviors and symptoms observed during the interview that suggest a dissociative symptomatology and/or disorder. Thirteen items are listed in this section of the SCID-D. The interviewer is to take both verbal statements and the patient's visual appearance into account to complete this section. In this particular assessment, the interviewer did notice an alteration in the subject's demeanor and mood (when Gray emerged) (items 259–262). However, Carol was observed to refer to herself in the first person plural (item 264). Additionally, she often omitted pronouns altogether when talking about herself, suggesting confusion regarding self-reference. The patient also reported intra-interview internal dialogues (item 264). Carol exhibited intra-interview amnesia (item 265), particularly when answering chronicity questions. She gave many responses such as "I do not know" or "I do not remember" to basic questions (item 268). In addition, the patient gave ambivalent responses to questions about dissociative symptoms (item 269) as seen in her pausing, her comments that "someone" was telling her not to answer, and her occasional "uh-oh's," as if she were unsure of the safety of being honest during the interview. Moreover, Carol responded with a significant degree of emotion to questions regarding dissociative symptoms (item 270), as indicated by her sad mood, lengthy pauses, and occasional sighs. No hypnotic eye movements were observed (item 271); however, she did have a slight trancelike or glassy-eyed appearance (item 272).

Diagnostic Assessment

1. Does the patient appear to have a dissociative disorder, past or present?   This patient suffers from all five dissociative symptoms at a high level of severity: she has endorsed severe amnesia, severe depersonalization, severe derealization, severe identity confusion, and severe identity alteration. In the course of administering the follow-up section, the interviewer learns more about her severe identity fragmentation—the existence of different people within her that have different sets of memories, behaviors, and feelings. Carol describes these entities as separate in some sense from her core self rather than as integral components of her basic identity. She also regards them as competing for control over her external behavior. Carol does appear to have a dissociative disorder: "The essential feature of the Dissociative Disorders is a disruption in the usually integrated functions of consciousness, memory, identity, or perception of the environment" (American Psychiatric Association 1994, p. 477).

2. Which of the dissociative disorders should be included in the differential diagnosis? Because of the presence and high severity level of all five dissociative symptoms in this patient, the differential diagnosis includes DID and DDNOS. (See Figure 15–1 and Figure 12–5 for a summary visual representation of the differential diagnosis.) Although Carol did initially meet the initial criteria for dissociative amnesia, dissociative fugue, and depersonalization disorder, the presence of severe identity confusion and identity alteration rule these dissociative disorders out. She is more likely to be suffering from DID or DDNOS, both of which would subsume dissociative amnesia, dissociative fugue, and depersonalization disorder. What is required for further resolution is whether the patient's identity alteration is severe enough to meet DSM-IV criteria for DID.

3. Which dissociative disorder does this patient have? DSM-IV (American Psychiatric Association 1994, p. 487) criteria for DID are as follows:

A. The presence of two or more distinct identities or personality states (each with its own relatively enduring pattern of perceiving, relating to, and thinking about the environment and self).

B. At least two of these identities or personality states recurrently take control of the person's behavior.
C. Inability to recall important personal information that is too extensive to be explained by ordinary forgetfulness.
D. The disturbance is not due to the direct physiological effects of a substance (e.g., blackouts or chaotic behavior during Alcohol Intoxication) or a general medical condition (e.g., complex partial seizures). **Note:** In children, the symptoms are not attributable to imaginary playmates or other fantasy play.

Patient data from the identity confusion, identity alteration, associated features, and follow-up sections of the SCID-D fully satisfy criteria A and B. Carol's severe amnesia rating from the amnesia section satisfies criterion C. Finally, her abstinence from alcohol or drugs and the fact that she is an adult satisfy criterion D. Based on this assessment interview, this patient meets the criteria for a diagnosis of DID. The diagnosis of DID clearly subsumes the DDNOS disorders involving cases similar to DID but lacking some defining features. More inclusively, DID, being the most severe dissociative syndrome, subsumes any and all of the other dissociative disorders.

4. Is there any reason why a dissociative disorder should be excluded in this patient?   No. There is no evidence of a psychotic disorder such as schizophrenia, and Carol's reality testing appears intact. Furthermore, the patient denies use of drugs and alcohol. Although she did report a history of temporal lobe epilepsy and one incident of minor head injury (without loss of consciousness), her dissociative symptoms do not appear to be caused by these factors.

5. The Summary Score Sheet.   Finally, the interviewer possesses all the necessary information to complete the Summary Score Sheet (Figure 15–3), which is found on the last page of the SCID-D booklet. The severity of each dissociative symptom has already been noted, and the form needs only the final indication, "meets criteria for a dissociative disorder," and DID. This sheet is a concise synopsis of the patient's interview results and diagnosis. At a glance, one can see severity ratings of each of the five symptoms as well as the type of dissociative disorder, if present.

6. Forensic considerations.   As was mentioned at the beginning of this chapter, the SCID-D is a diagnostic tool that can also be helpful to clinicians involved in the diagnostic assessment of patients being evaluated for competency to stand trial, especially in cases in which there is a suspicion of DID. The patient in the foregoing sample case study was not involved in a criminal case; however, the SCID-D offers some specific advantages to clinicians working with patients with dissociative disturbances who are thus implicated. In the first place, the SCID-D Summary Score Sheet could be offered as evidence in courtroom proceedings as a form of symptom documentation. Because DID complicates evidentiary issues (Lewis and Bard 1991), the Summary Score Sheet offers an additional form of documentation that is less controversial than videotaping, amobarbital interviews, or hypnosis.

Second, the SCID-D's good-to-excellent interrater reliability for the assessment of dissociative symptoms allows for reasonable confidence in findings regarding evaluation of a patient by more than one examiner. In cases in which an accused person is transferred from one jurisdiction to another, the SCID-D can be administered without prejudice to the accused.

Figure 15–2 shows the distinction between primary and secondary dissociative symptoms that can be applied to the four major possibilities for secondary symptomatology in criminal cases:

1. The suspect has dissociative symptomatology secondary to drug or alcohol abuse, such that the crime was committed under the influence of the mood-altering substance(s).
2. The suspect has dissociative symptoms secondary to a personality disorder (e.g., antisocial personality disorder) or disorders of impulse control such as intermittent explosive disorder.
3. The suspect has developed dissociative symptoms as a reaction to the commission of a particularly gruesome or offensive

crime. Dietz (1992) has observed that "offenders are sometimes so stressed or traumatized by their offenses that they develop mental disorders. The most common among these are dissociated and depersonalized states .... Evaluators sometimes mistake such a result of crime for its cause" (p. 549). Because the SCID-D allows an interviewer to situate a suspect's dissociative symptoms within the context of his or her life history, not just the circumstances immediately surrounding the crime, it can help to differentiate between reactive and preexistent dissociative symptoms (Steinberg et al., in press).

4. The suspect is malingering or suffering from Ganser's syndrome.

Patient Education

Educating patients about the nature and prognosis of their symptoms is an important dimension of any treatment plan for recovery from a dissociative disorder. Precisely because these disorders are distinctive among psychiatric disturbances in that they have good prognoses in most cases, clinicians should be careful to inform patients in appropriate ways of their correct diagnosis. This is particularly important when the patient has a lengthy history of trauma. Because of the social consequences of dissociative symptomatology (i.e., patients' frequent difficulties with employment and intimate relationships), accurate information concerning the nature and severity of the symptoms is necessary for improvement on the interpersonal as well as the intrapsychic level. Carol's case is particularly instructive in its reflection of the contribution of negative reactions from family and friends to the patient's general attitude of depression and personal inadequacy. Consequently, it is also a useful example of the critical position of patient education in the recovery process.

The feedback interview that followed administration of the SCID-D is a remarkable illustration of a patient's first tentative steps toward empowerment and self-affirmation. At first skeptical of the interviewer's estimation of her as "bright," Carol proceeds to take a number of conversational initiatives in the course of the interview, asking questions about the necessity of recovering painful memories and of allowing her alters to identify themselves to her therapist, about the significance of her episodes of self-cutting, about the possible presence of dissociative disturbances in other family members, and about ways and means of explaining her disorder to her family. That all these insights and inquiries have arisen in her mind within a week of the SCID-D's administration is an indication of the interview's effectiveness as an educational tool as well as a diagnostic instrument. Although her low self-esteem and underestimation of her intelligence cannot be expected to dissipate overnight, it is evident from her genuine curiosity and desire to understand herself better, together with her active engagement with the interviewer, that she is on the path to recovery of confidence in her mental capacities as well as cognitive integration of them.

Treatment Planning

Carol had been referred to the author for a consultative assessment by her therapist and neurologist to rule out the presence of dissociative disorder. After the assessment and feedback interviews, the author was able to advise a course of treatment designed to alleviate her dissociative symptoms.

Accurate diagnosis is the primary step toward effective treatment of dissociative disorders. Following diagnosis, proper treatment must take account of the defensive nature of the dissociative symptoms, the sensitivity of memories of abuse and trauma, the need to reintegrate these memories, and the need to heal the patient's fragmented consciousness.

The SCID-D is also useful to clinicians in screening for specific symptoms because it allows them to monitor the patient's progress with regard to them. It is then possible to set specific treatment goals of diminishing the severity of each of the five dissociative symptoms. The reader is referred to Appendix 2 for an example of a SCID-D diagnostic report that can be filed with a patient's records.

CHAPTER 16

Conclusion

As a group, the dissociative disorders are a relatively recent addition to the literature of human suffering. Compared with the victims of some of the more headline-grabbing disasters—war, famine, plague, natural catastrophes—those who suffer from dissociative disturbances rarely make the news in terms of their primary disorder. Some people with DID may run afoul of the criminal justice system if one of their alters has a taste for violent or lethal behavior; some who turn to substance abuse to numb the distress arising from their dissociative symptoms may find themselves in a detox center or general hospital. For the most part, however, this population suffers in silence.

The suffering inflicted by dissociation is intense, not only because it is so often unspoken but because it represents a twofold insult to a person's basic sense of humanity. In the first place, the mechanism that breaks the links of memory between past and present, and between different levels of perception in the present, is experienced as an assault on a person's fundamental appreciation of his or her identity and integrity. The genuine distress that people experience as they anticipate an interviewer's possible judgment has been described at a number of points in this book: to have one's sanity or rationality questioned is to be symbolically cast out of membership in a species that defines itself by virtue of its ability to think, reason, and remember.

Second, dissociation is a silent witness in the present to abuse endured in the past. It is a mechanism that begins to operate unbidden in childhood, when a young person subjected to trauma in the family of origin learns to split off experiences of unspeakable pain. In later life, dissociative symptoms reappear when the stressors of adult existence—completing one's education or vocational training, establishing a family of one's own, planning one's future, coping with aging, and the like—reopen the scar tissue of the past. These symptoms are the wordless reemergence of the inarticulate cries of an injured child. It is hoped that this book will equip clinicians to better understand and interpret this secret language.

It is obvious that, in spite of the progress that has been made in the identification, classification, and diagnosis of the dissociative disorders, much work remains to be done. This concluding chapter will summarize a few of the areas requiring further investigation by researchers or consideration by the helping professions as a whole.

■ New Directions for Future Research

The bulk of the material in this book is intended to introduce persons in the medical and allied helping professions to the comprehensive assessment of dissociative symptoms and disorders as evaluated by the SCID-D (Steinberg 1993b) interview, as well as to the clinical applications of this diagnostic instrument. However, its format and its tested discriminant validity for the dissociative disorders commend it to researchers in a variety of disciplines.

Sociology and Cross-Cultural Studies

Although the SCID-D and some less intensive self-administered questionnaires have been drawn up in the past decade to assess the presence of dissociative symptoms and disorders, their full implementation as reliable instruments for sociological studies awaits future research. The social dimension, in its simplest terms, concerns the ways in which mental health or pathology are defined for individuals by their reference groups (i.e., the families, institutions, and other collectivities to which they belong). As Michael Kenny has observed, therapists are in the process of "engaging culturally specific problems with culturally specific tools" (Kenny 1986). At present we do not know the extent to which the dissociative disorders, at their present level of incidence, are a by-product of certain problems and stressors in the wider society and, if so, whether these problems affect all groups and classes equally. Hollingshead and Redlich (1958) demonstrated over three decades ago that social class, race, and income level very definitely affect not only the quality of treatment that persons receive within American mental health facilities but, in many cases, the diagnosis as well. With respect to the dissociative disorders in particular, the SCID-D promises to be a useful instrument in the study of the sociology of mental illness. At present we do not know whether the sex-ratio imbalance in diagnosis reflects a higher overall level of traumatic stressors in the lives of girls and women, sex-specific biochemical responses to trauma in early childhood, or patterns of sex socialization that permit women to seek therapy more readily than men. Nor do we know at present whether there is a racial imbalance in the incidence of this group of disorders. These issues deserve further attention (Lukoff et al. 1992).

It is true that DSM-IV (American Psychiatric Association 1994) has included some explicit guidelines concerning this sociological dimension of psychiatric illness. The editors include the following under the heading "Ethnic and Cultural Considerations":

Diagnostic assessment can be especially challenging when a clinician from one ethnic or cultural group uses the DSM-IV Classification to evaluate an individual from a different ethnic or cultural group. A clinician who is unfamiliar with the nuances of an individual's cultural frame of reference may incorrectly judge as psychopathology those normal variations in behavior, belief, or experience that are particular to the individual's culture. . . . The provision of a culture-specific section in the DSM-IV text, the inclusion of a glossary of culture-bound syndromes, and the provision of an outline for cultural formulation are designed to enhance the cross-cultural applicability of DSM-IV. It is hoped that these new features will increase sensitivity to variations in how mental disorders may be expressed in different cultures and will reduce the possible effect of unintended bias stemming from the clinician's own cultural background. (pp. xxiv–xxv)

With regard to the dissociative disorders, DSM-IV has introduced the category of *dissociative trance disorder* as a subcategory of dissociative disorder not otherwise specified (DDNOS), specifically to include culture-specific dissociative pathologies that might otherwise be misdiagnosed as psychosis. The SCID-D has been designed to evaluate trance disorder as well as to facilitate the study of possession states; the ninth follow-up section for optional use at the end of the interview deals specifically with possession. Moreover, the SCID-D has been translated into a Spanish-language version for use in the American Hispanic population. This version of the instrument is being field-tested for cross-cultural conceptual adequacy as well as for literal correctness of the translation. It is hoped that future SCID-D research will be able to address questions of differential *incidence* of dissociative symptoms and disorders in various racial, ethnic, occupational, or economic categories. A few current studies of dissociative symptomatology in different populations and subcultures indicate that some of the behavioral manifestations of dissociation may vary in superficial details. For example, Putnam's recent research involving African American, inner-city male adolescents discusses some culture-specific forms of dissociative symptomatology in this population, such as the use of "rap" during interviews (Putnam 1993). However, because the SCID-D is intended to assess the patient's subjective experiences of dissociation as well as external behavior, research to date indicates that it is a reliable instrument for data collection in cross-cultural or multicultural studies. The SCID-D has already been translated into Dutch, Italian, Norwegian, and Spanish, and additional translations are in press.

Longitudinal Studies

The temporal dimension of mental health issues operates on two levels: the human life cycle and the broader stream of evolution across history. On the human life cycle level, the differences between children and adults with respect to dissociative symptoms was mentioned in Chapter 2. One subject that needs further investigation is the incidence of specific dissociative symptomatology and its severity at different points in the life cycle. At present there is no way to accurately assess the actual age at onset of dissociative symptoms when patients present with long-standing, previously undiagnosed dissociative disorders. However, because the SCID-D can be used in adolescents, it is possible to evaluate patients as young as 13 (A. Steinberg and M. Steinberg 1994; M. Steinberg and A. Steinberg, in press). It is hoped that future research in the dissociative disorders will benefit from data compiled through routinized administration of instruments such as the SCID-D (Steinberg 1994b), DDIS (Ross et al. 1989), and screeners such as the DES (Bernstein and Putnam 1986), Mini-SCID-D (Steinberg, in press [b]), and the QED (Riley 1988). In addition, future studies based on the SCID-D will supplement and expand the pioneering work of Coons (1985) on intergenerational incidence of DID and Kluft (1985c) on the natural history of DID. Although it is known that DID begins in childhood, Kluft has noted that "the degree of agreement has been more substantial than the evidence marshalled to support it" (Kluft 1985b, p. 168). Moreover, although present findings support the hypothesis that the incidence of dissociative pathology or DID is transgenerational, the studies are based on retrospective evidence without the use of control groups. The need for prospective collection and interpretation of family history data is widely recognized (Braun 1985).

History of Medicine/Intellectual History

In addition to research on the incidence of the dissociative disorders across generations and within the individual's life cycle, further investigation is needed of the wider historical context of these disorders. The relationship between broadly based historical changes in the larger society and changes in the incidence of psychiatric disorders first came to the attention of the professional community after World War II, when a new generation of clinicians noticed that the classical disorders described by Freud were being displaced by a statistical increase in narcissistic and borderline disturbances. These statistics raised the question as to whether major shifts in object relations within the family were taking place or whether the popularization of psychological concepts and terminology was affecting people's self-concepts and subsequent symptom presentation. Michael Kenny has interpreted the rise in reported cases of DID precisely in terms of this circular pattern of interaction between publication and public reaction. He reported that "one psychiatric authority who has seen a considerable cohort of multiples remarks that 'naive' patients are now hard to find. Popular psychology has begun a feedback process between theory and clinical reality that produces through resonance a heightened incidence of multiple personality" (Kenny 1986, p. 164). In addition, the history of psychiatry indicates the presence of fluctuations in intellectual trends and fashions not unlike those in the humanities and social sciences. For example, Greaves' (1993) concise account of the history of DID pinpoints a number of occasions in which now-classic clinical studies "fell through the cracks" because they were published when studies of DID were not considered to be part of mainstream research. The same ebb and flow of interest marks the history of trauma studies, as Kluft (1993b) has recently observed. Although the connection between childhood trauma and dissociative disturbances in later life is generally accepted, no one can state definitely whether the incidence of child abuse is higher than it was in previous centuries, whether dissociative symptoms are more likely to be recognized by professionals in the present cultural context as an indication of disturbance, or whether abuse survivors themselves are more likely to realize that their experiences and behavior are abnormal and more likely to speak out. All that can be said for certain is that there is definitely a reciprocal interaction between the dissemination of psychological models and concepts, and people's ways of thinking and speaking about themselves. Writers as diverse as Philip Rieff and Charles Taylor have charted the ways in which the conceptual framework of Freud and his successors have become part of the mental furniture of educated men and women. For the future, researchers will want to use the SCID-D for longitudinal studies assessing the incidence of the dissociative disorders across time. Whether these disorders will continue to manifest at their present rate in their present form is a question for historians of medicine in the next generation.

Treatment Protocols and Outcome Studies

Because the SCID-D is the first tool that allows clinicians and researchers to evaluate the *severity* of specific dissociative symptom
areas, its development has opened up a new area of investigation
for researchers interested in pharmacological treatments of the dissociative disorders, as well as for researchers conducting comparative studies of pharmacotherapy and the psychotherapies. It is
likely that a variety of drugs will prove effective in treating recurrent depersonalization as well as the other dissociative symptoms.
Several researchers have reported on the potential benefits of a
variety of antianxiety and antidepressant medications (Hollander
et al. 1989; Loewenstein et al. 1988; Noyes et al. 1987; Nuller 1982;
Stein and Uhde 1989; Walsh 1975). At present, no controlled double-blind studies have been done comparing either the relative efficacy of pharmacotherapy and psychotherapy in the treatment of
dissociation, or the relative efficacy of different forms of psychotherapy. Because recent reports are anecdotal or contain small samples, controlled double-blind studies with larger patient samples
are needed before definite recommendations can be made regarding specific agents or treatment regimens. Because the SCID-D
summary score sheet can be used to record the severity as well as
the presence of dissociative symptoms, it is an effective tool for the
establishment of patients' baselines prior to medication trials, as
well as facilitating the matching of patient groups for comparative
studies. At present, it is recommended that therapeutic trials of
medications for the dissociative disorders include 1) accurate assessment of the patients' symptoms and their severity; 2) matching
of subjects in different treatment groups for comparable levels of
symptom severity; 3) systematic ratings of the five dissociative
symptoms recorded at baseline (prior to medication trials) and at
several intervals throughout the clinical trial; and 4) systematic
outcome measures, including symptom ratings. The reliability of
the SCID-D now allows researchers in these areas to evaluate the
relative efficacy of various forms of treatment, using pre- and post-
treatment assessments of symptom severity as measured by the
instrument.

▌ Reclassification of Existing Diagnostic Categories

The issue of change across history leads us to the second major area of considerations for the future: the medical profession's periodic need for reassessment of the adequacy of diagnostic nomenclature, criteria, and taxonomy. Just as epidemiologists are aware that pathogens can mutate and alter the symptoms of a disease to the point that renaming is necessary, so also psychiatrists with a knowledge of history are sensitive to the possibility that new disorders of the mind are replacing the older forms. Increasing recognition of the prevalence of the dissociative disorders and the high level of misdiagnosis of patients has led a number of researchers to speculate that dissociation may be a more inclusive concept than was previously thought. As was mentioned in Chapter 14, SCID-D research is compiling data in support of PTSD as a dissociative disturbance rather than an anxiety disorder and so may merit reclassification.

It is not unprecedented in the history of medicine for a diagnostic instrument that was drawn up to assess the incidence of a particular disorder to cause researchers to recognize the need for classificatory modifications. As the introduction to the DSM-IV indicates, field trials of new diagnostic tools were one source of data collection for evaluating revisions in classification.

Clinicians who use the SCID-D for routine screening and assessment will be contributing to increased understanding of the dissociative disorders by recording data that would be available to future researchers.

▌ Cost-Benefit Analysis

The study of cost-benefit analysis in the mental health care field is still in its early stages. Although further work in this area will obviously benefit clinicians as well as hospital administrators, it is noteworthy that one current research project concerning early diagnosis of DID estimates that proper diagnosis and treatment of this particular dissociative disorder would have saved taxpayers an average of $84,900 per patient for the first 10 years following diagnosis (Ross and Dua 1993). Given researchers' findings that an average of 7–10 years elapses between initial assessment of patients with undetected dissociative disorders and proper diagnosis (Coons et al. 1988; Kluft 1987a; Putnam et al. 1986), one can readily understand that routine screening of patients from populations known to be at risk for the dissociative disorders, such as trauma survivors, is highly cost-effective. Although the full SCID-D requires 2–3 hours of the interviewer's time, the costs of its administration are minor compared with the systemic costs of misdiagnosis and misdirected treatment. The SCID-D's cost-effectiveness is corroborated by another recent study focusing on the cost differential between inpatient and outpatient treatment for DID patients. The report estimates that the weekly cost for such patients, *when chronically hospitalized prior to the correct diagnosis,* ranges from $883–$3,176. After diagnosis, the weekly cost for appropriate outpatient treatment drops to $188 (Quimby et al. 1993). Moreover, as was mentioned in Chapter 15, patients typically find that the open-ended format of the SCID-D represents the beginning of the actual therapeutic process for them, as well as the establishment of their correct diagnosis. For many individuals, the SCID-D's questions about their experiences and reactions provide them with a new understanding of their symptoms and a less negative self-image; thus their recovery period *after* diagnosis may be effectively shortened as well.

▌ Interprofessional Education and Cooperation

The SCID-D has been designed for use by health care professionals to facilitate proper diagnosis and treatment of a specific group of mental disorders. However, because of the growing recognition that human life cannot be neatly subdivided into physical and nonphysical components, and that individuals' conditions cannot be evaluated for treatment apart from the social and kinship networks to which they belong, this book is also addressed to members of the helping professions outside the practice of medicine. As our understanding of the incidence and implications of the dissociative disorders improves, it is hoped that all professionals who come in contact with this patient population will find this book helpful in their respective fields.

Social Work

Although proper administration of the SCID-D requires that interviewers have some specific clinical training, it is not necessary that they be medical practitioners or psychiatrists. Social workers whose clients include a high percentage of persons with histories of trauma or substance abuse may find training in the administration of the SCID-D useful in evaluating clients for referral to therapy. In addition, social workers are particularly well placed to identify children at risk for intrafamilial abuse and the development of DID. To the extent that good mental health care includes prevention as well as treatment, social work professionals have an important role to play in reducing the incidence of dissociative disorders in the next generation.

Clergy and Institutional Chaplains

Religious professionals have been increasingly involved in the assessment and treatment of mental and emotional disturbances since World War II, partly because clinical pastoral education programs including psychiatric rotations are now mandatory for ordinands in mainstream Christian and Jewish traditions in the United States. Most hospitals have some form of resident chaplaincy or religious ministry and allow visiting privileges to the patients' own clergy. In addition, clergy still function as a source of referrals to clinical therapists (Bowman 1989); one recent survey found that a majority of the American population still turns to a religious professional first when confronted with a personal crisis. As a result of this pattern, a growing number of clergy are interested in continuing education programs that will help them improve their skills in distinguishing between spiritual problems and disturbances requiring psychiatric evaluation.

The dissociative disorders are particularly significant because they occupy one of the border areas between religion and psychiatry (Bowman 1993). As was mentioned earlier, because some dissociative symptoms are difficult to describe, patients who are practicing members of a religious tradition may use its language to relate their experiences. It should be noted that DSM-IV includes religious beliefs and practices in its enumeration of cross-cultural differences that clinicians must take into account in differential diagnosis (Lukoff et al. 1992). Second, certain religious practices such as prayer and meditation may occasionally induce dissociative states or experiences in patients who are vulnerable because of previously unsuspected histories of trauma. Although the risk of hallucinations or similar manifestations of dissociated material is small, one widely respected spiritual director (de Mello 1984) has acknowledged that some spiritual exercises are not profitable for people with a tendency to dissociate. Because of the growing interest in spirituality among ministerial candidates, as well as the increasing number of such persons who know themselves to be trauma survivors, most seminaries in the major traditions now have at least one faculty member in the field of psychology of religion. Clinicians who are treating patients who use religious language extensively in describing their experiences, or who are reluctant to confide in a secular therapist, may wish to consult these professionals for information or referral.

Lastly, religious professionals can help clinicians in providing or designing rituals to assist the patient's recovery. Because the majority of patients diagnosed as having a dissociative disorder are trauma survivors, those who have some form of religious commitment often find a healing ritual to be an important part of their therapy. Vesper (1991) has provided an example of a ceremony for the healing of a woman with DID who had been involved in a Druidic cult and was tormented by memories of the cult and its rituals. This particular ritual was a highly individualized ceremony that was planned by the patient and therapist together. Patients who are members of the liturgical Christian churches (Eastern Orthodox, Roman Catholic, Lutheran, and Anglican) may not be aware that these bodies have recently approved rituals for the healing of emotional trauma as well as the traditional sacraments for physical healing. Persons who are recovering from memories of traumas inflicted by men may benefit from consultation with ordained women in their respective traditions.

Law and Law Enforcement

As the introduction to DSM-IV points out, forensic medicine is a complicated subject because of "the imperfect fit between the questions of ultimate concern to the law and the information contained in a clinical diagnosis" (p. xxiii). More specifically, issues of personal responsibility for behavior are defined differently in the two fields. (For a comprehensive review of issues related to DID and criminal responsibility, see Saks 1992). However, because of a number of recent developments in law enforcement focusing attention on the dissociative disorders, a better understanding of them will be helpful to legal professionals as well as clinicians. The first has to do with the increased frequency of criminal cases in which DID has been the basis of a plea of diminished responsibility. As Crabtree's (1985) summary of the 1977 case of Billy Milligan indicates, experts in forensic psychiatry still disagree as to whether DID is a bona fide condition in which a normally law-abiding individual could have a homicidal alter personality, or whether it is simply a pseudocondition that a clever deceiver can invoke to avoid responsibility for crimes committed against society. The availability of new tools such as the SCID-D should facilitate further research with prisoners who manifest dissociative symptoms as well as with patients outside the criminal justice system. In addition, clinicians who may be involved with the legal system as expert witnesses should be aware that the SCID-D can be used to document symptoms in forensic evaluations. The SCID-D and Summary Score Sheet have been designed to be filed with patient records and can be submitted in court as documentation. (For a detailed description of the responsibilities of an expert witness, see Scheflin and Shapiro 1989). Figure 15–3, Differential Diagnosis of Dissociative Symptoms, in Chapter 15 has been included as an example of the instrument's applicability to differential diagnosis involving forensic cases.

The second development is the FBI's expansion of statistical analysis and "profiling" of serial murderers and other violent criminals within the last decade. As data compiled from administration of the SCID-D continues to accumulate, future studies of the incidence of dissociative disorders will be of interest to law enforcement professionals as well as clinicians. One account of the FBI's work in this area, written by the retired chief of the division, indicates that many of the criminals who are profiled by the FBI have dissociative symptoms (Ressler 1992). Moreover, because the legal profession has an interest in the prevention of criminal behavior as well as the administration of justice, an improved understanding of the dissociative disorders will help in this direction. For example, Hall (1989) reports a case in New Jersey in which a man with undiagnosed DID and years of misdirected therapy committed a homicide. In addition, the hypothesis that the present statistical disproportion between women and men diagnosed as dissociative can be accounted for by a large population of undiagnosed men in prison suggests not only the necessity of further research but the selective assessment of juvenile offenders with a history of trauma or substance abuse.

■ Improvements in Planning and Implementation of Therapy for the Dissociative Disorders

The SCID-D is a diagnostic instrument rather than a guide to therapeutic strategies and interventions as such. However, its semi-structured format, together with the optional sets of follow-up questions and its measurement of symptom severity, allow the therapist to plan treatment strategies that are tailor-made for each patient. The interviewer can conveniently assess the particular symptoms that are causing the most distress or the greatest dysfunction in the patient's life, document these symptoms on the summary score sheet for record-keeping purposes, and assist the patient to set appropriate goals for recovery. To return to the example of the patient cited in Chapter 15, the interviewer decided on the basis of symptom assessment that treatment goals should include reduction of the patient's amnesia and an increase in cooperation among the conflicting alter personalities. Moreover, the SCID-D questions provided the interviewer with a basis for educating the patient about the nature and specific symptoms of her disorder. Because patient education is an important dimension of recovery for persons with dissociative disorders, clinicians will find the SCID-D useful in this respect as well.

In addition, the fact that the patient is helped by the SCID-D to recognize that she or he is not "crazy" or "weird" usually lowers the patient's anxiety level within a short period of time. Clinicians will also discover that use of the SCID-D often strengthens the therapeutic alliance; because effective work between patient and therapist depends on the patient's level of trust in the therapist, the patient's discovery that the interviewer will not dismiss his or her experiences as incredible or confabulated helps to build the necessary trust. Lastly, SCID-D assessment may be useful to therapists whose professional orientation might influence them to interpret patients' self-descriptions in terms of symbolic categories (e.g., the alter personalities of a person with DID are not simply eruptions of archetypes or unassimilated *Gestalten*).

■ Summary

The SCID-D's most significant contribution to improved effectiveness in the actual treatment of patients is its provision of hope for recovery. Without hope, any person with symptoms of any form of mental disturbance will find it hard to take the next step forward. Although studies in the monetary cost-effectiveness of early diagnosis of the dissociative disorders have their rightful place in influencing the allocation of institutional resources, the ultimate high cost of misdiagnosis is the wasted years of patients' lives and the emotional burdens of unrelieved hopelessness. With regard to dissociative disturbances, Kluft has pointed out that patients with undiagnosed dissociative disorders do not improve with the simple passage of time. Unlike some forms of depression and other psychiatric disturbances, the dissociative disorders do not resolve spontaneously. Kluft (1985c) noted that "the earlier the condition is diagnosed, the more readily and rapidly it responds to treatment" (p. 200). Although therapy in adults can be prolonged and arduous, the prognosis for recovery is nonetheless good (Kluft 1984c). As Spiegel (1993) has observed, the dissociative disorders belong to the category of "the few serious psychiatric illnesses for which a record of success with appropriate psychotherapy is developing" (p. 88). Given the SCID-D's tested effectiveness in identifying previously undetected dissociative disorders, its unquestioned contribution to numbers of inpatients and outpatients alike is the benefit of a good prognosis for restoration to a full and productive life, once the correct diagnosis allows for the implementation of appropriate therapy. It is hoped that this book will help to guide clinicians in the effective use of an instrument designed to improve treatment, through the earliest possible diagnosis of a group of disorders whose victims suffer too often and too long in silence.

Severity Rating Definitions of Individual Dissociative Symptoms

1. Amnesia—A specific and significant block of time that has passed but that cannot be accounted for by memory.	SCID-D items

MILD
- Occasional forgetfulness (lasting seconds to minutes) of a minor nature or amnesia for very early childhood.

MODERATE   (ONE OF THE FOLLOWING)

• Recurrent brief episodes of amnesia (if prolonged amnesia, rate as severe).	1–16
• Frequent difficulty with memory. May be described as "gaps" in memory.	1–16
• Two or more episodes of amnesia or "blank" spells lasting from 30 minutes up to several hours.	3–5
• Up to two "blank spells" or brief amnestic periods during interview.	265
• Frequent loss of time, or time feels discontinuous.	1–16
• Episodes (1–4) of memory difficulties/amnesia that (ONE OF THE FOLLOWING)	
• produce impairment in social or occupational functioning.	21
• are not precipitated by stress.	22
• are prolonged (over 4 hours).	3–5
• are associated with dysphoria.	23

SEVERE   (ONE OF THE FOLLOWING)

• Subject experiences persistent episodes of amnesia (lasting several hours or longer).	3–5
• Subject experiences episodes of amnesia, brief or prolonged (or time feels discontinuous), most of the time.	1–16
• Subject has recurrently found self in a place away from home and is unaware of	7

how or why he/she went there.
- Subject experiences an episode of amnesia in which   3–5,
  he/she has a large memory gap for a time in his/her
  life (after age 6).
- Subject shows inability to recall important   15–16
  personal information that is too extensive to
  be explained by ordinary forgetfulness.
- Subject has abilities and/or talents that   1–16,
  he/she cannot recall learning, or subject   135
  intermittently forgets previous skills
  (e.g., subject was a skilled pianist for years,
  and states he/she "forgot" how to play the piano).
- Subject experiences significant intra-interview   265
  amnesia (e.g., subject has amnestic episode
  during interview, becomes disoriented, and is
  unaware of who he/she is or who the interviewer is).
- Frequent (more than 4) episodes of amnesia that
  (ONE OF THE FOLLOWING)
  - produce impairment in social or
    occupational functioning.   21
  - do not appear to be precipitated by stress.   22
  - are prolonged (over 4 hours).   3–5
  - are associated with dysphoria.   23

Note. The Severity Rating Definitions are not an inclusive list. The purpose of these definitions is to give the rater a general description of the parameters of the spectrum of dissociative symptoms and their severity.
Source. Reprinted with permission from Steinberg M: *Interviewer's Guide to the Structured Interview for DSM-IV Dissociative Disorders (SCID-D), Revised.* Washington, DC, American Psychiatric Press, 1994. Copyright © 1994, Marlene Steinberg, M.D.

Severity Rating Definitions of Individual Dissociative Symptoms *(continued)*

2. Depersonalization—Detachment from one's self, e.g., a sense of looking at one's self as if one is an outsider.	SCID-D items

MILD

- Single episode or rare (total of 1–4) episodes of depersonalization that are brief (less than 4 hours) and are usually associated with stress or fatigue.   38–47, 54, 55, 64

MODERATE   (ONE OF THE FOLLOWING)

- Recurrent (more than 4) episodes of depersonalization. (May be brief or prolonged. May be precipitated by stress.)   38–47, 54, 55, 64
- Episodes (1–4) of depersonalization that (ONE OF THE FOLLOWING)
  - produce impairment in social or occupational functioning.   63
  - are not precipitated by stress.   64
  - are prolonged (over 4 hours).   55
  - are associated with dysphoria.   65

SEVERE   (ONE OF THE FOLLOWING)

- Persistent episodes of depersonalization (24 hours and longer).   38–47, 55
- Episodes of depersonalization occur daily or weekly. May be brief or prolonged.   38–47, 54
- Frequent (more than 4) episodes of depersonalization that (ONE OF THE FOLLOWING)
  - produce impairment in social or occupational functioning.   63
  - do not appear to be precipitated by stress.   64
  - are prolonged (over 4 hours).   55
  - are associated with dysphoria.   65

Note. The Severity Rating Definitions are not an inclusive list. The purpose of these definitions is to give the rater a general description of the parameters of the spectrum of dissociative symptoms and their severity.

Source. Reprinted with permission from Steinberg M: *Interviewer's Guide to the Structured Interview for DSM-IV Dissociative Disorders (SCID-D), Revised.* Washington, DC, American Psychiatric Press, 1995. Copyright 1994. Copyright © 1994, Marlene Steinberg, M.D.

Severity Rating Definitions of Individual Dissociative Symptoms *(continued)*

3. Derealization—A feeling that one's surroundings are strange or unreal. Often involves previously familiar people.	SCID-D items

MILD
- Single episode or rare (total of 1–4) episodes of derealization that are brief (less than 4 hours) and are usually associated with stress or fatigue.

79–86

MODERATE   (ONE OF THE FOLLOWING)
- Recurrent (more than 4) episodes of derealization. (May be brief or prolonged. May be precipitated by stress.)

79–86

- One or few episodes of derealization that (ONE OF THE FOLLOWING)
  - produce impairment in social or occupational functioning.

91

  - are not precipitated by stress.

92

  - are prolonged (over 4 hours).

86

  - are associated with dysphoria.

93

SEVERE   (ONE OF THE FOLLOWING)
- Persistent episodes of derealization (24 hours and longer).

79–86

- Episodes of derealization occur daily or weekly. May be brief or prolonged.

79–86

- Frequent (more than 4) episodes of derealization that (ONE OF THE FOLLOWING)
  - produce impairment in social or occupational functioning.

91

  - are not precipitated by stress.

92

  - are prolonged (over 4 hours).

86

  - are associated with dysphoria.

93

Note. The Severity Rating Definitions are not an inclusive list. The purpose of these definitions is to give the rater a general description of the parameters of the spectrum of dissociative symptoms and their severity.

Source. Reprinted with permission from Steinberg M: *Interviewer's Guide to the Structured Interview for DSM-IV Dissociative Disorders (SCID-D), Revised.* Washington, DC, American Psychiatric Press, 1995. Copyright 1994. Copyright © 1994, Marlene Steinberg, M.D.

Severity Rating Definitions of Individual Dissociative Symptoms *(continued)*

4. Identity Confusion—Subjective feelings of uncertainty, puzzlement, or conflict about one's identity.	SCID-D items

MILD
- Single episode or rare (total of 1–4) episodes of confusion and/or uncertainty as to sense of self and/or who one is. Episodes are brief (less than 3 hours) and may be associated with stress.   101–112
- Single episode or rare (1–4) isolated episodes of identity crisis, characterized by uncertainty of one's role. (Often associated with life-stage transition.)   101–112

MODERATE   (ONE OF THE FOLLOWING)
- Recurrent episodes of confusion and/or uncertainty as to sense of self and/or who one is.   101–112
- Recurrent transient internal struggle regarding who one is.   102–103
- Recurrent confusion regarding one's sexual identity.   102–103
- Episodes (1–4) of identity confusion (not limited to adolescent years) that (ONE OF THE FOLLOWING)
  - produce impairment in social or occupational functioning.   110
  - are not precipitated by stress.   111
  - are prolonged (over 4 hours).   106
  - are associated with dysphoria.   112

SEVERE   (ONE OF THE FOLLOWING)
- Persistent internal struggle or uncertainty as to who one is.   102–103
- One or more episodes of complete loss of one's identity (with or without the assumption of a new identity).   11–13, 101–112
- Recurrent episodes associated with dysphoria (not limited to adolescent years).   112
- Frequent (more than 4) episodes of identity confusion (not limited to adolescent years) that (ONE OF THE FOLLOWING)

- produce impairment in social or   110
  occupational functioning.
- are not precipitated by stress.   111
- are prolonged (over 4 hours).   106
- are associated with dysphoria.   112

Note. The Severity Rating Definitions are not an inclusive list. The purpose of these defini-
tions is to give the rater a general description of the parameters of the spectrum of dis-
sociative symptoms and their severity.
Source. Reprinted with permission from Steinberg M: *Interviewer's Guide to the Structured
Interview for DSM-IV Dissociative Disorders (SCID-D), Revised.* Washington, DC, American
Psychiatric Press, 1995. Copyright 1994. Copyright © 1994, Marlene Steinberg, M.D.

Severity Rating Definitions of Individual Dissociative Symptoms *(continued)*

5. Identity Alteration—Objective behavior indicating the assumption of different identities, much more distinct than different roles.	SCID-D items

MILD

- Subject reports that he/she plays different roles or exhibits different demeanors, but is aware of this, and states that this is under his/her control (subject may refer to this as "acting"). Generally not associated with dysphoria. — 114–116, 131

MODERATE   (ONE OF THE FOLLOWING)

- Subject reports alterations in identity (acting like two different people). However, it is unclear whether these identity alterations take control of his/her behavior or it is unclear whether these alterations in identity represent distinct personalities. The alterations in identity are not always in his/her control. — 114–117, 234–244
- Subject spontaneously refers to self in first-person plural ("we") or third person ("he/she"). — 263
- Subject has internal dialogues between different aspects of self, which have unique characteristics such as age, visual appearance, etc. — 134–158, 202–211
- INTRA-INTERVIEW CUES of moderate identity alteration, i.e., several of the following: subtle changes in voice, speech, behavior, demeanor, movement characteristics, or general style of responding. — 259–272

SEVERE   (ONE OF THE FOLLOWING)

- Subject has experienced alterations in identity representing distinct personalities that appear to take control of his/her behavior. — 113–117, 234–244
- Subject has serious indicators of alteration in identity (such as the use of several names). — 118–121
- Subject has considered having or has had a sex-change operation. — 101–112

- Subject has referred to self by several names, or
  others have referred to him/her by different
  names (not only nicknames, and not for
  antisocial reasons only).

  118–121

- Subject has been told frequently that he/she acts
  like a completely different person or frequently
  feels as if he/she has led completely different lives,
  and is unaware of why that has occurred.

  114–117

- Subject feels as if there are one or more people
  inside of him/her who influence his/her behavior.

  114–117, 124

- Subject feels as if there is a child inside of him/
  her, which takes control of his/her behavior and/
  or speech.

  113, 212–222

- Subject has a history of spontaneous age regressions.

  113, 136, 223–233

- INTRA-INTERVIEW CUES of severe identity
  alteration, i.e., several of the following:
  distinct changes in voice, speech, behavior,
  demeanor, movement characteristics, or
  general style of responding.

  259–272

Note. The Severity Rating Definitions are not an inclusive list. The purpose of these definitions is to give the rater a general description of the parameters of the spectrum of dissociative symptoms and their severity.

Source. Reprinted with permission from Steinberg M: *Interviewer's Guide to the Structured Interview for DSM-IV Dissociative Disorders (SCID-D), Revised.* Washington, DC, American Psychiatric Press, 1995. Copyright 1994. Copyright © 1994, Marlene Steinberg, M.D.

Sample SCID-D Diagnostic Report for Inclusion in Patient Records

[letterhead]

[date]

Summary of evaluation: Carol Smith

Dates of evaluation: 2/20/93, 2/27/93, with Carol.

Referral sources: Martin Stone, M.S.W.; Jane Doe, M.D. (neurologist)

Reason for referral: Diagnostic evaluation, suspects presence of dissociative symptoms that cannot be accounted for by patient's history of epilepsy.

Information obtained from: Carol, current therapist, and referring neurologist

Brief summary: Carol Smith is a 25-year-old part-time secretary in Palm City, CA, and residing with her parents in Los Santos, CA. Carol was referred for diagnostic evaluation due to dissociative symptoms that her neurologist felt were not due to her petit mal epilepsy. She has a history of self-destructive behaviors, including self-cutting and the swallowing of household cleaners. She is currently in treatment with Mr. Stone on a once-weekly basis. She has reported instances of "coming to" in other cities on the West Coast, such as Seattle and San Diego, as well as finding herself in shopping malls, bars, etc. These episodes are unrelated to substance abuse or epileptic seizures and have been occurring over a period of years. The patient also mentioned several traumatic sexual experiences, including a gang rape at age 22 and an abortion at age 23.

Psychiatric history: Hospitalization for 3 weeks at Grove Village Hospital in 1990, followed by individual therapy with Mr. Stone.

See reports from Grove Village Hospital for further details. Mr. Stone reports that he thinks the patient's current diagnosis is Borderline Personality Disorder.

Family history: Carol described being subjected to verbal and sexual abuse in childhood and referred to alcohol abuse on the part of both parents beginning when she was 10. She mentioned that her parents were separated for a year at this time due to the requirements of the father's employment. Carol is the youngest of three children and has an older sister and an older brother. During the second interview on 2/27, the patient reported that her mother and sister manifest a variety of dissociative and compulsive symptoms. She indicated at that time that her family is not supportive of her problems, not well disposed toward psychotherapy in general, and inclined to ridicule or criticize her frequently.

SCID-D evaluation summary: In addition to performing a routine diagnostic evaluation, I administered the Structured Clinical Interview for DSM-IV Dissociative Disorders (SCID-D; Steinberg 1993b) to systematically evaluate posttraumatic dissociative symptoms and the presence of dissociative disorders. The SCID-D interview was then scored according to the guidelines described in the Interviewer's Guide to the SCID-D (Steinberg 1993a). A review of the significant findings from the SCID-D interview includes the following:

Carol is suffering from severe amnestic episodes that occur on a daily or weekly basis and involve losses of significant periods of time, including unexplained journeys and unaccountable purchases. She also experiences recurrent episodes of depersonalization that include feeling that her body does not belong to her, that "someone else" touches her, and that she is like an observer sitting on her own shoulder. In addition, Carol endorses severe recurrent derealization and identity confusion, particularly confusion regarding her sexual identity. She reports episodes of identity alteration that include childlike behavior, mood swings that are confusing to her boyfriend and other friends, referring to herself by different names, including Vinnie, Jamie, Carol, and Gloria, and receiving mail addressed to these names. She also endorsed feeling controlled by these entities and experiencing them as separate from herself. Carol was able to describe several examples of their control of her behavior, including speaking to her therapist and instances of self-cutting.

Mental status exam: Carol was casually dressed in a conservative dress, was calm and cooperative. She spoke clearly and intelligently, and answered questions with relevant replies. She denied having any psychotic symptoms. Based on information obtained from the SCID-D interview, Carol has suffered for many years from posttraumatic dissociative symptoms, including severe amnesia, depersonalization, derealization, identity confusion, and identity alteration. She acknowledged intermittent feelings of depression that did not last for more than 2 weeks at a time; she also had episodic feelings of anxiety and panic. She felt that her moods were not in her control. Carol has also had intermittent suicidal ideation and a history of self-destructive behaviors, including self-cutting, for which she has been amnestic. She denied acute suicidal or homicidal ideation.

Assessment: Based on this evaluation, Carol's symptoms and history of trauma are consistent with a primary diagnosis of a dissociative disorder. More particularly, her experiences of severe amnesia, depersonalization, derealization, identity confusion, and identity alteration consisting of the presence of several different alters who exist within her and assume executive control of her behavior, are consistent with a diagnosis of Dissociative Identity Disorder (formerly Multiple Personality Disorder). She is also suffering from a coexisting seizure disorder.

Recommendation: I would recommend intensive individual therapy focused on treatment of the dissociative symptoms. I would recommend specifically that the course of treatment include educating the patient about the nature of her symptoms and helping her to identify the specific stimuli that trigger her amnesia, depersonalization, derealization, and identity alteration. This should be done to reduce the frequency and severity of her symptoms. Furthermore, I would recommend exploration of the conflicts among her alter personalities to facilitate cooperation among them and to reduce the patient's self-destructive and self-mutilating behavior.

[signature]

References

Ackner B: Depersonalization; I: aetiology and phenomenology. Journal of Mental Science 100:838–853, 1954

Akhtar S, Brenner I: Differential diagnosis of fugue-like states. J Clin Psychiatry 40:381–385, 1979

Ambrosino SV: Phobic-anxiety-depersonalization syndrome. N Y State J Med 73:419–425, 1973

American Psychiatric Association: Diagnostic and Statistical Manual of Mental Disorders, 3rd Edition. Washington, DC, American Psychiatric Association, 1980

American Psychiatric Association: Diagnostic and Statistical Manual of Mental Disorders, 3rd Edition, Revised. Washington, DC, American Psychiatric Association, 1987

American Psychiatric Association: Diagnostic and Statistical Manual of Mental Disorders, 4th Edition. Washington, DC, American Psychiatric Association, 1994

American Psychiatric Association Board of Trustees: Statement on Memories of Sexual Abuse, December 1993

Anderson EW: Prognosis of the depressions of later life. Journal of Mental Science 82:559–588, 1936

Arlow JA: Depersonalization and derealization, in Psychoanalysis: A General Psychology. Edited by Loewenstein RM, Newman LM, Schur M. New York, International Universities Press, 1966, pp 456–478

Augustine: Confessions. Translated by Pine-Coffin RS. Harmondsworth, UK, Penguin Books, 1961

Bagley C: The prevalence and mental health sequels of child sexual abuse in a community sample of women aged 18 to 27. Canadian Journal of Community Mental Health 10:103–116, 1991

Baker AW, Duncan SP: Child sexual abuse: a study of prevalence in Great Britain. Child Abuse Negl 9:457–467, 1985

Bear DM, Fedio P: Quantitative analysis of interictal behavior in temporal lobe epilepsy. Arch Neurol 34:454–467, 1977

Bellah RN, Madsen R, Sullivan WM, et al: Habits of the Heart: Individuality and Commitment in American Life. Berkeley, University of California Press, 1985

Benson DF: Amnesia. South Med J 171:1221–1227, 1978

Berkow I: The Burden of Unhealed Memory. The New York Times. August, 15, 1993, pp 1–9

Bernstein E, Putnam FW: Development, reliability and validity of a dissociation scale. J Nerv Ment Dis 174:727–735, 1986

Bingley T: Mental symptoms in temporal lobe epilepsy and temporal lobe gliomas. Acta Psychiatrica et Neurologica 33 (suppl 120):1–151, 1958

Blackmore S: Out of body experiences in schizophrenia: a questionnaire survey. J Nerv Ment Dis 174:615–619, 1986

Bliss EL: Multiple personalities, related disorders, and hypnosis. Am J Clin Hypn 26:114–123, 1983

Bliss EL: Spontaneous self-hypnosis in multiple personality disorder. Psychiatr Clin North Am 7:136–137, 1984

Bliss E: Multiple Personality, Allied Disorders and Hypnosis. New York, Oxford University Press, 1986

Bliss EL, Jeppsen EA: Prevalence of multiple personality among inpatients and outpatients. Am J Psychiatry 142:250–251, 1985

Bliss EL, Clark LD, West CD: Studies of sleep deprivation: relationship to schizophrenia. Arch Neurological Psychiatry 81:348–359, 1959

Bok S: Lying: Moral Choice in Public and Private Life. New York, Random House, 1978

Bonime W: Depersonalization as a manifestation of evolving health. J Am Acad Child Adolesc Psychiatry 1:109–123, 1973

Boon S, Draijer N: Diagnosing dissociative disorders in The Netherlands: a pilot study with the Structured Clinical Interview for DSM-III-R Dissociative Disorders. Am J Psychiatry 148:458–462, 1991

Booth L: When God Becomes A Drug. New York, Jeremy P. Tarcher, 1991

Bourne DJ: Truth beyond history: pitfalls and challenges. Psychiatric Annals 24:155–159, 1994

Bowman ES: Clinical and spiritual effects of exorcism in fifteen patients with multiple personality disorder. Dissociation 6:222–231, 1993

Bowman ES: Understanding and responding to religious material in the therapy of multiple personality disorder. Dissociation 2:231–238, 1989

Bradshaw J: Healing the Shame that Binds You. Deerfield Beach, FL, Health Communications, 1988

Brauer R, Harrow M, Tucker G: Depersonalization phenomena in psychiatric patients. Br J Psychiatry 117:509–515, 1970

Braun BG: Towards a theory of multiple personality and other dissociative phenomena. Edited by Braun BG. Psychiatr Clin North Am 7:171–194, 1984

Braun BG: The transgenerational incidence of dissociation and multiple personality disorder: a preliminary report, in Childhood Antecedents of Multiple Personality. Edited by Kluft RP. Washington, DC, American Psychiatric Press, 1985, pp 128–150

Braun BG: Treatment of Multiple Personality Disorder. Washington, DC, American Psychiatric Press, 1986

Braun BG: The BASK (Behavior, Affect, Sensation, Knowledge) model of dissociation. Dissociation 1:4–23, 1988

Braun BG: Dissociative disorders as sequelae to incest, in Incest-Related Syndromes of Adult Psychopathology. Edited by Kluft RP. Washington, DC, American Psychiatric Press, 1990, pp 227–245

Braun BG, Sachs RG: The development of multiple personality disorder: predisposing, precipitating, and perpetuating factors, in Childhood Antecedents of Multiple Personality. Edited by Kluft RP. Washington, DC, American Psychiatric Press, 1985, pp 37–65

Breuer J, Freud S: Studies on Hysteria (1893–1895). New York, Basic Books, 1955

Briere JN: Child Abuse Trauma: Theory and Treatment of the Lasting Effects. Newbury Park, CA, Sage, 1992

Briere J, Conte J: Self-reported amnesia for abuse in adults molested as children. Journal of Traumatic Stress 6:21–31, 1993

Brown LM, Gilligan C: Meeting at the Crossroads: Women's Psychology and Girls' Development. Cambridge, MA, Harvard University Press, 1992

Bryer JB, Nelson BA, Miller JB, et al: Childhood physical and sexual abuse as factors in adult psychiatric illness. Am J Psychiatry 144:1426–1430, 1987

Cameron P, Proctor K, Coburn W, et al: Child molestation and homosexuality. Psychol Rep 58:327–337, 1986

Cassano GB, Petracca A, Perugi G, et al: Derealization and panic attacks: a clinical evaluation on 150 patients with panic disorder/agoraphobia. Compr Psychiatry 30:5–12, 1989

Castillo RJ: Depersonalization and meditation. Psychiatry 53:158–168, 1990

Cattell JP, Cattell JS: Depersonalization: psychological and social perspectives, in American Handbook of Psychiatry, 2nd Edition. Edited by Arieti S. New York, Basic Books, 1974, pp 766–799

Chernin K: The Hungry Self: Women, Eating and Identity. New York, Times Books, 1985

Chopra H, Beatson J: Psychotic symptoms in borderline personality disorder. Am J Psychiatry 143:1605–1607, 1986

Christianson S, Nilsson L-G: Functional amnesia as induced by a psychological trauma. Memory and Cognition 12:142–155, 1984

Christodoulou GN: Role of depersonalization-derealization phenomena in delusional misidentification syndromes. Bibl Psychiatr 164:99–104, 1986

Chu JA: On the misdiagnosis of multiple personality disorder. Dissociation 4:200–204, 1991

Chu JA, Dill DL: Dissociative symptoms in relation to childhood physical and sexual abuse. Am J Psychiatry 147:887–892, 1990

Clary WF, Burstin KJ, Carpenter JS: Multiple personality and borderline personality disorder. Psychiatr Clin North Am 7:89–100, 1984

Cohen SI: The pathogenesis of depersonalization: a hypothesis (letter). Br J Psychiatry 152:578, 1988

Cohen BM, Giller E, Lynn W: Multiple Personality Disorder From the Inside Out. Lutherville, MD, The Sidran Press, 1991

Coleman SM: Misidentification and non-recognition. Journal of Mental Science 79:42–51, 1933

Confer WN, Ables BS: Multiple Personality: Etiology, Diagnosis and Treatment. New York, Human Sciences Press, 1983

Coons PM: The differential diagnosis of multiple personality: a comprehensive review. Psychiatr Clin North Am 12:51–67, 1984

Coons PM: Children of parents with multiple personality disorder, in Childhood Antecedents of Multiple Personality. Edited by Kluft RP. Washington, DC, American Psychiatric Press, 1985, pp 151–165

Coons PM: Treatment progress in 20 patients with multiple personality. J Nerv Ment Dis 174:715–721, 1986

Coons PM: Iatrogenesis and malingering of multiple personality disorder in the forensic evaluation of homicide defendants. Psychiatr Clin North Am 14:757–768, 1991

Coons PM, Bowman ES: Dissociation and eating (letter). Am J Psychiatry 150:171, 1993

Coons PM, Milstein V: Psychosexual disturbances in multiple personality: characteristics, etiology, and treatment. J Clin Psychiatry 47:106–110, 1986

Coons PM, Milstein V: Self-mutilation associated with dissociative disorders. Dissociation 3:81–87, 1990

Coons PM, Milstein V: Psychogenic amnesia: a clinical investigation of 25 cases. Dissociation 5:73–79, 1992

Coons PM, Bowman ES, Milstein V: Multiple personality disorder: a clinical investigation of 50 cases. J Nerv Ment Dis 176:519–527, 1988

Crabtree A: Multiple Man: Explorations in Possession and Multiple Personality. New York, Praeger, 1985

Croft PB, Heathfield KWG, Swash M: Differential diagnosis of transient amnesia. BMJ 4:593–596, 1973

Dietz PE: Mentally disordered offenders: patterns in the relationship between mental disorder and crime. Psychiatr Clin North Am 15:539–551, 1992

de Mello A: Sadhana: A Way to God: Christian Exercises in Eastern Form. New York, Image Books, 1984

Deisenhammer E: Transient global amnesia as an epileptic manifestation. J Neurol 225:289–292, 1981

Devinsky O, Putnam F, Grafman J, et al: Dissociative states and epilepsy. Neurology 39:835–840, 1989

Dixon JC: Depersonalization phenomena in a sample population of college students. Br J Psychiatry 109:371–375, 1963

Dwyan J, Bowers K: The use of hypnosis to enhance recall. 222:184–185, 1983

Edwards G, Angus J: Depersonalization. Br J Psychiatry 120:242–244, 1972

Eichenbaum L, Orbach S: Understanding Women: A Feminist Psychoanalytic Approach. New York, Basic Books, 1983

Ellenberger HF: The Discovery of the Unconscious: The History and Evolution of Dynamic Psychiatry. New York, Basic Books, 1970

Ellerstein N, Canavan JW: Sexual abuse of boys. Am J Dis Child 134:250–257, 1980

Emslie GJ, Rosenfelt A: Incest reported by children and adolescents hospitalized for severe psychiatric problems. Am J Psychiatry 140:708–711, 1983

Endicott J, Spitzer RL: A diagnostic interview: the Schedule for Affective Disorders and Schizophrenia. Arch Gen Psychiatry 35:837–844, 1978

Ensink BJ: Confusing Realities: A Study on Child Sexual Abuse and Psychiatric Symptoms. Amsterdam, VU University Press, 1992

Erickson MH: A special investigation into altered states of consciousness with Aldous Huxley. Am J Clin Hypn 8:14–32, 1965

Erikson EH: Identity: Youth and Crisis. New York, WW Norton, 1968

Farmer S: Adult Children of Abusive Parents. Walnut Creek, CA, Launch Press, 1989

Fast I, Chethik M: Aspects of depersonalization-derealization in the experience of children. International Review of Psychoanalysis 3:483–490, 1976

Fewtrell WD: Depersonalization: a description and suggested strategies. British Journal of Guidance and Counseling 14:263–269, 1986

Fine CG: Thoughts on the cognitive perceptual substrates of multiple personality disorder. Dissociation 1:5–10, 1988

Fine CG: The cognitive sequelae of incest, in Incest-Related Syndromes of Adult Psychopathology. Edited by Kluft RP. Washington, DC, American Psychiatric Press, 1990, pp 161–182

Fink DL: The core self: a developmental perspective on the dissociative disorders. Dissociation 1:43–47, 1988

Finkelhor D, Hotaling G, Lewis IA, et al: Sexual abuse in a national survey of adult men and women: prevalence, characteristics, and risk factors. Child Abuse Negl 14:19–28, 1990

Fishel R: The Journey Within. Deerfield Beach, FL, Health Communications, 1987

Fleiss J, Gurland BJ, Goldberg K: Independence of depersonalization-derealization. J Consult Clin Psychol 43:110–111, 1975

Fletcher LY: Again, in She Who Was Lost Is Remembered. Edited by Wisechild LM. Seattle, WA, The Seal Press, 1991, p 52

Flor-Henry P: Epilepsy and psychopathology, in Recent Advances in Clinical Psychiatry. Edited by Granville-Grossman K. Edinburgh, Churchill Livingstone, 1976

Follette VM: Marital therapy for sexual abuse survivors, in Treating Victims of Child Sexual Abuse. Edited by Briere J. San Francisco, CA, Jossey-Bass, 1991, pp 61–71

Fontana VJ: Somewhere a Child Is Crying: Maltreatment—Causes and Prevention, Revised Edition. New York, Mentor Books, 1992

Frances A, Sacks M, Aronoff M: Depersonalization: a self relations perspective. Int J Psychoanal 58:325–331, 1977

Frankel FH: Hypnotizability and dissociation. Am J Psychiatry 147:823–829, 1990

Frankel FH: Adult reconstruction of childhood events in the multiple personality literature. Am J Psychiatry 150:954–958, 1993

Freud S: The aetiology of hysteria (1896), The Standard Edition of the Complete Psychological Works of Sigmund Freud, Vol 3. Translated and edited by Strachey J. London, Hogarth Press, 1962, pp 191–221

Freud S: Beyond the pleasure principle (1920), in The Standard Edition of the Complete Psychological Works of Sigmund Freud, Vol 18. Translated and edited by Strachy J. London, Hogarth Press, 1920

Freud S: Introductory Lectures on Psychoanalysis (1922). New York, WW Norton, 1966

Frischholz EJ: The relationship among dissociation, hypnosis, and child abuse in the development of multiple personality disorder, in Childhood Antecedents of Multiple Personality. Edited by Kluft RP. Washington, DC, American Psychiatric Press, 1985, pp 99–126

Fritz GS, Stoll K, Wagner NN: A comparison of males and females who were sexually molested as children. J Sex Marital Ther 7:54–59, 1981

Gabel S: Dreams and dissociation theory: speculations on beneficial aspects of their linkage. Dissociation 3:38–47, 1990

Galdston I: On the etiology of depersonalization. J Nerv Ment Dis 105:25–39, 1947

Gale J, Thompson RJ, Moran T, et al: Sexual abuse in young children: it's clinical presentation and characteristic patterns. Child Abuse Negl 12:163–170, 1988

Ganaway GK: Historic versus narrative truth: clarifying the role of exogenous trauma in the etiology of MPD and its variants. Dissociation 2:205–220, 1989

Garbarino J, Guttman E, Seeley J: The Psychologically Battered Child: Strategies for Identification, Assessment and Intervention. San Francisco, CA, Jossey-Bass, 1986

Garcia FO: The concept of dissociation and conversion in the new edition of the International Classification of Diseases (ICD-10). Dissociation 3:204–208, 1990

Gelinas DJ: The persisting negative effects of incest. Psychiatry 46:312–332, 1983

Gergen K: The Saturated Self: Dilemmas of Identity in Contemporary Life. New York, Basic Books, 1991

Ghadirian AM, Gauthier S, Bertrand S: Anxiety attacks in a patient with a right temporal lobe meningioma. J Clin Psychiatry 47:270–271, 1986

Gil E: Outgrowing the Pain: A Book For and About Adults Abused as Children. San Francisco, CA, Launch Press, 1984

Gil E: Treatment of Adult Survivors of Childhood Abuse. Walnut Creek, CA, Launch Press, 1988

Gilbert GJ: Transient global amnesia: manifestation of medial temporal lobe epilepsy. Clinical Electroencephalogr 9:147–152, 1978

Glass JM: Shattered Selves: Multiple Personality in a Postmodern World. Ithaca, NY, Cornell University Press, 1993

Glover J: I: The Philosophy and Psychology of Personal Identity. London, Allen Lane, Penguin Press, 1988

Goff DC, Olin JA, Jenike MA, et al: Dissociative symptoms in patients with obsessive-compulsive disorder. J Nerv Ment Dis 180:332–337, 1992

Goldman RJ, Goldman JD: The prevalence and nature of child sexual abuse in Australia. Australian Journal of Sex, Marriage and Family 9:94–106, 1988

Good MI: Substance-induced dissociative disorders and psychiatric nosology. J Clin Psychopharmacol 9:88–93, 1989

Goodwin J: Credibility problems in multiple personality disorder patients and abused children, in Childhood Antecedents of Multiple Personality. Edited by Kluft RP. Washington, DC, American Psychiatric Press, 1985, pp 1–19

Goodwin JM: Applying to adult incest victims what we have learned from victimized children, in Incest-Related Syndromes of Adult Psychopathology. Edited by Kluft RP. Washington, DC, American Psychiatric Press, 1990, pp 55–74

Goodwin JM, Attias R: Eating disorders in survivors of multimodal childhood abuse, in Clinical Perspectives on Multiple Personality Disorder. Edited by Kluft RP, Fine CG. Washington, DC, American Psychiatric Press, 1993, pp 327–341

Greaves GB: Multiple personality: 165 years after Mary Reynolds. J Nerv Ment Dis 168:577–596, 1980

Greaves GB: A history of multiple personality disorder, in Clinical Perspectives on Multiple Personality Disorder. Edited by Kluft RP, Fine CG. Washington, DC, American Psychiatric Press, 1993, pp 355–380

Green H: I Never Promised You a Rose Garden. New York, Holt, Rinehart, & Winston, 1964

Greenberg MS, van der Kolk BA: Retrieval and integration of traumatic memories with the "painting cure," in Psychological Trauma. Edited by van der Kolk BA. Washington, DC, American Psychiatric Press, 1987, pp 191–215

Grigsby JP: Depersonalization following minor closed head injury. International Journal of Clinical Neuropsychology 8:65–68, 1986

Grigsby JP, Johnston CL: Depersonalization, vertigo and Meniere's disease. Psychol Rep 64:527–534, 1989

Gunderson JG: Borderline Personality Disorder. Washington, DC, American Psychiatric Press, 1984

Gunderson JG, Kolb JE, Austin V: The Diagnostic Interview for Borderline Patients. Am J Psychiatry 138:896–903, 1981

Gutheil TG: True or false memories of sexual abuse? A forensic psychiatric view. Psychiatric Annals 23:527–531, 1993

Guttmann E, Maclay W: Mescalin and depersonalization. Journal of Neurological Psychopathology 16:193–212, 1936

Hall P, Steinberg M: Systematic assessment of dissociative symptoms and disorders in a clinical out-patient setting: three cases. Dissociation 7:21, 1994

Hall P: Multiple Personality Disorder and Homicide: Professional and Legal Issues. Dissociation 2:110–115, 1989

Hammond C: Handbook of Hypnotic Suggestions and Metaphors. New York, WW Norton, 1990

Harper M, Roth M: Temporal lobe epilepsy and the phobic anxiety-depersonalization syndrome. Compr Psychiatry 3:129–151, 1962

Havenaar J, Boon S, Tordoir C: Dissociative symptoms in patients with eating disorders in the Netherlands: a study using a self rating scale (DES) and a structured clinical interview (SCID-D). International Conference on Multiple Personality/Dissociative States. Rush-Presbyterian–St. Luke's Medical Center, Rush North Shore Medical Center, Skokie, Illinois, 1992

Helzer J, Robins L, McEvoy L: Post-traumatic stress disorder in the general population. N Engl J Med 317:1630–1634, 1987

Herman JL: Father-Daughter Incest. Cambridge, MA, Harvard University Press, 1981

Herman J, Schatzow E: Recovery and verification of memories of childhood sexual trauma. Psychoanal Q 4:1–14, 1987

Hewlett SA: When the Bough Breaks: The Cost of Neglecting Our Children. New York, Basic Books, 1991

Hicks R: Failure to Scream. Nashville, TN, Thomas Nelson Publishers, 1993

Hilgard ER: Divided Consciousness: Multiple Controls in Human Thought and Action, Expanded Edition. New York, Wiley, 1986

Hollander E, Fairbanks J, Decaria C, et al: Dr. Hollander and associates reply (comment). Am J Psychiatry 146:401, 1989

Hollingshead AB, Redlich FC: Social Class and Mental Illness: A Community Study. New York, Wiley, 1958

Horevitz RP, Braun BG: Are multiple personalities borderline? Psychiatr Clin North Am 7:69–87, 1984

Horowitz M: Hallucinations: an information processing approach, in Hallucinations. Edited by Siegel RK, West LJ. New York, Wiley, 1975, pp 163–195

Hornstein NL, Tyson S: Inpatient treatment of children with multiple personality/dissociative disorders and their families. Psychiatr Clin North Am 24:631–648, 1991

Horton P, Miller D: The etiology of multiple personality. Compr Psychiatry 13:151–159, 1972

Hovec FJM: Hypnosis to facilitate recall in psychogenic amnesia and fugue states: treatment variables. Am J Clin Hypn 24:7–13, 1981

Hunter M: Abused Boys: The Neglected Victims of Sexual Abuse. New York, Fawcett Columbine, 1990

Husain A, Chapel JL: History of incest in girls admitted to a psychiatric hospital. Am J Psychiatry 140:591–593, 1983

Imlah N: Unusual effect of fenfluramine. BMJ 2:178–179, 1970

Institute of Psychiatry and Maudsley Hospital: Psychiatric Examination: Notes on Eliciting and Recording Clinical Information in Psychiatric Patients. New York, Oxford University Press, 1987

Jacobson E: Depersonalization. J Am Psychoanal Assoc 7:581–610, 1959

Jacobson A, Richardson B: Assault experiences of 100 psychiatric inpatients: evidence of the need for routine inquiry. Am J Psychiatry 144:908–913, 1987

Jacobson A, Herald C: The relevance of childhood sexual abuse to adult psychiatric inpatient care. Hosp Community Psychiatry 41:154–158, 1990

Jaffe R: Dissociative phenomena in former concentration camp inmates. Int J Psychoanal 49:310–312, 1968

James W: Principles of Psychology. New York, Dover Publications, 1890

Janet P: The Major Symptoms of Hysteria. New York, Macmillan, 1907

Janet P: Psychological Healing, Vols 1 & 2. New York, Macmillan, 1925

Karasek R, Theorell T: Healthy Work: Stress, Productivity, and the Reconstruction of Working Life. New York, Basic Books, 1990

Kaushall PI, Zetin M, Squire LR: A psychosocial study of chronic, circumscribed amnesia. J Nerv Ment Dis 169:383–389, 1981

Keller R, Shaywitz BA: Amnesia or fugue state: a diagnostic dilemma. Developmental and Behavioral Pediatrics 7:131–132, 1986

Kelly L: Surviving Sexual Violence. Minneapolis, University of Minnesota Press, 1988

Kempe CH, Helfer R: The battered child syndrome. JAMA 181:17–24, 1962

Kenna J, Sedman G: Depersonalization in temporal lobe epilepsy and the organic psychoses. Br J Psychiatry 111:293–299, 1965

Kennedy RBJ: Self-induced depersonalization syndrome. Am J Psychiatry 133:1326–1328, 1976

Kenny M: The Passion of Ansel Bourne: Multiple Personality in American Culture. Washington, DC, Smithsonian Institution Press, 1986

Kercher G, McShane M: The prevalence of child sexual abuse victimization in an adult sample of Texas residents. Child Abuse Negl 8:495–501, 1984

Kernberg OF: Severe Personality Disorders: Psychotherapeutic Strategies. New Haven, CT, Yale University Press, 1984

Keshaven MS, Lishman WA: Prolonged depersonalization following cannabis abuse. British Journal of Addiction 81:140–142, 1986

Kiersch TA: Amnesia: a clinical study of ninety-eight cases. Am J Psychiatry 119:57–60, 1962

Kihlstrom JF: Conscious, subconscious, unconscious: a cognitive perspective, in The Unconscious Reconsidered. Edited by Bowers KS, Meichenbaum. New York, Wiley, 1984

Kihlstrom JF: The cognitive unconscious. Science 237:1445–1452, 1987

Kihlstrom JF: Dissociative and conversion disorders, in Cognitive Science and Clinical Disorders. Edited by Stein DJ, Young J. Orlando, FL, Academic Press, 1992

Kihlstrom JF, Hoyt I: Repression, dissociation, and hypnosis, in Repression and Dissociation: Implications for Personality Theory, Psychopathology and Health. Edited by Singer JL. Chicago, IL, University of Chicago Press, 1990, pp 181–208

Kirshner LA: Dissociative reactions: an historical review and clinical study. Acta Psychitr Scand 49:698–711, 1973

Kluft RP: An introduction to multiple personality disorder. Psychiatric Annals 14:19–24, 1984a

Kluft RP: Multiple personality in childhood. Psychiatr Clin North Am 7:121–134, 1984b

Kluft RP: Treatment of multiple personality: a study of 33 cases. Psychiatr Clin North Am 7:9–29, 1984c

Kluft RP: Childhood Antecedents of Multiple Personality. Washington, DC, American Psychiatric Press, 1985a

Kluft RP: Childhood multiple personality disorder: predictors, clinical findings and treatment results, in Childhood Antecedents of Multiple Personality. Edited by Kluft RP. Washington, DC, American Psychiatric Press, 1985b, pp 167–196

Kluft RP: The natural history of multiple personality disorder, in Childhood Antecedents of Multiple Personality. Edited by Kluft RP. Washington, DC, American Psychiatric Press, 1985c, pp 197–238

Kluft RP: First rank symptoms as a diagnostic clue to multiple personality disorder. Am J Psychiatry 144:293–298, 1987a

Kluft RP: Making the diagnosis of multiple personality disorder, in Diagnostics and Psychopathology. Edited by Flach FF. New York, Norton, 1987b, pp 207–225

Kluft RP: An update on multiple personality disorder. Hosp Community Psychiatry 38:363–373, 1987c

Kluft RP: The dissociative disorders, in The American Psychiatric Press Textbook of Psychiatry. Edited by Talbott J, Hales R, Yudofsky S. Washington, DC, American Psychiatric Press, 1988a, pp 557–585

Kluft RP: The phenomenology and treatment of extremely complex multiple personality disorder. Dissociation 1:47–57, 1988b

Kluft RP: Treating the patient who has been sexually exploited by a previous therapist. Psychiatr Clin North Am 12:483–500, 1989

Kluft RP: Incest and subsequent revictimization: the case of therapist-patient sexual exploitation, with a description of the sitting duck syndrome, in Incest-Related Syndromes of Adult Psychopathology. Edited by Kluft RP. Washington, DC, American Psychiatric Press, 1990a, pp 263–287

Kluft RP: On the apparent invisibility of incest: a personal reflection on things known and forgotten, in Incest-Related Syndromes of Adult Psychopathology. Edited by Kluft RP. Washington, DC, American Psychiatric Press, 1990b, pp 11–34

Kluft RP: Multiple personality disorder, in American Psychiatric Press Review of Psychiatry, Vol 10. Edited by Tasman A, Goldfinger SM. Washington, DC, American Psychiatric Press, 1991, pp 161–188

Kluft RP: Basic principles in conducting the psychotherapy of multiple personality disorder, in Clinical Perspectives on Multiple Personality Disorder. Edited by Kluft RP, Fine CG. Washington, DC, American Psychiatric Press, 1993a, pp 19–50

Kluft RP: Foreword: on paradigms and the legitimization of myopia, in Rediscovering Childhood Trauma: Historical Casebook and Clinical Applications. Edited by Goodwin JM. Washington, DC, American Psychiatric Press, 1993b, pp xv–xxii

Kluft RP, Braun BG, Sachs RG: Multiple personality, intrafamilial abuse, and family psychiatry. International Journal of Family Psychiatry 5:283–301, 1984

Kluft RP, Steinberg M, Spitzer RL: DSM III-R revisions in the dissociative disorders: an explanation of their observation and rationale. Dissociation 1:39–46, 1988

Knoepfler PT, Knoepfler GS: Beyond true and false answers: a continuum approach to diagnosing symptoms of sexual abuse. Psychiatric Times, May 1994, pp 24–25

Kohan MJ, Pothier P, Norbeck JS: Hospitalized children with history of sexual abuse: incidence and care issues. Am J Orthopsychiatry 57:258–264, 1987

Kopelman MD: Amnesia: organic and psychogenic. Br J Psychiatry 150:428–442, 1987

Krener P: After incest: secondary prevention? J Am Acad Child Adolesc Psychiatry 24:231–234, 1985

Krizek GO: Derealization without depersonalization (comment). Am J Psychiatry 146:401, 1989

Krugman S: Trauma in the family: perspectives on the intergenerational transmission of violence, in Psychological Trauma. Edited by van der Kolk BA. Washington, DC, American Psychiatric Press, 1987, pp 127–151

La Rue A: Memory loss and aging: distinguishing dementia from benign senescent forgetfulness and depressive pseudomentia. Psychiatr Clin North Am 5:89–103, 1982

Langer LL: Holocaust Testimonies: The Ruins of Memory. New Haven, CT, Yale University Press, 1991

Lehman L: Depersonalization. Am J Psychiatry 131:1221–1224, 1974

Lerner HG: Women in Therapy. New York, Jason Aronson, 1988

Levi P: Voices, in Against Forgetting: Twentieth-Century Poetry of Witness. Edited by Forché C. New York, WW Norton, 1993, p 377

Levy JS, Wachtel PL: Depersonalization: an effort at clarification. Am J Psychoanal 38:291–300, 1978

Lewis DO, Bard JS: Multiple personality and forensic issues. Psychiatr Clin North Am 14:750–756, 1991

Linton PH, Estock RE: The anxiety phobic depersonalization syndrome: role of the cognitive-perceptual style. Diseases of the Nervous System 38:138–141, 1977

Livingston R: Sexually and physically abused children. J Am Acad Child Adolesc Psychiatry 16:413–415, 1987

Loewenstein RJ: Psychogenic amnesia and psychogenic fugue: a comprehensive review, in American Psychiatric Press Review of Psychiatry, Vol 10. Edited by Tasman A, Goldfinger SM. Washington, DC, American Psychiatric Press, 1991, pp 189–222

Loewenstein RJ, Hornstein N, Farber B: Open trial of clonazepam in the treatment of post-traumatic stress symptoms in MPD. Dissociation 1:3–11, 1988

Lower RB: Affect changes in depersonalization. Psychoanal Rev 59:565–577, 1972

Ludwig AM: Altered states of consciousness. Arch Gen Psychiatry 15:225–233, 1966

Ludwig AM: The psychobiological functions of dissociation. Am J Clin Hypn 26:93–99, 1983

Lukianowicz N: "Body image" disturbances in psychiatric disorders. Br J Psychiatry 113:31–47, 1967

Lukoff D, Lu F, Turner R: Psychoreligious and psychospiritual problems. J Nerv Ment Dis 180:673–682, 1992

MacNeice L: Prayer before birth, in Against Forgetting: Twentieth-Century Poetry of Witness. Edited by Forché C. New York, WW Norton, 1993, p 249

Marcum JM, Wright K, Bissell WG: Chance discovery of multiple personality disorder in a depressed patient by amobarbital interview. J Nerv Ment Dis 174:489–492, 1985

Mayer R: Through Divided Minds: Probing the Mysteries of Multiple Personalities. New York, Avon Books, 1988

Mayer-Gross W: On depersonalization. Br J Med Psychol 15:103–126, 1935

McGee R: Flashbacks and memory phenomena: a comment on "Flashback Phenomena—Clinical and Diagnostic Dilemmas." J Nerv Ment Dis 172:273–278, 1984

McGlynn TJ, Metcalf HL: Diagnosis and Treatment of Anxiety Disorders: A Physician's Handbook. Washington, DC, American Psychiatric Press, 1989

McKinney K, Lange M: Familial fugue: a case report. Can J Psychiatry 28:654–656, 1983

Mesulam M-M: Dissociative states with abnormal temporal lobe EEG: multiple personality and the illusion of possession. Arch Neurol 38:176–181, 1981

Miller A: Prisoners of Childhood. New York, Basic Books, 1981

Miller A: For Your Own Good: Hidden Cruelty in Child-Rearing and the Roots of Violence. New York, Farrar, Straus, Giroux, 1983

Miller A: Thou Shalt Not Be Aware: Society's Betrayal of the Child. New York, Meridian, 1984

Miller A: The Untouched Key: Tracing Childhood Trauma in Creativity and Destructiveness. New York, Doubleday, 1988

Miller JW, Petersen RC, Metter EJ, et al: Transient global amnesia: clinical characteristics and prognosis. Neurology 37:733–737, 1987

Minsky M: K-lines: a theory of memory. Cognitive Science 4:117–133, 1980

Moran C: Depersonalization and agoraphobia associated with marijuana use. Br J Med Psychol 59:187–196, 1986

Myers D, Grant G: A study of depersonalization in students. Br J Psychiatry 121:59–65, 1972

Myers MF: Physical and sexual abuse histories of male psychiatric patients (letter). Am J Psychiatry 148:399, 1991

Nathanson DL: Understanding what is hidden: shame in sexual abuse. Psychiatr Clin North Am 12:381–388, 1989

Neisen JH, Sandall H: Alcohol and other drug abuse in a gay/lesbian population: related to victimization? Journal of Psychology and Human Sexuality 3:151–168, 1990

Nemiah JC: Dissociative amnesia: a clinical and theoretical reconsideration, in Functional Disorders of Memory, 14th Edition. Edited by Kihlstrom JF, Evans FJ. Hillsdale, NJ, Lawrence Erlbaum Associates, 1979

Nemiah JC: Dissociative disorders, in Comprehensive Textbook of Psychiatry, 4th Edition. Edited by Kaplan H, Sadock B. Baltimore, MD, Williams & Wilkins, 1985, pp 942–957

Nemiah JC: Dissociative disorders (hysterical neurosis, dissociative type), in Comprehensive Textbook of Psychiatry, 5th Edition. Edited by Kaplan H, Sadock B. Baltimore, MD, Williams & Wilkins, 1989a, pp 1028–1044

Nemiah JC: Dissociation, conversion, and somatization, in American Psychiatric Press Review of Psychiatry, Vol 10. Edited by Tasman A, Goldfinger S. Washington, DC, American Psychiatric Press, 1991, pp 248–260

Nietzsche F: On the Advantage and Disadvantage of History for Life (1874). Translated by Peter Preuss. New York, Hackett, 1980

North CS, Ryall J-EM, Ricci DA, et al: Multiple Personalities, Multiple Disorders, Psychiatric Classification and Media Influence. New York, Oxford University Press, 1993

Noyes R, Kletti R: Depersonalization in the face of life-threatening danger: an interpretation. Omega: The Journal of Death and Dying 7:103–114, 1976

Noyes R Jr, Kletti R: Depersonalization in response to life-threatening danger. Compr Psychiatry 18:375–384, 1977a

Noyes R Jr, Kletti R: Panoramic memory: a response to the threat of death. Omega: The Journal of Death and Dying 8:181–194, 1977b

Noyes RJ, Hoenk P, Kuperman S, et al: Depersonalization in accident victims and psychiatric patients. J Nerv Ment Dis 164:401–407, 1977

Noyes RJ, Kuperman S, Olson S: Desipramine: a possible treatment for depersonalization disorder. Can J Psychiatry 32:782–784, 1987

Nuller YL: Depersonalisation: symptoms, meaning, therapy. Acta Psychiatr Scand 66:451–458, 1982

Oberndorf C: Role of anxiety in depersonalization. Int J Psychoanal 31:1–5, 1950

Ogata SN, Silk KR, Goodrich S, et al: Childhood sexual and physical abuse in adult patients with borderline personality disorder. Am J Psychiatry 147:1008–1013, 1990

Parfit D: Reasons and Persons. Oxford, UK, Oxford University Press, 1983

Pessoa F: The Book of Disquiet. Translated by MacAdam A. New York, Pantheon, 1991

Pope H, Jonas J, Hudson J, et al: An empirical study of psychosis in borderline personality disorder. Am J Psychiatry 142:1285–1290, 1985

Pulse: child abuse. The New York Times, May 1, 1994, p B1

Putnam FW: Dissociation as a response to extreme trauma, in Childhood Antecedents of Multiple Personality. Edited by Kluft RP. Washington, DC, American Psychiatric Press, 1985, pp 65–97

Putnam FW: Diagnosis and Treatment of Multiple Personality Disorder. New York, Guilford, 1989a

Putnam FW: Disturbances of "self" in victims of childhood sexual abuse, in Incest-Related Syndromes of Adult Psychopathology. Edited by Kluft RP. Washington, DC, American Psychiatric Press, 1990, pp 113–131

Putnam FW: Dissociation in the inner city, in Clinical Perspectives on Multiple Personality Disorder. Edited by Kluft RP, Fine CG. Washington, DC, American Psychiatric Press, 1993, pp 179–200

Putnam FW, Loewenstein RJ, Silberman EK, et al: Multiple personality disorder in a hospital setting. J Clin Psychiatry 45:172–175, 1984

Putnam FW, Guroff J, Silberman E, et al: The clinical phenomenology of multiple personality disorder: 100 recent cases. J Clin Psychiatry 47:285–293, 1986

Quimby LG, Andrei A, Putnam FW Jr: The deinstitutionalization of patients with chronic multiple personality disorder, in Clinical Perspectives on Multiple Personality Disorder. Edited by Kluft RP, Fine CG. Washington, DC, American Psychiatric Press, 1993, pp 201–225

Reber AS: The Penguin Dictionary of Psychology. London, Penguin Books, 1985

Reed G: The Psychology of Anomalous Experience. Buffalo, NY, Prometheus Books, 1988

Reed GF, Sedman G: Personality and depersonalization under sensory deprivation conditions. Percept Mot Skills 18:659–660, 1964

Reiser MF: Memory in Mind and Brain: What Dream Imagery Reveals. New York, Basic Books, 1990

Ressler RK: Whoever Fights Monsters. New York, Saint Martin's Press, 1992

Richards D: A study of the correlations between subjective psychic experiences and dissociative experiences. Dissociation 4:83–91, 1991

Riley K: Measurement of dissociation. J Nerv Ment Dis 176:449–450, 1988

Risin LI, Koss MP: The sexual abuse of boys: prevalence and descriptive characteristics of childhood victimization. Journal of Interpersonal Violence 2:309–323, 1987

Roberts W: Normal and abnormal depersonalization. Journal of Mental Science 106:478–493, 1960

Rosenbaum M: The role of the term schizophrenia in the decline of the diagnoses of multiple personality. Arch Gen Psychiatry 37:1383–1385, 1980

Ross CA, Norton G: Multiple personality disorder patients with a prior diagnosis of schizophrenia. Dissociation 1:39–42, 1988

Ross CA, Dua V: Psychiatric health care costs of multiple personality disorder. Am J Psychother 47:103–112, 1993

Ross CA, Heber S, Norton GR, et al: The Dissociative Disorders Interview Schedule: a structured interview. Dissociation 2:169–189, 1989

Ross C, Ryan L, Voigt H, et al: High and low dissociators in a college student population. Dissociation 3:147–151, 1991

Roth G: When Food is Love: Exploring the Relationship Between Eating and Intimacy. New York, Penguin Books, 1992

Roth M: The phobic anxiety-depersonalization syndrome. Proc Roy Soc Med 52:587–595, 1959

Roth M: The phobic anxiety-depersonalization syndrome and some general aetiological problems in psychiatry. J Neuropsychiatry 1:293–306, 1960

Roth M, Harper M: Temporal lobe epilepsy and the phobic anxiety-depersonalization syndrome; II: practical and theoretical considerations. Compr Psychiatry 3:215–226, 1962

Roth M, Argyle N: Anxiety, panic, and phobic disorders: an overview. J Psychiatr Res 22:33–54, 1988

Rowan AJ, Rosenbaum DH: Ictal amnesia and fugue states. Adv Neurol 55:357–367, 1991

Ruedrich SL, Chu C-C, Wadle CV: The Amytal interview in the treatment of psychogenic amnesia. Hosp Community Psychiatry 36:1045–1046, 1985

Russell DEH: The incidence and prevalence of intrafamilial and extrafamilial sexual abuse of female children. Child Abuse Negl 7:133–146, 1983

Russell DEH: Sexual Exploitation: Rape, Child Sexual Abuse, and Workpace Harassment. Beverly Hills, CA, Sage, 1984

Russell DEH: The Secret Trauma: Incest in the Lives of Girls and Women. New York, Basic Books, 1986

Rutter P: Sex in the Forbidden Zone: When Men in Power—Therapists, Doctors, Clergy, Teachers, and Others—Betray Women's Trust. New York, Jeremy P Tarcher, 1991

Saks ER: Multiple personality disorder and criminal responsibility. UC Davis Law Review 25:384–461, 1992

Sandberg DN: The child abuse-delinquency connection: evolution of a therapeutic community. J Psychoactive Drugs 18:215–220, 1986

Sanders B: Dr. Sanders replies. Am J Psychiatry 149:1127, 1992a

Sanders B: The imaginary companion experience in multiple personality disorder. Dissociation 5:159–162, 1992b

Sansonnet-Hayden H, Haley G, Marriage K, et al: Sexual abuse and psychopathology in hospitalized adolescents. J Am Acad Child Adolesc Psychiatry 26:753–757, 1987

Saperstein JL: On the phenomenon of depersonalization. J Nerv Ment Dis 110:236–251, 1949

Sarlin CN: Depersonalization and derealization. Journal of the American Psychiatric Association 10:784–804, 1962

Schachtel E: On memory and childhood amnesia. Psychiatry 10:1–26, 1947

Schacter DL, Kihlstrom JF: Functional amnesia, in Handbook of Neuropsychology. Edited by Boller F, Grafman J. Elsevier, 1989, pp 209–231

Schacter DL, Kihlstrom JF, Kihlstrom LC, et al: Autobiographical memory in a case of multiple personality disorder. J Abnorm Psychol 98:508–514, 1989

Scheflin AW, Shapiro JL: Trance on Trial. New York, Guilford, 1989

Schenck L, Bear DM: Multiple personality and related dissociative phenomena in patients with temporal lobe epilepsy. Am J Psychiatry 138:1311–1326, 1981

Schetky DH: A review of the literature on the long-term effects of childhood sexual abuse, in Incest-Related Syndromes of Adult Psychopathology. Edited by Kluft RP. Washington, DC, American Psychiatric Press, 1990, pp 35–54

Schoenewolf G: Jennifer and Her Selves. New York, Dell Publishing, 1991

Schreiber FR: Sybil. Chicago, IL, Henry Regnery, 1973

Schultz R, Braun BG, Kluft RP: Multiple personality disorder: phenomenology of selected variables in comparison to major depression. Dissociation 2:45–51, 1989

Schuman DC: Psychodynamics of exaggerated accusations: positive feedback in family systems. Psychiatric Annals 17:242–247, 1987

Schwartz JI, Moura RJ: Severe depersonalization and anxiety associated with indomethacin. South Med J 76:679–680, 1983

Sedman G: Theories of depersonalization: a reappraisal. Br J Psychiatry 117:1–14, 1970

Sedman G, Kenna JC: Depersonalization and mood changes in schizophrenia. Br J Psychiatry 109:669–673, 1963

Shainess N: Sweet Suffering: Woman as Victim. New York, Bobbs-Merrill, 1984

Sheldon H: Child sexual abuse in adult female psychotherapy referrals: incidence and implications for treatment. Br J Psychiatry 152:107–111, 1988

Shimizu M, Sakamoto S: Depersonalization in early adolescence. Jpn J Psychiatry Neurol 40:603–608, 1986

Shorvon HJ, Hill JD, Burkitt E, et al: The depersonalization syndrome. Proceedings of the Royal Society of Medicine 39:779–792, 1946

Shraberg D: The phobic anxiety-depersonalization syndrome. Psychiatric Opinion 14:35–40, 1977

Siomopoulos V: Derealization and déjà vu: formal mechanisms. Am J Psychother 26:84–89, 1972

Slater E, Beard AW, Glitheroe E: The schizophrenia-like psychoses of epilepsy. Br J Psychiatry 109:95–150, 1963

Sno HN, Linzen DH: The déjà vu experience: remembrance of things past? Am J Psychiatry 147:1587–1595, 1990

Spiegel D: Multiple personality as a posttraumatic stress disorder. Psychiatr Clin North Am 7:101–110, 1984

Spiegel D: Dissociation, double binds, and posttraumatic stress in multiple personality disorder, in Treatment of Multiple Personality Disorder. Edited by Braun B. Washington, DC, American Psychiatric Press, 1986, pp 61–77

Spiegel D: Hypnosis in the treatment of victims of sexual abuse. Psychiatr Clin North Am 12:295–305, 1989

Spiegel D: Trauma, dissociation, and hypnosis, in Incest-Related Syndromes of Adult Psychopathology. Edited by Kluft RP. Washington, DC, American Psychiatric Press, 1990, pp 247–261

Spiegel D: Dissociation and trauma, in American Psychiatric Press Review of Psychiatry, Vol 10. Edited by Tasman A, Goldfinger SM. Washington, DC, American Psychiatric Press, 1991, pp 261–275

Spiegel D: Multiple posttraumatic personality disorder, in Clinical Perspectives on Multiple Personality Disorder. Edited by Kluft RP, Fine CG. Washington, DC, American Psychiatric Press, 1993, pp 87–99

Spiegel D, Cardeña E: Disintegrated experience: the dissociative disorders revisited. J Abnorm Psychol 100:366–378, 1991

Spitzer RL, Endicott J, Robins E: Research Diagnostic Criteria. Arch Gen Psychiatry 35:773–782, 1978

Spitzer RL, Williams JBW, Gibbon M, et al: Structured Clinical Interview for DSM-III-R. Washington, DC, American Psychiatric Press, 1990

Stein MB, Uhde TW: Depersonalization disorder: effects of caffeine and response to pharmacotherapy. Biol Psychiatry 26:315–320, 1989

Steinberg A, Steinberg M: Systematic assessment of multiple personality disorder in an adolescent who is blind. Dissociation 7:117–128, 1994

Steinberg M: The spectrum of depersonalization: assessment and treatment, in American Psychiatric Press Review of Psychiatry, Vol 10. Edited by Tasman A, Goldfinger SM. Washington, DC, American Psychiatric Press, 1991, pp 223–247

Steinberg M: Interviewer's Guide to the Structured Clinical Interview for DSM-IV Dissociative Disorders (SCID-D). Washington, DC, American Psychiatric Press, 1993a

Steinberg M: Structured Clinical Interview for DSM-IV Dissociative Disorders (SCID-D). Washington, DC, American Psychiatric Press, 1993b

Steinberg M: Interviewer's Guide to the Structured Clinical Interview for DSM-IV Dissociative Disorders (SCID-D), Revised. Washington, DC, American Psychiatric Press, 1994a

Steinberg M: Structured Clinical Interview for DSM-IV Dissociative Disorders (SCID-D), RevisedWashington, DC, American Psychiatric Press, 1994b

Steinberg M: Systematizing dissociation: symptomatology and diagnostic assessment, in Dissociation: Culture, Mind and Body. Edited by Spiegel D. Washington, DC, American Psychiatric Press, 1994c, pp 59–88

Steinberg M: Assessing posttraumatic dissociation with the SCID-D, in Assessing Psychological Trauma and PTSD: A Handbook for Practitioners. Edited by Wilson J, Keane T. New York, Guilford (in press [a])

Steinberg M: The Mini-Structured Clinical Interview for DSM-IV Dissociative Disorders (Mini-SCID-D). North Tonawanda, NY, Multi-Health Systems (in press [b])

Steinberg M, Steinberg A: Systematic assessment of MPD in adolescents using the SCID-D: three case studies. Bull Menninger Clin (in press)

Steinberg M, Rounsaville R, Cicchetti DV, et al: NIMH field trials of the Structured Clinical Interview for DSM-III-R Dissociative Disorders (SCID-D). New Haven, CT, Yale University School of Medicine, 1989–1992

Steinberg M, Kluft RP, Coons PM, et al: Multicenter field trials of the Structured Clinical Interview for DSM-IV Dissociative Disorders (SCID-D). New Haven, CT, Yale University School of Medicine, 1989–1993

Steinberg M, Rounsaville BJ, Cicchetti DV: The Structured Clinical Interview for DSM-III-R Dissociative Disorders: preliminary report on a new diagnostic instrument. Am J Psychiatry 147:76–82, 1990

Steinberg M, Bancroft J, Buchanan J: Multiple personality disorder in criminal law. Bull Am Acad Psychiatry Law 21:345–365, 1993

Steinberg M, Cicchetti DV, Buchanan J, et al: Distinguishing between multiple personality disorder (dissociative identity disorder) and schizophrenia using the Structured Clinical Interview for DSM-IV Dissociative Disorders. J Nerv Ment Dis 182:495–502, 1994

Stern CR: The etiology of multiple personalities. Psychiatr Clin North Am 7:149–160, 1984

Stewart W: Report of panel on depersonalization. J Am Psychoanal Assoc 12, 1964

Stone MH: Individual psychotherapy with victims of incest. Psychiatr Clin North Am 12:237–255, 1989

Stone MH: Incest in the borderline patient, in Incest-Related Syndromes of Adult Psychopathology. Edited by Kluft RP. Washington, DC, American Psychiatric Press, 1990, pp 183–204

Surrey J, Swett C, Michaels A, et al: Reported history of physical and sexual abuse and severity of symptomatology in psychiatric outpatients. Am J Orthopsychiatry 60:412–417, 1990

Sutcliffe FP, Jones J: Personal identity, multiple personality and hypnosis. Int J Clin Exp Hypn 10:231–269, 1988

Swanson JM, Kinsbourne M: State-dependent learning and retrieval: methodological cautions and theoretical considerations, in Functional Disorders of Memory. Edited by Kihlstrom JF, Evans FJ. Hillsdale, NJ, Lawrence Erlbaum, 1979, pp 275–299

Swett C, Surrey J, Cohen C: Sexual and physical abuse histories and psychiatric symptoms among male psychiatric outpatients. Am J Psychiatry 147:632–636, 1990

Szymanski HV: Prolonged depersonalization after marijuana use. Am J Psychiatry 138:231–233, 1981

Taylor C: The Making of Modern Identity. Cambridge, MA, Harvard University Press, 1989

Terr LC: What happens to early memories of trauma? A study of twenty children under age five at the time of documented traumatic events. J Am Acad Child Adolesc Psychiatry 27:96–104, 1988

Terr LC: Too Scared to Cry: Psychic Trauma in Childhood. New York, Harper & Row, 1990

Terr LC: Childhood traumas: an outline and overview. Am J Psychiatry 148:10–20, 1991

Terr LC: Unchained Memories: True Stories of Traumatic Memories, Lost and Found. New York, Basic Books, 1994

Thigpen CH, Cleckley H: The Three Faces of Eve. New York, McGraw-Hill, 1957

Thomas T: Men Surviving Incest. Walnut Creek, CA, Launch Press, 1989

Threlkeld ME, Thyer BA: Sexual and physical abuse histories among child and adolescent psychiatric outpatients. Journal of Traumatic Stress 5:491–496, 1992

Timsit-Berthier M, de Thier D, Timsit M: Electrophysiological and psychological aspects of the derealization state induced by nitrous oxide in nine control subjects. Advances in Biological Psychiatry 16:90–101, 1987

Torch EM: The psychotherapeutic treatment of depersonalization disorder. Hillside Journal of Clinical Psychiatry 9:133–143, 1987

Torem M: Dissociative states presenting as eating disorders. Am J Clin Hypn 29:137–142, 1986

Torem MS: Covert multiple personality underlying eating disorders. Am J Psychother 65:357–368, 1990

Trueman D: Anxiety and depersonalization and derealization experiences. Psychol Rep 54:91–96, 1984a

Trueman D: Depersonalization in a non-clinical population. J Psychol 116:107–112, 1984b

Tucker G, Harrow M, Quinlan D: Depersonalization, dysphoria, and thought disturbance. Am J Psychiatry 130:702–706, 1973

Turner P: Sex and the single life. First Things 3:15–21, 1993

Tyson GM: Childhood MPD/dissociation identity disorder: applying and extending current diagnostic checklists. Dissociation 5:20–28, 1992

Ulman R, Brothers D: The Shattered Self: A Psychoanalytic Study of Trauma. Hillsdale, NJ, Analytic Press, 1988

van der Kolk BA: The trauma spectrum: the interaction of biological and social events in the genesis of trauma response. Journal of Traumatic Stress 1:273, 1988 van der Kolk BA: Compulsion to repeat the trauma: re-enactment, revictimization, and masochism. Psychiatr Clin North Am 12:389–411, 1989

van der Kolk BA, Kadish W: Amnesia, dissociation, and the return of the repressed, in Psychological Trauma. Edited by van der Kolk BA. Washington, DC, American Psychiatric Press, 1987, pp 173–190

van der Kolk BA, van der Hart O: Pierre Janet and the breakdown of adaptation in psychological trauma. Am J Psychiatry 146:1530–1540, 1989

van der Kolk BA, Blitz R, Burr W, et al: Nightmares and trauma: a comparison of nightmares after combat with lifelong nightmares in veterans. Am J Psychiatry 141:187–190, 1984

Vesper JH: The use of healing ceremonies in the treatment of multiple personality disorder. Dissociation 4:109–114, 1991

Walsh RN: Depersonalization: definition and treatment. Am J Psychiatry 132:873–874, 1975

Waltzer H: Depersonalization and the use of LSD: a psychodynamic study. Am J Psychoanal 32:45–52, 1972

Watkins M: Invisible Guests: The Development of Imaginal Dialogues. Hillsdale, NJ, Analytic Press, 1986

Watkins HH, Watkins JG: Ego-state therapy in the treatment of dissociative disorders, in Clinical Perspectives on Multiple Personality Disorder. Edited by Kluft RP, Fine CG. Washington, DC, American Psychiatric Press, 1993, pp 277–299

Wiesel E: The Fifth Son: A Novel. New York, Summit Books, 1985

Wilbur CB: Multiple personality and child abuse. Psychiatr Clin North Am 7:3–8, 1984a

Wilbur CB: Treatment of multiple personality. Psychiatric Annals 14:27–31, 1984b

Wilbur CB: The effect of child abuse on the psyche, in Childhood Antecedents of Multiple Personality. Edited by Kluft RP. Washington, DC, American Psychiatric Press, 1985, pp 21–35

Williams LM: Recall of childhood trauma: a prospective study of women's memories of child sexual abuse. J Consult Clin Psychol 1994

Wineburg E, Straker N: An episode of acute, self-limiting deper-
    sonalization following a first session of hypnosis. Am J Psy-
    chiatry 130:98–100, 1973

Wise ML: Adult self-injury as a survival response in victim-survi-
    vors of childhood abuse. Special issue: aggression, family vio-
    lence and chemical dependency. Journal of Chemical
    Dependency Treatment 3:185–201, 1989

World Health Organization: International Statistical Classification
    of Diseases and Related Health Problems, 10th Revision (ICD-
    10). Geneva, Switzerland, World Health Organization, 1992

INDEX

*Page numbers in **boldface** type refer to tables or figures.*